With POWER of each BREATH

A DISABLED WOMEN'S ANTHOLOGY

Susan E. Browne, Debra Connors
and Nanci Stern

CLEIS PRESS
Pittsburgh • San Francisco

Published in the United States by Cleis Press, A Women's Publishing Company, PO Box 8933, Pittsburgh, PA 15221 and PO Box 14684, San Francisco, CA 94114.

10 9 8 7 6 5 4

Cover Design: Cecilia Brunazzi
Typesetting: Coming Up! Graphics
ISBN: 0-939416-06-9
Library of Congress Catalog Card Number: 85-71206

Printed in the United States.

This book is available on tape from the Womyn's Braille Press, PO Box 8475, Minneapolis, MN 55408.

Deborah Abbott: "This Body I Love" first appeared in *Matrix Newsmagazine*. Mary Ambo: "Speaking Out" first appeared in *Valley Women's Voice*. Anne Finger: "Claiming All of Our Bodies" first appeared in *Test-Tube Women*, published by Routledge & Kegan Paul. Anne Finger: "Like the Hully-Gully But Not So Slow" first appeared in *13th Moon*. Edwina Franchild: "Beginning With My Life" first appeared in *Lesbian Contradictions*. Frances Lynn: "Waiting Again" first appeared in *The Disability Rag*. Victoria Ann Lewis: "The Great Outdoors" appeared in a shortened version in *Ms Magazine*. Robyn Miller: "Taking Leave" first appeared in *Voice Magazine*. Jill Sager: "'Just Stories" first appeared in *Feminary*. Nanci Stern: "This Script is Very Private" first appeared in her book *Visions Incognito*. Naomi Woronov: "A -See-by-Logic Life" first appeared in the Columbia University Teachers College *Record*.

The publishers wish to thank all the people at *Creative Growth Art Center* who helped us find the wonderful artwork of Carrie Oyama, the cover artist. *Creative Growth* is a pioneering Art Program in Oakland, California, serving over 125 disabled adults. *Creative Growth* is dedicated to the idea that all people, no matter how severely disabled, physically, mentally, or emotionally, have the right to creative expression and can produce work of high artistic merit.

Title: *With the Power of Each Breath* is from Susan Hansell's poem, "The Wolf".

We dedicate this book to
disabled women everywhere.

Name of Book
With the Power of Each Breath

Date Due	Date Due

TABLE OF CONTENTS

CHAPTER 4
Invisible and On Center Stage
Who Do We Think We Are Anyway
page 173

CHAPTER 5
This Body I Love -
Finding Ourselves
page 246

CHAPTER 6
Becoming Mothers - Raising Our Children
page 274

CHAPTER 7
Finding Our Friends
page 308

CHAPTER 8
United We Stand, Sit, and Roll -
Finding Each Other
page 330

Acknowledgments

We would like to thank all those who have envisioned a need for this book and have given us support in putting it together.

A special thanks to the more than 300 women who sent us their contributions. All the work received helped create this book.

Thanks to our readers Toni Pebbles, Liza Reilly, Joey Finkelstein, Eugenia Franco, Susan Browne, Debi Connors, and all the contributors who sent their articles on tape.

We received editorial assistance from Patricia Smith, Leslie Bergson, Catherine G. Nelson, April A. Sinclair, Abigail Abbuehl, Carol A. Park, Anne Finger, Deborah Lieberman, Felice Newman and Frederique Delacoste.

We thank JoAnn Eggstaff for her personal contribution and for introducing us to Rebecca Grothaus and Donna Hyler. Thanks to Eugenia Franco for proofreading manuscripts.

We would like to give thanks to all our friends, roommates, lovers and therapists who gave us moral support, put up with us, and helped us with the task of putting together the book.

Everyone who has touched our lives has helped to create this book.

The Wolf*

by susan hansell

I

i write
    when it hurts

    last night i dreamt
        there were tubes in my back
    my body
            hooked
    to machines
           this morning i couldn't bend over

i write
    when it hurts

    last night i dreamt
           the soles of my feet split
      i walked on bare bones
           glass splinters grinding in my joints

*i have a chronic illness called Lupus, which is the latin word for Wolf.
Lupus causes my immune system to make anti-bodies against my own
DNA. this means my body is literally devouring itself.

i write
    when it hurts

my mind pouring out through my fingertips
        relieved
my body melting into images i create
            relieved
the words
    tie me to a past
        to a future
           where our lives are re/lived
         over and over

write it down
    write it all down

push
    the pencil
        across
           the page

i write
    when it hurts

searching for words
    to tell
        how it feels

II

in a dream i am walking alone at night   i come to an
intersection of wide streets   i stop to peer in every
direction   i am very careful   i begin to cross   then
a car drives   speeding heading right for me
i can't run away   i can't run   i'm not able to run
somehow i jump onto the hood   this life still in me
i curse   make fists   and pound   against the windshield
but there is no one to hear me   there is no one driving

i wake
    to the cries of a wolf
  circling my brain

my mind spins into the day
        while my body lags behind
      rocking
                licking the wounded legs
                    the swollen joints

if the pain controlled me
    i might tear through my flesh
            and pull open the back bones
                    spine by spine

if time controlled me
    i might never sleep
            there's so much left undone

but i have learned the power of each breath
      in and out

III

i dream i have 10 days to live
i flee the city for the earth's edge
    where water turns mountains to sand
and lie naked
      under yellow cliffs
         spilling salty currents
      into the sea
rivers run from my pores
    until i float
on my own dusty bones
    will you
        take me

    take me
      turn my body
        into smooth round stones
          and scatter me
            across the shore

Introduction

At the moment, we can't remember a time when we didn't meet at least twice a week over our caffeinated and non-caffeinated cups. We have come to regard morning diabetic check-ins as a fact of life.

"I got up at 3:30 a.m. and my blood sugar was 40."

"Oh yeah? I bet you feel about as bad as I do. Mine was 300 this morning." We exchange tips on good restaurants, talk about our attempts to manage stress. and praise ourselves for the work we've accomplished.

We found each other through the commonalities of our personal histories, in a support group. In what has become feminist tradition, we shared our stories of growing up and living daily with chronic physical illness, our feelings about it, and personal information about managing it. Through this process we became stronger, more self-affirming and, in very important ways, less alone.

When we decided to do a workshop on disability together, we found that we had learned far more about ourselves by talking with each other than we ever had by reading literature, whether traditional or feminist. As we realized the importance of our connecting, we began to fantasize a book for, by, and about disabled women.

Meanwhile, at Cleis Press, women with the same vision were looking for editors for this anthology, and our dream became a possibility.

As contributions began pouring into our mailboxes, the need for *With the Power of Each Breath* became overwhelmingly clear. The first letters repeatedly spoke of the pain each woman felt in going deeply into herself to write her story and of the relief this searching gave her. We were moved to tears and laughter, given strength, and prompted to face deeper issues. These letters affirmed that disabled women have long awaited the opportunity to reach inside and open our hearts to ourselves and one another.

There were many moments along the way of creating this book in which we had serious doubts that it would ever be completed. The complexities of doing the work in ways that maximized each of our individual strengths, and, at the same time, acknowledged our human limitations and specific disability-related needs were staggering.

The material we received had to be available in several forms to be accessible to us all. We needed taped and Braille versions, as well as printed, to communicate with each other. Major fluctuations in our disabilities required us to use different media at different times. The logistics of finding and scheduling readers to tape printed information was a continuous job. But with the help of contributors and friends, tapes, Braille and the telephone, we managed.

We all dealt with the daily ups and downs of diabetes, as well as major complications. Nanci was hospitalized with a diabetes-related infection, Debi lost all of her vision for several weeks, and Susan became acutely ill using an insulin infusion pump. And we not only faced our own disabilities and mortality. Susan's mother died, as did David, a life-long diabetic friend of Nanci, and Petunia, Nanci's sixteen-year-old cat, whose face she remembered from the time before she was totally blind. Several other friends became critically or terminally ill.

Fortunately, with three of us working together, we were able to encourage each other. And we had before us story after story by disabled women who were living full lives and determined to continue. So we survived all this and more. Nanci developed her counseling practice, Debi completed her bachelor's degree and has almost finished graduate school, and Susan completed her doctorate.

The three of us tend to view the world and disability from different perspectives. This has led to many intense discussions, frustrations and eventual openings to appreciation of the strength of having diverse perspectives from which to view complex problems and suggest alternative solutions. We are in constant process of evolving our own perspectives and theories based on our experiences and those of others. We hope that this anthology will create as much controversy and growth in those who read it as it has for those of us who have been involved in putting it together.

With the Power of Each Breath is a work of resistance against institutionalized silence. All of the fifty-four women who contributed to this anthology are disabled (with the exception of Bobbie-Jo Goff, Marsha Ablowitz and Tilly Schalkwyk who provided us with access to the words of Elaine Robidoux and the women of The Reminiscence Group). Our purpose is to bridge the gap that separates disabled women from one another and from the non-disabled world. This book is a tool we can use to examine and challenge our able-ism without defending it, and to demystify disability and the lives of disabled women.

These pages are a journey into our lives as we survive in an inaccessible society, express our anger, grow up in our families, live in our bodies, find our own identities, parent our children, and find our friends and each other. We challenge ourselves by looking at our pasts and presents to find ourselves and to accept our bodies, sexuality, and right to be parents. We explore the meaning of dependence, independence and control of our own lives to ourselves and to our relationships with others. We challenge the able-bodied world to examine their perceptions of us and their role in the social construction of disability. Our immediate needs for accessible role models, attendant care, housing, education, medical care and employment are made painfully clear. Common issues that unite us are identified and illustrated. Differences are recognized and acknowledged so that our diversity can become strengthening rather than divisive.

We began this work with a strong political commitment to produce an anthology representative of all disabled women. We wanted the impossible: that this collection would be *the* definitive statement by and about disabled women. It is not. Because of the willingness of many, we have been able to address a broad spectrum of disability issues. Our contributors cross the lines of race, age, class, sexual orientation, geographical location and type of disability. But we know there are more disabled women, young and old, third world and institutionalized, whose stories we need to hear.

Few contributors discussed our sexuality explicitly. Although its impact on our lives is woven through the book, there is a lot more that could be said. More exploration of alcoholism and drug abuse among disabled women is needed. And, although this anthology is not limited to physical disabilities, we recognize the need for a more comprehensive examination of emotional disabilities.

We planned to include a chapter on spirituality. Many women with disabilities seek spiritual assistance for strength and solace as we face the things that can't be fixed. But the articles we received did not represent a broad enough spectrum of what spirituality can mean for us.

It seems that we have written about those things most important in our lives right now: our immediate survival. Although about half of us will probably die as a result of our disabilities, we have written little about our own dying. Like other people of our culture, we have difficulty viewing death as part of the life cycle. For similar reasons, we received no contributions for a chapter we wanted to call "The Future on Our Own Terms". Perhaps once we share our past and present lives, we will be able to create fantasies of the future we want and explore feelings about our own deaths.

This is a beginning. Until each of us has related her experience, our story will not be told. In the meantime, we meet one fundamental need: that we, as disabled women, find each other. Together these works form a realistic picture of our lives, the struggles and rewards. With great joy, pride, celebration, and the power of each breath, we bring you these women.

1.

Shut In, Shut Out, Shut Up
— Surviving the System —

The needs and capabilities of disabled women are not taken seriously because of our gender as well as our physical or emotional differences. Inequitable education and employment opportunities reinforce our dependence on social service benefits, which are designed to be inadequate. Dependence and childishness are presumed to be the totality of our existence. This is most evident to us in our interactions with paternalistic social institutions.

Paternalism is the policy or practice of governing by providing for the needs of those deemed incapable of self-care. Social service becomes social control when our survival is threatened if we are perceived as being noncompliant toward our administrators. Disabled women have found that welfare agencies, the medical establishment, residential institutions, rehabilitators, employers and well-intentioned strangers have played this fatherly role in our lives. The services and facilities we have demanded and may need in order to live more self-managed lives work directly against that possibility. Our access to quality living is always contingent upon the political climate.

Accessibility is the common denominator of disabled women's demands. We are disabled more by barriers of access than from the specific conditions of our bodies. We expect the removal of communication, transportation and architectural barriers. To consider it a special privilege to use a telephone, ride a bus or use a public bathroom is absurd. While curb-cuts and telephone amplification devices are essential, interpretations of accessibility remains narrow. By accessibility we mean access to the same choices accorded able-bodied people. Attitudinal and functional barriers work in concert. Both must be eliminated. Our requirements should be built into the fabric of society and considered routine.

A radical change in perspective is needed. We are encouraged to see our needs as specific to us, rather than system-wide issues. In reality, the entire society benefits from increased accessibility. Curb-cuts, for example, make traveling easier for women in wheelchairs and those pushing baby carriages and pulling shopping carts. Flexible work schedules benefit everyone including chronically ill women and women with small children. Moreover, when the strengths of disabled women go unacknowledged or remain underdeveloped because we do not have access to basic resources, society suffers the loss of our participation, resourcefulness and creativity.

Infusing Blues

by susan e. browne

i have been an insulin-dependent diabetic for twenty-two of
my thirty seven years. At first this meant taking one or two
shots a day, checking the amount of sugar in my urine and trying to follow a strict diet. It also meant feeling very alone, isolated,
afraid and ashamed of what was wrong with my body. From reading
everything I could find about diabetes I learned that after having
it for twenty years, there was a good chance I could develop all sorts
of terrible complications, such as blindness, amputations, kidney
failure, heart disease, strokes and nerve disease. I got no encouragement to talk about my feelings, so I did what I had to and tried not
to think about it. Later in my career as a nurse, I cared for many
diabetics with severe complications. I came to realize that many other
health professionals believed that diabetics who develop complications were a "bad lot" who had basically brought it upon themselves,
and my isolation continued. But I also wanted to believe that if only I took good enough care of myself, the complications wouldn't
happen to me. At the same time, deep inside, I knew that I was not
able to do enough things to keep my body from acting diabetic. Still
sugar was often in my urine, a sign of diabetes. One of my most terrifying fantasies was that I would become blind as a result of diabetes.
Diabetes is, in fact, the leading cause of new blindness in adults in
the U.S. I didn't share my fears about the disease for fear of being
judged. It was eighteen years before I talked with other diabetics
about what our lives are really like.

After many years of checking my urine for sugar, I learned of
a new development. I could now check my own blood sugar levels
at home, and know at any time what was happening. I started checking my blood sugars immediately and learned that it was often too
high or too low. Even after a variety of insulin regimens, strict

dieting, and exercise, I still had not hit on a combination that was very helpful in stabilizing my blood sugars.

As I approached my twentieth year with diabetes, my doctor discovered diabetic changes starting to happen in my eyes. I felt desperate about my future. I had recently become friends with several other diabetics who were very supportive to me emotionally. Some of my friends already had worse complications than I did. That brought home to me on a very personal level the reality and impact of diabetic complications. I was ready to try almost anything, when my doctor told me about a new device that might help me control my diabetes better, an insulin pump.

In a very precise way, this pump would push insulin from a syringe through tubing and a needle into the fatty tissue of my body. I would change the needle and tubing every one to three days and program the pump for appropriate doses of insulin based on the results of frequent blood sugar tests. I would have to wear the pump all the time. A small maintenance dose of insulin would go in continuously, and then I could just push a button to take an extra dose before meals. Since the body needs a base-line dose of insulin all the time for normal metabolism and extra to use the nutrients from meals, this system made perfect sense to me. I was attracted to the theory behind the insulin pump. I knew it would be a big adjustment to wear a needle in my flesh all the time, and have a box strapped to my waist, but I wanted desperately to control my blood sugars, and this idea offered me hope. After careful consideration of the pros and cons, I decided to try the pump.

I rented the first pump I used. It was large, heavy and strange looking, but I noticed that my blood sugars were much more stable than they had been while I was taking shots. However, when I bought a different brand of pump, smaller and more sophisticated, my blood sugars became erratic again.

Once, shortly after starting on the new pump, the needle slipped from the fatty tissue into a blood vessel and blood backed up in the tubing. No alarm sounded, as it should have. I noticed other problems too. The tubing became easily kinked and vital connections were not protected by the case. I wrote down the problems I was having and suggestions for improvements and, at my doctor's suggestion, sent this information with her to a meeting the company was having about its pump. The company never acknowledged my letter, although my doctor told me that they had xeroxed several copies and found it very useful.

As my experience with the pump grew, I realized that I had a lot of information and thought I could be a useful resource to the company. I suggested they hire me as a consultant. They were not interested. They told me they had all the information they needed. Perhaps so, but I needed more. I was still having problems regulating my blood sugars with their pump.

There are many factors that can influence blood sugar, and I tried to control as many of them as I could. When I was doing all I knew how and my blood sugars were still erratic, I started to question the pump itself. This was frightening to do since it required a certain amount of trust to be able to continue hooking myself up to this piece of machinery every day. After a series of experiments, I figured out that there seemed to be something blocking up the needle, slowing and sometimes stopping the flow of insulin into my body.

I shared this information with the company, and asked if there were others having similar problems. They said I was the only one. They said they were not satisfied with the company making the tubing/needle sets and that the blockage could be due to the glue used to hold the needle in the tubing. My problems continued, and later when I repeated this conversation to them, they would not acknowlege it. From that interchange on, they revealed little to me about what they thought might be going on. I got the distinct feeling that they knew I would be trouble for them and would not give me information that could be used against them. They continued to tell me I was the only one having problems with blockages of the system, and suggested it might be a specific reaction between the insulin and/or the needle and my body fluids, or perhaps a piece of flesh blocking the end of the needle when it was first inserted. Both were apparently my responsibility. Obviously I could not change my bodily fluids and the "piece of flesh" theory made no sense since the blockages did not happen when the needle was first put in. They offered no specific solutions until I persisted. Finally they suggested I try diluting the insulin.

This idea seemed worth a try, but actually getting my hands on the special diluent was very difficult. Although their parent company manufactured it, the pump company refused to help me get it. I finally tracked some down through a local pharmacist, who later told me he could not continue to supply me because it was only authorized for experimental use. No one had ever mentioned that it was an experimental substance.

I tried diluting the insulin, but the blockages continued. Each blockage meant unnecessary blood sugar problems. Because the alarm system was not detecting them, it was only when my blood sugar rose without explanation that I would suspect the system was blocked. The only way to be sure was to take out the needle and watch what happened when I tried to run some insulin through it. Then I would have to put in a whole new needle. This was painful, stressful and time consuming. I was also running out of the tubing/needle sets. The pump was sold to me for $2000, which was supposed to include a year's worth of supplies, but they had estimated needing to change the set-up only every three days.

The company next suggested I change the sets more often. I told them that they would have to send me more sets. They refused to send them free of charge and claimed that nothing was wrong with the pump. I explained that if the connections between the pump and me didn't work, the pump was useless. I reread the warranty and found that indeed all of the syringes, needles and tubings were classified as "accessories" and were not covered. When I asked my doctor to help me deal with them, she called and they immediately sent me, at no cost, the equipment I had been asking for.

Meanwhile I got a form letter from the pump company to all pump users. After having told me I was the only one having problems, they acknowledged in this letter that blockages were the most common problem experienced by pump users. Although this made me feel less alone, I realized that I had been lied to, and there were more lies in the letter. They reassured us that blockages would be detected by the alarm system, and that partial blockages would not compromise the dose of insulin delivered. They knew from me that neither of these statements were totally true. They warned of other potential problems. "In rare cases" static electricity could reprogram the pump. They did not explain that this could be a deadly problem, causing the pump to deliver a massive overdose of insulin. Although I now knew to be suspicious of anything in this letter, what of the other pump users reading it?

I was very concerned about them, but I had to focus on my day-to-day survival. In spite of diluting the insulin and changing the sets every twenty four hours, they were still blocking up. After my persistent complaints, the company suggested I try a cannula (plastic tube inserted with a needle) instead of a needle. It was larger and might not block up so much. I was scared of the pain of sticking myself with an even larger needle, but agreed out of desperation. To my great relief the cannulas were more comfortable because they were flexible. And the blockages stopped!

But my worries were not over. The company could not send me more cannulas; I would have to figure out where to get them and pay for them myself. Also they required a different kind of tubing made by only one company. It seems that another pump company had bought up all the available tubings and were refusing to sell them to the manufacturer of my pump. I would have to try to buy them directly from the competition. I was advised not to tell what brand pump I would be using the tubings with or they might refuse to sell them to me. With the help of a friend, I found a supplier who was willing to sell me twenty five tubings for $70.

Meanwhile my pump company had made several broken promises about when they would be able to supply me with cannulas. I had no idea how much longer I could continue using the pump, because I did not know if and when I would be able to get the cannulas. They assured me they were just as upset about the cannula supply as I was, since they would not be available to display as a new product at the upcoming national convention of the American Diabetes Association.

In the midst of all this, several friends sent me copies of a clipping from a local paper, billed "Insulin Pump Probe — Mystery Deaths of 12 Diabetics." The National Center for Disease Control (CDC) in Atlanta was investigating the deaths of diabetics who had died while using insulin pumps and found that all but four of the deaths were possibly related to the insulin pumps. I had to to call my doctor to find out if she had more information. She told me the CDC was upset about all the sensational publicity. She accepted my pump company's reassurances that these deaths were probably the result of poor patient compliance rather than problems with the pump. I later heard the speaker from the CDC report their findings and conclude on shaky evidence that the pump was not responsible for any of the deaths. When I told the speaker my story, he said, "Now, if I were you, I wouldn't make too big a fuss with the FDA or they might take the pumps off the market."

By this time I was feeling pretty overwhelmed. Dealing with the pump had become my life. Doing all the work to handle diabetes is a big job anyway, but also having to deal with lies, supply problems, lack of help, and most recently, fears about the basic safety of the pump was just too much. It was clear that I didn't have access to the information I needed to make safe, informed choices about taking care of myself. Meanwhile my eyes started hemorrhaging frequently. I felt very powerless.

Since my doctor had been able to help me get what I needed before, I called on her again. This time it was quite a different story. She told me that the company had bent over backwards to help me. "Your needs, I would suspect, are quite unusual." she said. "This is your personal problem. You can't expect them to keep taking care of it." She suggested that since the pump had been so stressful for me I stop using it for a month, and perhaps I would appreciate it more at that time. I felt that she had totally missed the point, blamed me for the problems and was now siding with the pump company. My feelings of abandonment were overwhelming and we have not spoken since. She later told a friend of mine that she thought she and I had different ideas about the doctor-patient relationship. While I seemed to think it should be a collegial one, she thought it should be like a father-son relationship. She was also upset that I had not been making appointments to see her, but had asked her to write letters for me *and* pay the postage herself.

Fortunately, I had other sources of information available to me. One was the National Women's Health Network, a feminist organization working to safeguard the health of women. I read in their newsletter of the United States Pharmacopeal Convention, an independent non-governmental group (although funded by the FDA) for reporting problems with medical devices. I filed a report and got an immediate response that, as promised, they had informed the FDA as well as the pump manufacturer of my problems. I also wrote the FDA to ask what specific research had been done on this pump before they approved it and what the standards were for approval of medical devices. The form letter I got in return ignored both of these questions. I understood why when three months later I read again in the NWHN newsletter, "FDA Fails to Protect Public from Defective Devices." A 1976 law required the FDA to establish a system for reporting problems with medical devices, to rate devices according to their potential hazards, and to establish standards of safety and effectiveness of devices. As of 1983, this had, for the most part, not been done. It is no wonder my questions to the FDA went unacknowledged and unanswered.

Meanwhile I received an urgent recall notice from the pump company about cracked tubings, and a separate warning about how the pump could accidentally deliver either insufficient insulin or all the insulin at once. This came one year and eight months after I had bought and started using the pump.

The next time I called the pump company to find out when they would be sending me my cannulas, I was told, "Since you made your report to the FDA, we have to do a barrage of tests on everything before we send it out. That includes the cannulas." Although I doubted that my individual report had had so much power, I was glad they were finally going to test equipment before selling it. Eventually they stocked the cannulas as a standard item. This put an end to my supply problems, but unfortunately not to my problems with the pump.

One day, I got quite ill, with my blood sugar climbing high in spite of my taking extra insulin. Eventually I discovered an almost invisible crack in the cannula. Most of the insulin had been leaking out, rather than going into me. I was sicker from high blood sugar than I had ever been in twenty two years of being diabetic. I put in a new cannula and went through the same process *again* when I found that the second cannula was also cracked! In trying to get my blood sugar back down, I gave myself too much insulin and had one of the worst insulin reactions of my life. I stopped using the pump that day.

After a few days of recovering my physical strength, I consulted with two feminist lawyers about all I had been through. Although they agreed that I had been wronged, they recommended that I not sue. I would be taking on a very rich and powerful company and would probably not win since it would be too hard to prove damages. The only such cases that were winning in the courts were ones of wrongful death.

Well, I am still alive, and wiser. I survived three years of problems with equipment performance, lack of acknowledgement of the seriousness of the problems, and being blamed for problems in the product and the whole system. I was offered superficial solutions with no help in carrying them out. Vital information was withheld from me as well as other pump users.

It has been very difficult for me to tell this story. I feel challenged on every front. Not only had my experiences been discounted and disbelieved by those in power over me, but I had to acknowledge that what I wanted to believe was not happening. I wanted to believe that the pump could work for me, and that I could trust the company to make it work.

Each time I got on the phone to try to get what I needed, I hoped that this time I would come away satisfied — that someone would finally say, "You have been wronged. This has all been a terrible mistake, and we will make it up to you. We don't want to sell or prescribe a product that is not safe, so we have stopped until we figure out what is happening."

This never happened. It was not a mistake, but consistent attempts to maintain the status-quo of powerful, profit-making institutions — from the medical profession to the companies that make the tools of the profession, to the agencies that determine the availability of these tools.

I have learned, as have many other women, that there is powerful truth in what we are learning about how these institutions jeopardize our health. I have learned to trust feminist sources of information, and to trust myself. I have learned that I cannot take on the system myself, and that I must be selective in the battles that I fight. I must conserve my energy and know who my allies are — the people who will continue to be critical of the status-quo and keep questioning the system and not just blaming the victims. I have learned the value of women's voices and of having places where we can speak our truths. It is vitally important that we tell our stories to heal ourselves, and to build connections between us so that we can keep working for change.

Read Into A System: And Thrive!

by tzipporah benavraham

his is a brief description of my 27 readers, where I find them and how I organize my time. As a college student, I am provided with $500 a year for readers. That does not go far, but I have found persons willing to read for me for two dollars an hour. One of these readers is a woman with multiple sclerosis. She lives in a motorized wheelchair, has a Master's degree in Primary Education and feels bored and unproductive. I provide her with blank cassettes, a tape recorder, the material I need read and baggies to keep things organized. Every two weeks when I go to the medical center near where she lives, I pick up the individual bags containing the print pieces with the recorded cassettes, and leave her more material. She started to tell her other friends about me and they started to read for me also. I bought an inexpensive tape recorder for each reader from my student financial aid. I also buy cheap cassettes, 300 at a time. They are not the best quality but for voice they are fine. Sometimes I have specialized reading done. I work for a legislator and must keep up with bills and the laws. For instance, I needed to work on a computer literacy bill draft, when I knew nothing of computers or of drafting bills. I needed help to get this information. Here is what I did.

I got five by seven file cards and a large print typewriter. Although I cannot see at all, at least the cards would be noticeable to the sighted. I typed on the cards BLIND STUDENT WORKING FOR A POLITICIAN NEEDS READER. Anyone interested contact.... . I sent these to the student councils of law schools and asked they be posted on bulletin boards. How did I find the law school addresses? I have a phone loop that tapes from the phone to my tape recorder. I called my local public library information service, asked for the names and addresses of law schools in my area, taped the information on the phone loop and later typed it onto envelopes using the tape as a "dictaphone".

Dealing with law students is interesting. Since I work with an elected official, they often will read *only* if I can get a letter on the politician's letterhead to thank them for their volunteer work. It bodes them well to have such a letter, especially if they are aspiring to be politicians.

When students come here to read for me, I give them a meal. I also do this for some unemployed bachelors in the neighborhood. This way I have readers and occasionally sighted guides, and they get food to take home.

Once I had to draft a bill concerning food stamps. I brought the current foodstamp law and a recording to my grocer and asked him to tape it between customers. I listened to the clanging cash register and trucks outside along with my grocer's familiar voice reading the law that concerned his food operations, and my future bill draft. He felt he had done a good deed and I got the information I needed.

My readers come from other places, too. The women who work at the local photocopy store read my mail for me occasionally. The New York State Assembly Correspondence Unit has Brailled my bill draft and taped proposed regulations I needed. A local volunteer group for the disabled often provides "hit and run" readers. They will come over once or twice and leave. They think they are wonderful to be helping a blind lady, and I get something else read. A friend of mine with cerebral palsy goes to the Midtown Manhattan Public Library to use the Kurzweil machine, a computer that reads print aloud. I give him some of my articles and papers, and he tapes what the machine "reads". He gets books read for his college classes and so do I.

My newest readers are three homebound frail elderly people. I help them with some concrete service and they tape things for me. We all enjoy the visits. Sometimes friends help me with reading. I have also gotten readers from a directory of volunteer reading groups in the United States and from Recording for the Blind.

Dealing with needing is not always easy for me. One difficulty I face with readers is training them to do what my eyes used to do. It is not easy. Some people think they must fill the tape with their own messages if it is not full. Others cough into the recorder. Some have thick accents, or are clearly bored with what they are reading. I just sit there and say, "they're human and I am human." I make bonds with my readers and we help each other.

This is how I have a network of 27 readers. I find them everywhere. I go with cheap cassettes, tape recorders, bags and labels in hand, and get my print accessed.

How the Rhino Got Its Flaky Skin

by emily levy

I am a prototype of the next generation.
I am a warning to society to change its ways.
I am a tree standing beside a super-highway;
I am the water downstream.
I have been poisoned by industrialism.

*a*bout a year ago I went to a workshop on disability awareness, figuring it would help me better understand my
disabled father. I never expected to leave that workshop with
the knowledge that I am also disabled.

I have a chronic condition called environmental illness. It's also
called immune system dysregulation, complex allergy syndrome,
acute systemic poisoning, and pollution sickness. Clinical ecologists,
the doctors of western medicine who diagnose and treat environmental illness (EI) assert that the disease is a result of a shortage or
dysfunction of certain white blood cells. The symptoms that result
can be similar to allergic reactions. But EI-induced toxic reactions
occur in response to a broader range of substances and create a
broader range of symptoms than do typical allergic reactions. Environmentally ill people usually react to dozens, if not hundreds, of
chemicals, foods, and inhalants. Symptoms include asthma, arthritis,
nasal congestion, laryngitis, skin rashes, vomiting, migraine
headaches, constipation, diarrhea, menstrual cramps and anaphylactic shock.[1] Brain-related symptoms, which are often difficult to
recognize, are also common. These include hyperactivity, addictions,
loss of memory or concentration, and learning disabilities.

EI is generally contracted through exposure to toxins in the environment. Some people become environmentally ill suddenly, in response to a massive poisoning incident. I was diagnosed two and a half years ago, at age twenty. I am aware of no specific incident when I was exposed to extremely high levels of toxic materials. I became ill gradually, probably as a result of high levels of toxins, a few "moderate" chemical exposures, and a family history of allergies. It strikes me as ironic that I'm considered sick because I react to the poisons in the environment as if they were poison.

More women than men are diagnosed as having EI. I suspect that this is because society gives women more permission than men to pay attention to our bodies, and to acknowledge when something is wrong. Yet because women's analyses and intuitions about our bodies are not generally taken seriously by the medical profession, and because environmental illness is not yet widely recognized, many women who report the unusual symptoms are diagnosed as mentally ill. (I'm sure this happens to men also, but less frequently.) Some allergists believe that over 50% of patients now in mental hospitals in the United States suffer mainly from "brain allergies."[2]

Most people with environmental illness go undiagnosed or untreated because of lack of money and the privilege that money buys in a capitalist system. Upper middle class white privilege has clearly affected my health situation. It was because my family had money that I could afford to weave through the maze of medical referrals until I found a physician who recognized my condition. Again it was money that enabled me to go through the testing process, receive treatment, and later seek alternative treatment from an acupuncturist. It was access to money that allowed me the flexibility to alter my living situation until I found a tolerable one, and to leave for the country when my condition was most severe. And it is my current money situation that has allowed me to set up a work situation conducive to my health needs. Many chronically ill and disabled people have no choice but to work at full time jobs, even when the job is the cause of their illness or disability.

Because few people are familiar with EI, those suffering from it often say we have "allergies." I am coming to realize that this works to our disadvantage. Allergies are perceived (often inaccurately) as minor and isolated problems. A few sneezes. Inability to eat seafood. Having to use nasal spray. Environmental illness extends well beyond being either minor or isolated. Like others with EI, I find that it affects nearly every facet of my life.

It affects my social life because I can't go to bars or cafes or dances or shows or ballgames without being sickened by tobacco smoke or perfume.

It affects my diet because there are so many foods I cannot eat. Citric acid, for example, is not only present in fruits and fruit juices, but is often used as a preservative in canned and packaged products. "Natural flavorings" on a list of food ingredients could mean lemon juice or rind. Citric acid is only one of the many food ingredients that I must completely avoid.

It affects my appearance because skin rash often leaves my hands cracked and bloody. My face is often swollen and red. Like others with EI, I have "allergic shiners" under my eyes. Formaldehyde fumes, synthetic fibers, and other antigens severely limit my clothing selection and access to clothing stores.

It affects my relationships with my pet-owning friends because animal hair and dander make their houses and cars inaccessible to me. Because it forces them to choose between being with their animals and being with me. It hurts to be excluded from camping trips again and again because I can't travel with a dog.

It affects my mobility because buses are full of exhaust, scented products, and tobacco. Because toxic fumes make driving in traffic lethal.

It affects my political activity because the stress involved in the organizing I used to do and want to do now aggravates my illness.

It affects my ability to earn a living because dust or formaldehyde or tobacco smoke or fluorescent lights or carpets or petrochemical fumes or air fresheners or plastics or stress or all of these things permeate most workplaces.

It affects my ability to live without working a regular job because I spend $300.00 a month on health care.

It affects my spontaneity because I always need to take care of my health first.

It affects my sexuality because warmth and wetness on my skin makes it itch, and I scratch and scratch and scratch instead of lying peacefully with my lover.

It affects my relationships with my roommates because they must avoid exposing me to the things that spark toxic reactions. Because we can't use a flea bomb or a can of Ajax. Because their friends can't smoke in the house. Because they can't have their wool rugs on the living room floor. Because they have to do my share of the dishes and rinse them extra well. Because they have to watch for foods I can't eat when they cook or go shopping. Because they have to understand. (And I'm afraid that if I lived alone I'd go into anaphylactic shock and there would be no one there to keep me from suffocating or tearing off my skin).

It affects my ability to decide where I want to live because hot weather aggravates my condition, and in cold places wool is prevalent. Wool has triggered some of my worst reactions.

It affects my sense of self-worth because I can't accomplish as much as my colleagues whose bodies can handle stress better than mine can.

It affects my ability to trust myself because so many people have told me that it's all in my head that sometimes I believe it.

It affects my fantasies for the future when reality butts in and asks, "Will you be healthy enough?"

It affects my leisure time because all of my favorite activites either involve the use of allergenic materials or require the use of my hands, which are often incapacitated by skin rash.

It affects my relationships with my mother, sister, and brother because I can't always trust them to be sensitive about my limitations.

It affects my relationship with my father because he just can't seem to remember what it is I react to, and just can't seem to believe it when he does remember.

My father never mentioned to me that my grandmother used to cover his legs with sand when they went to the beach. His legs were "ugly" and she didn't want anyone to see her child was crippled. He never mentioned that he was incontinent as a child and always smelled of pee and shit. He was the stinky kid who had to sit by the teacher so he wouldn't offend the other students. And I'm sure Dad never told me that he has no sensation in his feet or lower legs. He certainly never said a word about the pain he must have felt growing up with the word "cripple" painted by his mother across his life. I've been told — though not by Dad — that my grandmother blamed him for my grandfather's death. My grandfather died of a stroke after shovelling snow that my father apparently would have shovelled had he been a "normal" ten-year-old.

I like to think that it would have made a difference if I had known these things. I like to think I wouldn't have resented his requests for a sweater from upstairs, or his anger at family outings that couldn't be hikes. But I really don't know.

I do know that to have been able to talk about those things would have meant a big change for him. Dad, who walked on crutches for four years after an unsuccessful operation before allowing himself to be convinced to get a special disabled license plate for his car. Dad, who became armchair coach to a super-athletic son because he couldn't play ball as a kid. Dad, who at age fifty-three has not yet found peace with his body.[3]

I am angry at my grandmother for doing this to my father. I am angry at my father for continuing to let the word "cripple" echo inside his head, and for fighting it only by denying that he is disabled.

When I became disabled I began to understand my father better. I began to see how physical difference and its resultant pain can force its way into every crevice of one's life. I also came to realize that he will not understand or accept my disability until he comes to terms with his own.

It has been painful to find that he is one of the people in my life least sensitive to my disability, that the issue has become another point of conflict between us rather than a patch of common ground.

It is becoming increasingly clear that I follow him in some ways on this issue. It took me longer than it should have to realize that I was disabled. I, too, mistakenly focus much of my anger on my body. I sometimes deny my limitations, although I am learning to accept and then challenge them. I blame myself for my pain and expect others to use my disability as a scapegoat. But I am proud to say that I also lead my father on this issue. I lead him by learning to discuss my disability honestly. I lead him because I have used his experiences to learn more quickly how to live with my situation.

My father believes that I blame him for my disability. Maybe he blames himself. Sometimes parents forget that other forces act on their children's lives. I don't believe that he caused me to have environmental illness, nor that he is even the main factor involved in the development of my feelings about it.

Like other environmentally ill people, I am deeply affected by what seems to be the prevailing notion that I am not really sick. A local newspaper recently ran an article on environmental illness, announced by a blurb on the front page which began, "Are These People Truly Ill or Merely Crazy?"[4]. Many would like to label us "mentally ill" and forget us as quickly as possible.

Co-workers, family members, friends, and others often tell us that we are only imagining that we are sick. They deny that environmental illness exists because they fear its implications. If we with EI are simply some of the first to collapse under the weight of environmental pollution (and I believe this is the case), how much time remains before everyone is environmentally ill?

Unfortunately, denying the existence of the disease and those who suffer from it won't make it disappear. In fact, denial prevents action from being taken to eliminate the environmental contaminants that cause us to be ill.

The same masculine world view that promotes pollution through capitalism has instilled us with a false concept of the body and mind as separate from each other. This view adds to people's disbelief of EI. While feminist theory reunites the mind and body, it is difficult to escape the social conditioning to disconnect the two. This sometimes causes even feminists to forget that we know that disturbances in the body can cause emotional and intellectual troubles, and vice versa. Yet we know that nutritious meals make children more able to learn in school. We know that premenstrual irritability has physiological causes. We know that during and after high-stress times we often become ill, and that the illness exists on a physiological plane. Still, when I tell people that my principal reaction to tobacco smoke is that I suddenly become violent, or that when someone walks by me wearing perfume my mind becomes confused, I am often told that this cannot possibly be true. I am told that I am crazy and that my silly disease doesn't really exist.

It is clear to me and to the people around me that my toxic reactions are more frequent and more severe when I am under a lot of stress. People often mistake this *aggravating* factor for a *causal* factor, and again believe that my illness is a hoax. While reducing stress does make me feel better, it does not make me healthy.

Telling me, directly or indirectly, that I am crazy does not help. Telling me that I will become healthy ''as soon as I really want to'' is similarly destructive. This attitude asks me to believe erroneously that I am in control of my disability and my environment. It asks me to deny my toxic reactions. Denial can prevent me from avoiding the substances that cause my symptoms. And increased exposure leads to more severe reaction.

I once went into a public bathroom that had just been cleaned with ammonia. My reaction to ammonia is immediate diarrhea. The diarrhea prevented me from leaving the bathroom, yet staying increased my exposure to the allergen. Twenty minutes passed before I was able to escape.

Environmental illness is unusual in that an otherwise accessible situation can be made inaccessible simply by the entrance of one antigen-bearing person. You may not know anyone with EI, yet you could set off a reaction of the person behind you in line at the bank or next to you on the bus with your cigarette or your perfume. Thousands of people in every urban area react to these two things. It would make our lives much less painful if smoking and perfume wearing were only done in private. That change is not going to happen quickly. In the meantime, we all need to be sensitive.

I recently attended a slideshow at a lesbian/gay club where a non-smoking policy was announced. When a woman began to smoke, I approached her and politely asked her not to smoke in the room. (This is a dangerous endeavor, as it requires my getting very close to a burning cigarette.) The woman replied, ''I'm not smoking in here. I'm standing next to the door (which was closed) so I'm not smoking in here.'' I told here that I was ''allergic'' and that her smoke was making me feel sick from my seat a few yards away. She responded by blowing smoke directly in my face from a range of about one foot. My friends and I had to leave the show. My reaction lasted nearly 24 hours.

Often friends and family of environmentally ill people feel frustrated and helpless to relieve the discomfort of someone they love. Ironically, the expression of these feelings often resembles hostility and lack of support. As you can imagine, this is not helpful at all. While you can't make your friend's environmental illness go away, you can help make the illness a little easier to live with, at least when you and she are together. The following suggestions come from my personal experience with both folks who are helpful and those who are not. They are meant simply to inspire thought and discussion. Please don't assume that all environmentally ill people are the same or want to be treated the same way.

Don't be embarassed or intimidated about asking questions. It's true that I get tired of answering them, but incorrect assumptions hurt me more.

Please don't tell me that you understand what I'm going through because you have an allergy. Recognize that there is a level on which you will never understand what I'm coping with unless you contract EI yourself. Do your best to understand what you can.

Be sure you know what substances make me react. (For example, don't assume that incense, essential oils, or herbal cigarettes are ok because they're "natural.") Consider keeping a list so you won't have to trust your memory. Ask if you don't know.

If you smoke, don't assume that your smoke won't cause me to react if we're outside. Inside, don't assume that standing at the window or by the door will help keep the smoke away. The air coming in the window will actually blow the smoke *into* the room. A doorway is no barrier. Smokers carry smoke with them a long time after they've had their last cigarette. I react to that smoke, too, even though you probably can't smell it.

Ask me what you can do to make your house, car, body, etc. less likely to cause me a reaction. Do what you can to accomodate. Be honest with yourself and with me about what you can't do, and about what you can do without becoming resentful. But realize that I will probably use my sense of your cooperation to gauge how important our relationship is to you. (If it's more important to you to wear perfume than to be with me, I probably won't want to see you at all!)

Ask me how I want you to respond if you're with me when I have a severe reaction.

Please don't assume that I'm exaggerating descriptions of my reactions. Don't conclude that because I drank a half a glass of milk once, I'm lying if I tell you I can't drink milk today. Reactions are cumulative; the tar fumes I was exposed to this morning may cause milk to set off a massive reaction tonight. Only I can make the choices about what to risk when, and I may not always make the best choice! Sometimes it's worth it to go to a concert despite the smoke, but that doesn't make my toxic reaction to it any easier to handle. In such an instance it would be much more supportive to say, "These trade-offs must be really hard to make," than to say, "Cut the complaining. You knew you'd get sick if you came here."

Don't tell me that I dwell on my environmental illness. (How do you feel when a man tells you that you dwell on being a woman?) If I repeatedly bring up conflicts that I have with you about it, it's because I don't feel that they have been resolved, not because I want to goad you.

One of the biggest hassles for me is constantly having to ensure accessibility. When we're going out together, you could help by occasionally doing this for me. Call ahead and ask about a smoking policy. Ask people to stop smoking or to move away. When the toxicity level becomes intolerable, it would help if you'd offer to leave an event with me. It's difficult for me to ask you to leave and spoil your good time.

If I am prone to brain reactions, you can help me learn to recognize them by asking me if the sudden change in my mood could be a reaction. *Make sure you do this in a supportive way.*

If you get tired of always having to "deal with" my disability, remember that I have to deal with it even when you're not around. It's a lot more inconvenient to me than it is to you. I, as a disabled person, have no more innate ability to cope with constant hassle than you have. It's as frustrating and maddening to me to be disabled as it would be to you.

You probably do lots of things socially that I can't. This is hard for me, but it's something that I have to accept while we're working to make the community more accessible. It's important that we talk about how this makes us both feel, and how it affects our relationship.

Please don't start doing all of these things at once! I may not be able to handle it.

I realize that being aware, nurturing, and supportive of a difficult illness takes its toll on you, too. We need to talk about this. I don't want you to resent me for the inconveniences my illness causes you.

If you're organizing an event and trying to make it accessible to disabled people, remember that environmental illness is a common disability. While it is impossible to make an event completely accessible to all people with EI, there are a number of things you can do. *Publicize* and *enforce* a "no smoking" policy. (Lobbies and bathrooms should be smoke-free). Ask those attending not to wear scents (lotions, colognes, shampoos and detergents can all be as dangerous as perfume). Avoid recently painted rooms, rooms with carpets, and places that are dusty, musty (this indicates mold growth), or have poor ventilation. Childcare rooms should meet the same requirements, as many children are environmentally ill. If food will be served, investigate and have available foods that are least likely to cause reactions. Consult with environmentally ill people or written materials on EI for more details. Advertise both safe and unsafe features. If you are unable to follow all of these suggestions, consider eliminating scents and tobacco smoke as the top priorities.

Being a lesbian and part of the feminist community has made coping with my disability somewhat easier than it might otherwise be. The growing community awareness of disabled rights is refreshing and helpful. I have learned much from both disabled and able-bodied women about my rights to respect and accessibility. (Some allergens are actually easier to avoid — birth control products and perfumes, for example.) Support and nurturance are more highly valued by feminist culture than by the mass culture in this country. I am glad to be surrounded by a politically conscious community, as it is important to me that the political roots of my disability be seen clearly. Environmental illness need not exist. Only with a thorough understanding of both EI and the political conditions by which it is promoted can we work effectively toward abolishing it.

Notes:

1. Anaphylactic shock is characterized by extremely severe symptoms including swelling, difficulty breathing, a choking feeling, wheezing, nausea, rashes, abdominal pain and loss of consciousness.

2. "What's Eating You?" by Nick Gonzalez, published in *Family Health/Today's Health,* November 1977.

3. This is the best information I have about my father's life as a disabled person. Even while telling me that some of it is incorrect, he has not been able to share more accurate information, feelings, or stories with me.

4. *Pacific Sun,* week of August 5-11, 1983. Published by Pacific Sun Publishing Co., Inc. Mill Valley, CA.

Untangling the Web Of Denial

by edwina trish franchild

A beginning: a source, a horizon, a point of departure, lines of separation, lines of merging, an explanation of difference, a disclosure of sameness.

Whenever I speak or act in the world, part of me falls silent and afraid, and my full strength remains hidden and unused. I become confused and frightened by the implications of my past and present as a blind lesbian writer with a history of psychiatric incarceration. All this makes me a potent source of danger to the patriarchal establishment. For my own protection, I have kept much of myself cloaked in secrecy, even to myself. My hidden parts rebel and emerge from time to time; I now give them the freedom to remain in the open as my allies, and as allies to true feminist understanding and achievement. I begin to come to terms with the contradictions of my experience by claiming and remembering the wholeness of my life.

I was born in 1951, the first child of a registered nurse and a grade school teacher, in Georgia. My parents were from the Akron, Ohio area where my mother and I returned to live while my father served in the Korean "conflict". My only brother was born exactly nine months after my father returned home. When I was about two, a little before my brother Michael was born, my father's mother began to notice that when I walked, I walked into things a lot. "I don't think she sees too good," Grandma Sarah commented. That began endless rounds of visits to opthalmologists; my parents constantly, anxiously trying to find out what was "wrong" with my eyes.

Apparently, it was not obvious to these doctors that I had retinitis pigmentosa, a condition that caused me to have tunnel vision, night blindness, sensitivity to bright light, and slow adjustment to changes in light. The opthalmologists all managed to prescribe treatments for this unknown (to them) condition: glasses, eyedrops, patches, and looking games of all kinds. It all seemed mysterious to me. Why was I still being subjected to all this humiliation? What had I done wrong? My stomach still churns with fear and anger when I hear the question, "How many fingers am I holding up?" Gradually, an impression was built up in my family that if nothing could be found "wrong" with my eyes, it must be "psychosomatic"; after all, I could see *some* things. "She just sees what she wants to see" is a familiar assertion.

I was unable to use the term "blind" about myself, since my family avoided the word entirely. They would speak in hushed tones about my "vision problem". I first began hearing the word blind when I went to school. The other children, adept at learning the truth and zeroing in on those who were different, began to taunt me, "Are you *blind?* She's *blind.*"

I was quite aware that it was a disgrace to be unable to see. I covered up my blindness by nodding in agreement whenever anyone said, "Look at that!" or the like. My father used to jerk my head into the correct position, demanding, "*Now* can you see?" I did my best to convince him that I could, though I was usually too frightened by then to see anything at all.

My father is an artist, he loves beauty, and has always been concerned that things "look right." He often seems to confuse superficial appearances of people and things with the totality of their being. I was disappointing to him in two ways: I was physically unattractive, never a pretty little girl, and I had a hard time perceiving the surface of the world, the part of reality which he preferred. Later, I disappointed him in a third way: I publicly manifested, through "anti-social" behavior, the carefully hidden pain of my family's life.

Remembering... hearing my father tell me, over and over, what he heard a teacher of mine say: "She'll see better and better as she learns to use her eyes." He believes this means I'll be sighted, normal, if I will "use my eyes." For much of my life, even after I become an adult, he slaps my hand whenever I reach out with my hand to locate a dropped object, or to acquaint myself with the shape of anything. "Use your eyes!" he exclaims.

I now realize that for my father it was more important that I "look normal" by using a sense that was quite inadequate, rather than to shift to any alternative or "weird" way of relating to my environment. This meant I had added difficulty functioning in the world, and would appear to be clumsy, for which I was also ridiculed. He wanted desperately to have a "normal" daughter, but everything he did worked against that possibility.

Eventually, while I continued to believe that there was something indefinably wrong with me, I grew to understand that there was also something wrong with the way I was being treated. Some deep part of me must have known it was wrong to be humiliated and punished for something that was a natural and unchangeable part of my being. As parents, grandparents, teachers, and opthalmologists conferred about possible ways to "help" me, I began to sense the presence of a plot. Since I did not fit the acceptable category of "sighted" or even the less acceptable but still comprehensible category of "blind," I threw those who came into contact with me into confusion. I was a creature who existed between two concepts, and they strove hard to get me to fit into one or the other. "Blind" meant helplessness, irrationality, hopelessness, darkness, even an association with death itself. "Sighted" meant hope, rationality, capability, life. Given these choices, the adults around me tried to force me into the sighted mold. They did this partly by taking me to eye doctors who might be able to "cure" me, but mostly by simply denying that I could be anything but sighted. Thus, the whole reality of my experience was being denied, and I was told that it did not exist. Part of me believed that I must be crazy and deficient to perceive things so differently than they did. But an older, pre-language part of myself realized that they were trying to deny my existence and therefore my life itself. *They were trying to kill me!* I then hypothesized that there was a world-wide conspiracy that was trying to do away with me, for some completely unfathomable reason. This feeling of mine was expressed by fear of and endless rage at my parents; I had frequent tantrums and kept running away from home. My parents and the school authorities decided I was deeply disturbed; I was sent in now for a new round of testing: psychological. I was given every test imaginable, including a brain scan, to see if my brain was damaged. I was taken in for counseling at a "child guidance" center. When that did not seem to work my parents committed me to a state psychiatric hospital for children. The year was 1962, and I was ten years old.

Remembering... "What is the matter with you?" asks my father. His voice is tense, frightened, the day I took all my cherished glass and china horses and smashed them to bits in the bathroom sink. "You know better than I do," I tell him. I don't want to give away any information that might be used against me. This is one of my strong days. When I am feeling weak, I cry and beg the world — "Please, just tell me what you want of me! I'll do anything! I'll kill myself! Just tell me what you want and tell me why!"

Remembering... the morning of June 12, 1962. Awakened by my mother's cheerful voice, saying, "Get up, Tricia! It's time to take a little ride to Sagamore Hills!"

The drive was a long one, about an hour or more. While we drove, I became more and more fearful of what might await me. The day my mother had first mentioned Sagamore Hills to me, we had walked the single block to the park. I hung idly twirling on the swing while my mother spoke. "How would you like to go a special school this summer? One with lots of other kids and a swimming pool?" she asked. I shrugged, imagining a sort of summer camp, where kids got to be solid friends as they complained about a not-so-terrific school. "I suppose that would be alright," I said. Later, I became frightened, wanted to change my mind about going to this place. My mother only laughed.

When we arrived, I took a good look at Sagamore Hills State Psychiatric Hospital for Children, and knew it wasn't for me. The "front office" was glass, full-length windows, ugly plastic furniture, and the porous, pale green brick walls with which I was to become so familiar. Piped-in beautiful music gave the same feeling to your ear and soul as the ghastly walls gave to your eye.

When a couple of "child-care workers" came to take me back to "Ward B", I put up a struggle. It took several adults to drag off my ten-year-old body, screaming, biting, kicking. But when I finally arrived at the Ward, I was frightened into silence.

Ward B was the youngest girls' ward, where girls from the ages of seven through twelve were placed. There was a ward for younger children; Ward A had girls and boys from the ages of four through seven.

I found Ward B very boring; the girls there, though some were older than I was, seemed so young. And even while I refused to accept my captivity (I wrote desperate letters to aunts and grandparents, begging them to come and release me; I threw tantrums and so got locked in the "conference room") the place began to work on me. I began to learn the times for all the regimented activities of the hospital; I talked to the other girls, learning who the "nice" child-care workers were. All of the wards in the institution were identical. At one end was a locked, tiny kitchen, next to the living room area with a TV and a couple of green plastic and metal couches. A large plain dining table was in front of the kitchen door. In back of that there was an open area, which in some wards contained a ping-pong table, in others just a plain table for working puzzles or playing cards. These were two major activities at Sagamore Hills. The third was watching television. In the open areas were bathrooms with toilets and sinks and a staff office with windows to watch the activities on the ward. Next to that was the bizarrely named "conference room" — a room designed for patients who were "out of control". Towards the back of the ward were the bedrooms, a couple of single ones, and two huge four-bed dorms. The beds were covered in dark brown ribbed institutional bedspreads which we were taught to make with neat hospital corners. I was never very good at bed-making, and received lots of "gigs" or demerits, because of my sloppiness, though I really did try. (I'm still unable to make a really straight, smooth bed.)

I stayed on Ward B for only three weeks. (Actually, that wasn't such a short time; three weeks was the usual length of time that a child stayed at Sagamore Hills. I was to stay for precisely two years.) I was tranferred to Ward C, the ward for the girls aged twelve to fourteen. I stayed there for about a year and a half, and on my twelfth birthday was transferred to Ward J, the oldest girls' ward. Why I was continually placed with girls much older than I was I don't know.

I don't know how to describe the monotony of Sagamore Hills. Each day seemed precisely identical to the one before it, except for weekends which were much more boring since some patients were away on visits and there were fewer staff to take us outside.

Boredom and rage are the two feelings I most associate with my time at Sagamore Hills. I also did a lot of thinking. I would stare for hours at those ghastly green walls. I could imagine that those holes in the walls were all kinds of things — beings and people. I day-dreamed stories about those holes, and I thought: Was I sent to the hospital as punishment for coming so close to figuring out the world? Is that why we were all here? Were we in fact the sane ones, and were the folks running around on the outside the ones who were really crazy? It seemed so hopeless. Sometimes it still does.

Remembering... Being hungry for books, reading anything that comes to hand; quickly running out of things to read in the hospital library, waiting and hoping for books from outside. They never come often enough.

Remembering... I am small, before the hospital, my mother takes me to the Cuyahoga Falls Library, the Taylor Memorial Library, an old firetrap of a building that smells deeply and intoxicatingly of books. Its cool, comforting darkness, the incredible delight of having shelf after shelf of alluring books to choose from, the regret of only being able to take home three or four.

Remembering ... other ghosts. My own ghostly selves, the girl-turning-woman who reads everything she can find. Finding a strange little paperback book lying on a table in Ward J, when I moved there from Ward C on my twelfth birthday. The book is called Jane Eyre, *and I marvel that anyone can write a book with a heroine that seems so much like myself, and figuring that very few people would want to read such a book. Being shocked to learn years later that Charlotte Bronte's novel is considered a classic, read by millions*

Remembering... Beech Brook, the second institution I stay at, so much softer and easier to live with than Sagamore Hills. Originally, an orphanage, it was built on a circular road that curves through the grounds. The buildings where children live are grand old mansions, built, I think, just after World War I. The cottages and other buildings are all named after some wealthy Cleveland family who gave to build the orphanage — all with large back porches where we do the laundry with old-fashioned wringer washers and a kitchen where we cluster around and drink juice (what a luxury! We never had juice at the hospital), a pantry, a dining room, a living room, a sewing room, a big mud room with a big sink for washing hair, a bathroom downstairs, and another with showers upstairs. During the day the doors are unlocked, I can take a walk anytime my chores and homework are done, even as far as the near-

by woods, if I get permission from the houseparent on duty.

I was in the two psychiatric institutions, Sagamore Hills and Beech Brook, for a total of four years. While I was in Beech Brook, my mother committed suicide: she, too, was feeling the torment of conflicting realities.

I am back in Sagamore Hills now, a grown up little girl, crying in a green-walled hopelessly bare and locked room, waiting for myself, older and stronger and wiser now, to come and talk to me, to help me break away. Maybe that way my child-self and my grown-self can rescue each other... That's overly dramatic, I don't really need to be rescued, I'm doing fine. I do need to remind myself of that fact pretty often. I am doing okay now, but I would have liked to have known that then, because I didn't know if things would ever change. I had hopes and dreams, however.

Dreaming, fantasizing, daydreaming... I had always done a whole lot of that. Ever since I can remember I was spending lots of time in imaginary worlds. I loved it, and looked forward to times when I could be alone so that I wouldn't be interrupted in the middle of a story. It was important to be alone, because people could tell if I was daydreaming. I would get so carried away, and be so oblivious to my surroundings, that my hands would start moving, and would wave and flutter around my head, and this looked very strange to other people. My parents called it "twiddling". My father took to grabbing my hands whenever he caught me at it. I felt a lot of shame about my "twiddling" — people would often ask me what it meant, what was I doing, was I nervous? and so forth. I told people, but they never could get it, not even my parents; it was completely alien and beyond their comprehension, apparently. I felt the same kind of uneasiness about this behavior as I did about my blindness, and I must have felt, as others did, that it was related to my blindness and my general feeling of strangeness.

I now understand that my daydreaming was a way of having someplace else to go, where I wouldn't feel uncomfortable, or strange, or ugly. I eventually learned to daydream without any physical movement, and this made life a bit easier. Still, staying in the real world is a difficult task for me, and one I wish I were better at.

In my adult life, people continue to insist that I cannot exist as I really am, to deny my reality. Everywhere I go, those around me try to fit me into their concept of what a blind woman must be like (they often even have trouble with the idea that I can be blind *and* a woman), or they insist that I am not *really* blind, or that if I am, it must be my own damn fault somehow, or that my being blind means that I'm incapable of being their employee, colleague, friend or lover.

Remembering... It is early evening, and I am riding home on a city bus through my neighborhood on the near south side of Minneapolis. As we stop near one of the many bars along Franklin Avenue, a drunk man gets onto the bus and takes a seat in front of mine. He glances back at me, and notices my white cane. "HEY, blind girl," he calls out. "You know, you're not bad-looking for a blind girl."

Remembering... I am disembarking from an airplane in New York, changing planes as I return from a demonstration in New York City where blind people were protesting our treatment by a custodial agency "for the blind". A young male flight attendant asks me if I need any assistance in finding my way. I thank him and say that I don't need any help. "Okay," he says reluctantly. "But I have to tell you one thing. I really admire the way you people ski." I have never skied in my life, but I don't mention this.

Remembering... Walking down the street in downtown Minneapolis, coming to a corner, and waiting for the light to change, lost in my private thoughts. Out of nowhere, an absolute stranger is standing in front of me, loudly demanding, "How blind are you, anyway? You don't look blind. Who are you kidding?"

Remembering... Having just moved to Seattle, I am, as usual, looking for any kind of employment I can find. I show up at the office of Greenpeace, Seattle, to volunteer some time, wanting to aid in the work of saving the whales and the earth. I discover that the organization is hiring people to do door-to-door fundraising. Since I have done a lot of telephone fundraising, I thought I might try my hand doing the door-to-door canvassing. I call for an interview, and am told I sound very "verbal", and just right for the job. When I appear for the interview, I am told that a blind person, cannot possibly do this kind of work, because I would work after dark (?) and I might fall down some steps. The young man in charge of the canvassing operation proves his point with a further absurdity. "I know," he assures me, "because I can see, and even I fell down once." Of course, nothing can change his mind, and I do not get the job. I cease thinking of Greenpeace as a non-violent organization, and am unable to force myself to volunteer for them.

Remembering... I am in a lesbian bar in Seattle. A woman passing by says, "Hi, Edwina." I respond, "Hi, who is that?" "It's Jill," she says. "Oh, hi Jill," I reply. "Don't you remember me?" she asks. "I just didn't recognize your voice right away," I tell her. "If you would just learn to focus your eyes, you'd see better," she says. "What?!" I gasp in disbelief. "It works," she insists. "Jill, do you have any idea what you're talking about?" I demand. But she has walked away, and doesn't respond.

In my personal life, at the age of thirty-two, I am still struggling with my self-hate, learned early and still being daily reinforced. I am beginning to accept and feel worthy of pleasure, beauty, and happiness. The forces that opposed my survival when I was small are there to squash me still, but my own strength, and, I hope, the support of feminist friends, are with me. We need to unite to survive.

The Field is Full
Of Daisies
And I'm Afraid to Pass

by maureen brady

two ripe fruits, plump, ready, whole. This was our state when we met. Our bodies came together, fit, everywhere. We felt ourselves sail. We were on a strong sea. Our fingers danced to a new moon, and it seemed as if our feet would not come down to touch the ground. We felt too full to have a future.

The field is full of daisies, and I'm afraid to pass. I planned to go to work that day. This was part of a larger plan, my five year plan, which arrogantly assumed a long future. Reaching the flats, I waited for the woman in the car ahead of me to pass the truck. Waited and waited with the road stretching long and straight ahead through the meadow. Then decided to go. Then her car came moving into mine, into my side. I moved over and over and finally off the road and soared and thought I was gone.

We had just come back from Maine. From beach walking, loving in the tent; from watching the waves wash against the crevices and butts of the rocks. Then I lay flat on my back at the side of the road, the top of my head open. "Please, call this woman, Judith," I told the man. "Please, tell her to come." I gave the phone number. "Please." "Who is she?" he asked. "She is Judith... my very best friend." I closed my eyes. Willed my body only to struggle to clot the blood — not against the man. To live to come back to control.

The wheel went out from my hands. Spun and spun with my hands chasing. Spun and spun back the other way. I saw the field, the road, the field. No sound. Sight, no sound. The field. The road. Out of control. Often I'd read that in the newspaper, never quite sure what it meant. The car went out of control. Alone. No sound. The steering wheel, a broken toy. Here goes, I thought. Here goes. There must have been some noise, but I didn't hear it. I ducked my head before it hit the windshield, didn't even hear that.

"Can you get out?" a man, calling me. My deaf ears came out of the silence. His voice sounded far away, muffled. Who was I? Where was I? I was a person squatted rightside up on the roof of the back seat of a car, upside down. The field was full of daisies. The man was outside. I was birthing consciousness. I was fully innocent.

"Why don't you open the door?" I asked.

He was bent over so that his head was nearly upside down. "I can't. Can you get out?"

Don't rush me, I said to myself. Don't confuse me. My mind stuck on a cartoon of a character who had received a blow to the head and saw symbols floating in disarray. I noticed the blood dripping on my new briefcase — soft brown leather, pleasing to caress — also on the roof of my new car — blue interior, five payments made out of thirty-six. Such was the environment I was being born into. I looked above me for the source of the blood, finally felt the top of my head.

GET OUT, I told myself, panic overtaking dismay. Tried to roll the window down, which was actually up. JAWS OF LIFE they call the machine that comes to bite open the wrecked car. I'd seen that in the paper, too, always imagined the victim being mouthed between iron jaws. Didn't want that, would rather have the soundlessness. My head began to scream pain. I stuck it through the window and crawled out. The man helped me stand up and I felt thoroughly stunned, as if I had no history. "I have no idea what happened to me," I said.

"I saw," he said. "WOW. I saw through my rear view mirror." He watched my face. "Let's lie you down." He walked me a few feet from the car and put me down in the grass. "My head," I said. "My head is coming off." That's when I told him to call Judith.

I once studied neuroanatomy by dissecting a brain. I tried to remember the stiffness of its substance, a texture like tofu, but all

I could imagine was an intestinal mush seeping from the hole in my skull. My eyes were closed. A woman knelt beside me and said, "Please, please open your eyes. Please be okay. Please be okay." The hysteria in her voice worsened my headache. I opened my eyes. She sighed. "Oh God, didn't you see my blinker?"

My memory came into focus with her words. "You never put your blinker on," I said. "Never. I watched. I waited." I closed my eyes. I heard the man tell someone else to take her away. "Watch her, she's upset," he said.

SHE'S UPSET, my body responded. She's upset because I might die.

The first time Harold came to see about restoring the chimney, he was dazed with the loss of his daughter. All the time he measured, I followed him around and listened as he spoke out of the side of his mouth. "I ain't right yet, you know. I just can't figure why her. I take it you heard about what happened." I nodded, asked where the accident had occurred. "Over to the curve just before before the lake road. Nobody saw. Nobody knows what happened. Emergency squad picked her up, carried her in to the hospital, her jabbering all the way. I got the call on the CB. Wife and I rushed in. She was dead by the time we got there." He stood back in the yard and contemplated the chimney for a long time, desolate.

I could feel my face swell as if it were a marsh that water was trickling into. My lips were swelling to numbness and my eyes wanted to puff shut. It was hard to move my attention from my head and face, but when I remembered Harold's daughter, I decided to take a survey of my organs. I tried to think myself on a route around my abdomen, to feel for the sensation of bruising, rupture, hemorrhage. My heart beat harder as I thought of Harold's daughter chattering her fear as she rode to the hospital. Places on my legs burned, but I couldn't feel anything except panic where my liver should be, my pancreas, my stomach, my gall bladder, my intestines, my spleen. As soon as I thought about my blood pressure, I felt faint. I told the man, who brought a stool and elevated my legs. "I'm an emergency tech," he said. "I guess I'm lucky," I said. "Am I still bleeding?"

Why don't we teach comforting as an emergency technique? As the time stretched out I felt I might die for the lack of it. "Have you called Judith?" I asked. "What did she say?" someone asked. "About calling the girl, Judy." I felt diminished. "Judith," I said, with enough venom that they drew back from me. The waiting time was exhausting. I felt with each new minute I had to call up deeper reserves from within.

The emergency tech decided to wrap my head to try to stop the bleeding. He instructed another man to straddle me so he could stoop and lift my head with full support around my neck. I felt disgusted by his position; the enormity of his shoes at my sides seemed humiliating. After they finished wrapping me, I talked to them little. The blood on my face was hardening sticky and these two men took turns fanning away the flies that came to light on it. They kept looking off down the road for the amulance while I listened in the other direction for Judith. Enough time had passed that she would be arriving any minute, I thought, and then I would be able to relax and stop comforting myself. I could feel others who had stopped and gotten out of their cars to come and view me, watching, but I didn't let my eyes move to them. My rescuers were getting restless. They reminded me of my father, waiting for my mother to soothe the one of us who had caught her finger in the car door, pacing and jingling the change in his pocket as if life had stopped and would not resume until the crying was over and we could pull out of the driveway.

The emergency tech asked me how old I was.

"Thirty-five."

"You married?"

"No."

"Tsk, tsk, tsk. What's a pretty girl like you doing without a husband?"

I couldn't believe I had to have this confrontation lying beside a road, losing my blood through my head, my face feeling more and more like a sponge, my nose merging with my upper lip. I opened my eyes, made my voice steady, said, "I never wanted to be married."

"Sometimes I get too nosy," he admitted, looking down the road again.

"Yes," I agreed, closing my eyes. I regretted having already complimented him on his bandaging technique.

The Sherriff's deputy came, asked me questions and tested me for a sense of humor. Why do people think that humor gives comfort? And for whom? When I felt most like a cartoon character, I wanted least to be treated as one. They had failed to call Judith. I wanted to scream. They had waited for him, the authority, to come and decide if my request should be honored.

Finally, the ambulance. A skinny stretcher, metal tubing and hard mat. I would know if I had a broken neck, wouldn't I? My writing teacher who was quadraplegic said he'd felt his limbs melt away right after the accident. My legs burned in spots, my right thigh, my left shin.

As the road dipped, my stomach dropped an infinity, the feeling just past the top arc of the ferris wheel. I was dizzy. The man accompanying me looked scared, slightly dazed, enough that I was afraid to tell him I felt dizzy. I asked him where he worked instead. He'd just come off the night shift at the paper mill, gone to bed for the morning when the call came.

In the E.R. the nurse worked rapidly, covered me with a sheet, stripped me of my clothes. One inspected my body with cool eyes while the other began shaving my head along the scalp wound. The scrapes of the razor jaggedly cutting the hair nauseated me, and I shook with chills. "A blanket, please." Can't you see I'm cold? They covered me with another sheet and left.

An official woman arrived to ask me some questions. "Fine," I said, glad for someone to talk to. Name. Address. Insurance coverage. To think that I took comfort in these questions. I wanted her to stay. She scribbed on her clipboard and was gone. The room was large, stark, and the clock eyed me — 10:05. I had lived an hour. Where was Judith? Why should someone, anyone, ME, have to stay alone in that large, stark room, supervising her own LIFE until the doctor arrived?

10:15. I could not bear the isolation, but how to call out? All my years of working in a hospital as a physical therapist, wearing a white uniform, hearing patients call out to me, "Nurse, hey nurse," usually wanting the bedpan. Always I'd resented the depersonalization of the term as well as the inaccuracy. But if the nurses had introduced themselves, I didn't remember. Finally I called, "Nurse." I asked if she could call my home and she brought me a phone and dialed for me. My brother, who was visiting us that week, answered. I tried to explain the accident without making it sound horrible, without ruining his vacation. Judith was on her way. I closed my eyes and pictured her and tried to send her messages to drive carefully. When we first fell in love we commuted on weekends between New York City and Saratoga Springs. I remembered the urge to fly, the milestones of thruway rest stops marking the closing of the gap, the Friday nights of touching and touching, confirming our feelings were not just fantasies we had conjured up in our separation, saying, "Our lives have been building to this all these years."

She was not there and then suddenly she was — holding my hand, kissing my face, her eyes brimmed with tears, her presence filling the vast, stark room. I could see in her eyes how battered I looked. They were the first eyes that expressed a relationship to me.

Just then, almost as if they'd been waiting for her too, they whipped me off to X-ray. "Easy," I said, "No hurry," but they left my stomach in the E.R. Judith walked beside the stretcher. The pad they had covered the wound on my head with went flying. The attendant picked it up off the floor and fitted it back to my head. Again, I saw in Judith's eyes an honest response, a large wound. I moved to instruction on the cold, hard X-ray table for dozens of X-rays. My skull, my neck, my back, my legs. I thought of an article I had read which described the aging effects of ordinary diagnostic X-rays. I should be protesting this, I thought. I should permit only one view of each part. But I went on moving to instruction.

Trauma. The doctors would say my trauma took place in the car, then secondarily on the operating table as they cleaned out and closed up my scalp wound. But I saw a clear line of demarcation between trauma and comfort, and every act, every gesture, every spoken word fell into a place on one side of this line or the other. There is no neutral territory in an open wound.

Trauma: I asked the surgeon to position my neck carefully when he put me under. "Here's the anesthesiologist, tell him," he said.

"Doesn't he have a name?" I asked, wanting full accountability. They understood and were hostile in return. I felt them look at each other across my body. I was surprised at my power to threaten them, given my weakened state.

Trauma: 10:05. Leaving me with only the clock to watch over me. Trauma: They didn't call Judith when I asked them to. Trauma: Cold sheets, no blankets in the E.R. Trauma: the scrape of the razor. Trauma: The man wanting to know why I'm not married. The big shoes at my side; the flipping, the upside down, the wheel spinning, the field, the road, the silence, the here goes — no time.

Comfort: It would have been a painless death.

Trauma: The pain in my head screamed with an intensity that obliterated the possibility of completing a thought. Several times it occurred to me to ask the doctor when I could have something for the pain. "I have a question for you," I said repeatedly, then couldn't remember what it was. I said stupid things instead when people asked me how I was, like, "Glad to be here."

Comfort: That euphoria — still not sure I would live, would have memory, intelligence, clarity, but sure how much I wanted my life *to be.*

Trauma: That night after the surgery I told the nurse I wanted to look in a mirror. "I think maybe you should wait a few days," she said, her voice officious, stern. "It's still me," I said. "I think I'll recognize myself."

Comfort: I looked. I touched all over my swollen face with my cool hand. My head was fully wrapped in a white, gauze turban. I admired the colors of my black eyes, the deep purple lines. I recognized the feelings that had been fluttering in my belly: a deep vulnerability, a need for tenderness to touch every part of me. I held my cheeks and wept. Then I held the split open backs of my knuckles, then I held my neck. Then I felt my hot burning right thigh and spoke to my femur with pride in the strength and resilience of my bones.

I'll Never Walk Alone

by toni gardiner

i sat in the vet's office, tears streaming down my face. I had just heard a death sentence pronounced on my guide dog Flicka.

She had terminal cancer and with chemotherapy might live seven to fourteen months longer. The words cut through me like a sharp knife. I put my arms around my beloved dog and held her close to me. I went home to break the news to those many friends who dearly loved Flicka, an outgoing and friendly dog. Despite my grief, I had to make plans. I am a realist and feel that I must be in control of my life whenever possible. Since there are so many times that, as a blind person, I am dependent upon others, it is vital to me to be as independant as I can. I needed to make plans for my future.

I was born with limited sight, which I lost by the time I started college. At age twenty-two, I decided to get a guide dog, the most important decision I've ever made. I got Charm, my first Golden Retriever, from Guiding Eyes for the Blind in 1967. She was a magnificent, quiet and passive Golden. Having a guide dog made a tremendous difference in how I greeted the world. I found that when I travelled with Charm I never felt alone. I now had a companion to talk to when the subway was late. I am basically an outgoing person, but I feel stymied when meeting people if I don't know exactly where they are or who they might be. People would often approach me now that I had a guide dog. That gave me the opening I needed to make friends with many new people.

Walking with untrained pedestrians can be very frightening for a blind person. I found that when walking with Charm I was able to maintain my independence. I could allow the dog to follow strangers to destinations I could not find myself. I would ask for this help from strangers when looking for a particular track at a subway station, for a store or for an unfamiliar address.

Charm accompanied me through graduate school. During this time I learned that I had to fight for my rights as a blind person. I was placed as a graduate intern in an agency for the blind in New York. This agency had a policy that guide dogs had to be kenneled. Charm was very quiet and would have waited patiently under my desk, not interfering with my multi-handicapped blind clients. I chose not to passively accept this policy, but tried to have it changed through political channels. I was severely criticized by school authorities for doing so. I was accused of being rigid and unyielding, sent to a psychiatrist and a psychologist — and finally let into the program. At no time did the school or the agency see me as a competent graduate student with a real grievance. The humiliation of this issue, and the kenneling of my dog for that year made me a spokesperson for all guide dog users. Discrimination still abounds and blind people are a target of ignorance and misinformation. Whenever possible, I take legal action when verbal convincing does not do the job.

Charm was there to share my triumphs and, at times, to comfort my pain. When Charm died from complications of pneumonia in 1977 I felt at loose ends. A blind friend offered to train a Golden Retriever guide dog for me. Although this was an unorthodox method, he lent me his black Labrador while my new dog was being trained. I purchased a nine month old Golden Retriever and named her Flicka. My friend then began the arduous process of training her to be a guide dog. This process takes three or four months to complete. A guide dog must learn to stop at curbs and stairs, avoid obstacles, and watch for overhanging objects. All dogs are color blind, therefore, unable to follow traffic signals. It is the responsibility of the blind person, in partnership with the dog, to listen for traffic. The dog will disobey a command to cross if it is unsafe to do so. The training covers only the rudiments of guiding; becoming a real team takes many months of working together.

Flicka was so different from Charm in temperament, it took me a long time to adjust to her outgoing personality. It has been extremely difficult for me to make the adjustment from one dog to the next. It feels to me like changing lovers or spouses a few years into a good relationship. It takes time to develop a truly deep mutual working relationship.

Six years after meeting Flicka I was faced with making new life supporting decisions for myself. I wanted a third Golden Retriever as I find this breed most suited to my personality. There are a dozen guide dog schools scattered throughout the United States. I told them of my plight and asked about the possibility of getting a Golden Retriever. Guide dog schools are run by sighted individuals and are as patronizing, condescending and custodial as many other agencies which purport to help the blind. I was told that they, as professional trainers, would make the decision as to what breed of dog I would get when I got to their school. Flicka had so little time left in her life that I didn't want to leave her for a month to train with a new dog. In a state of grief and terror, I sought other alternatives. Stephen Kotun, who had trained Charm in 1967, after eighteen years as a trainer, was no longer with Guiding Eyes. I called him and asked if he would be interested in training a dog privately. He agreed and we set a training price of fifteen hundred dollars. I then selected my own Golden Retriever puppy by interviewing several available dogs. I chose Ivy, a beautiful, soft, playful Golden, to be my new guide. Initially, Ivy stayed with my supervisor's family from Monday night to Friday morning. She was able to relax, play with the family's two children, Tara and Joey, and just be a pet. On Friday morning my supervisor, Joe Fischetti, would bring Ivy to the psychiatric center where I work as a rehabilitation counselor and she would spend the day there. Ivy would then travel with Flicka and me from Long Island to Queens on the Long Island Railroad. In the beginning, Flicka was well enough to do the guiding and Ivy would walk along on my right, as a pet. Ivy would then return to work with me on Monday and she would go back to my supervisor's home until the following Friday morning. I taught her obedience work and Steve would come and teach her guide dog training. In the meantime, Flicka was receiving chemotherapy, and the next seven months were a rough time for both of us. As Ivy would receive training in a particular area, she would take over as the guide on the left, with Flicka walking as the pet on the right. Flicka was instrumental in training Ivy. When Ivy showed confusion, Flicka would take over the guiding and present to Ivy the right way to handle the situation. Ivy, with her playful puppy ways, was a stimulant to Flicka who was fading quickly on the chemotherapy. I was never prevented from taking two dogs with me on the railroad, on the subway, on public busses, or into restaurants. Although both were quiet and well trained, it is somewhat unorthodox for a blind person to be walking with two guide dogs.

The original time slot Steve and I had set appeared to be prophetic. Flicka died just as Ivy's training was completed. Did Flicka know, almost mystically, that Ivy would know how to take care of me? Did that put her mind at peace? I would like to believe so.

Throughout Flicka's illness, my vet, Dr. Jerald Tobias, was extremely supportive during the various crises in her treatment. He said repeatedly that I had to learn to take one day at a time. I am trying hard not to think about future guide dogs and future alternatives. Ivy is here with me now, I love her, and that will have to suffice for the present. It is the beginning of a new era. The era of my love and partnership with Ivy.

Smiles...

by norma james

Of course we smile.
What else is one to do?
Despair will not penetrate —
Defiance will not disintegrate
This glass wall that surrounds us
And hostility will only puzzle you.
This smile covers a multitude of things —
The frustration of short-circuited
    human contact,
The deep-seated pain on loss of
    a whispered word,
The hidden but utter rebellion
    against the gods.
Would crying help?
Of course we smile.
It is our defense against
The rest of you.

A Four-Wheeled Journey

by marjorie wagner

When I was in graduate school, training to be a psychotherapist, I suddenly found myself facing a major and traumatic change in my life.

I was 53 at the time — retired on disability and walking with crutches. I had had Muscular Dystrophy since early childhood and knew from the slow progression of the disease that someday I'd need to use a wheelchair. Some day in the far future, I thought, not then.

I believed that my recent falling was due to an injury. So when I saw my doctor and found out my muscles had become too weak to support me, that I had to stop walking or use braces and suffer future chronic pain from the undue stress on my joints, I was shocked. I couldn't believe this was happening. I always thought my arms were too weak to handle a wheelchair and didn't see how I could manage.

The doctor's assessment that my muscles had gotten too weak to support me caught me off guard, disarmed. It made sense and accounted for the problems I had, but I didn't want it to be true. I wanted a cure for my wobbly legs. I wanted to maintain my denial of what was happening to me. With a unexpected burst of tears I ushered in the next stage of my life.

A new phase of life, a transition, begins with the ending of an old one. Old ways didn't work for me anymore. Something was wrong. My body, my legs, were getting weaker. My walking had become increasingly precarious. I could only walk short distances. Getting out of bed became more and more difficult. If I sat too long I was too stiff to walk until I braced my legs against a chair to "lock" my knees.

As much as I had fought against the inevitable — by taking physical therapy, hydrotherapy, and by getting proper exercise and rest — the time had come for me to stop walking and use a wheelchair.

I disconnected from my old way of life before being committed to the new. I had to mourn the loss of using my legs before I could put energy into using a wheelchair instead.

Part of this process consisted of reviewing other episodes concerning my health, the falls I had as a child that left me feeling embarassed, the profound disappointment and confusion at age 14 when my leg operation didn't cure me, and the intensive year-long therapy I had in my 30's to recover from another operation before I could return to my job.

At times I wondered why I was singled out to have to go through this. Other people were strong for no apparent reason. Sometimes I was resentful, angry or depressed. Other times I realized that I could go through this if I would only try. I had overcome other disappointments and gone through other crises. I knew others, also, who lived satisfactory lives with severe physical limitations.

My first major task was to find an accessible apartment. My bathroom door was too narrow for a wheelchair. Within a few days Vocational Rehabilitation informed me that a previously requested van would be made available to me. This prompted my decision to leave San Francisco.

Facing all the changes I had to make left me full of anxiety, even panicky, much of the time. I was overwhelmed with thoughts of things to do and fears that I couldn't cope. How could I ever use a wheelchair with my weak arms? Where did I want to live? How could I find an apartment without any transportation of my own? How could I pack and move when I felt so tired all of the time?

My anxiety mounted until I chose the "right" city and then I felt better having made a decision. Soon, however, my panic increased again and I would decide to live somewhere else. I repeated this pattern several times before I finally moved to Walnut Creek. I had responded to an apartment ad in the paper, a friend checked it out for me and the San Francisco Independent Living Program arranged transportation for me to see it for myself. Then with help of friends and a moving company I packed and moved.

The week after I moved I entered Santa Clara Valley Medical Center for evaluation and wheelchair training. This consisted of physical therapy and occupational therapy sessions focusing on transferring, daily care and household skill training.

Returning "home" to my apartment was the hardest part. I felt very alone and isolated. My emotions fluctuated from depression to rage and despair. My anger over feeling helpless was displaced onto others, but nevertheless proportionate to the trauma I felt.

Once my attendant left without closing the window. In the middle of the night I awoke to hear the door rattling. In a flash my anger grew to such intense rage that I was alarmed, I felt so out of control. Suddenly my rage left as soon as it had come and I realized I was resentful at having to depend on someone else to do what I wanted to do for myself.

I was losing my old self — the way I controlled my body, the way I conducted my physical being. My daily routine — not only closing windows, but getting out of bed, getting dressed and washed, doing dishes, cooking and going to the john — seemed nearly impossible. I had taken for granted the old ways of doing things and only appreciated the simplicity now that drastic changes were necessary. Everything was an extreme effort. New patterns were not yet perfected. (Did you ever try putting on pants while sitting down? It took me weeks to accomplish this.)* Gone are the days when I can get up late and be out of the house in 15 minutes. It takes me that long to get out of bed now, and another hour to dress and wash. Like the bumper sticker says, "Disableds do it slower."

While planning the modifications for my apartment I felt like I was in a daze. My new home didn't seem like mine yet. I had a carpenter raise my kitchen floor (so I could reach the stove and sink), raise the patio deck with a redwood flooring (because a step made it inaccessible), build a ramp at the front doorstep and a bath platform over my tub, to use with my hand shower for bathing. I learned to use a raised toilet seat, a slideboard to transfer. I got a looped strap to lift my legs and reachers to pick things up from the floor.

As I became more proficient my frustration and anger gradually

---

*For me this is done while sitting on the (raised) toilet seat with one leg on my wheelchair and the other on my bath platform in front of it. I pull my pants up each leg as far as they will go. Then while stabilizing myself with one arm and leaning to that side, I pull my pants up under me on the other side with the opposite arm. I do this about three times on each side before I can get my pants up to my waist.

waned. As my daily care became easier I began to appreciate my accomplishments. Trade-offs became obvious. I might not be walking, but I was more mobile using the chair. I was no longer afraid of falling. I went places where I couldn't before because my walking was too precarious. I slipped into a comfortable routine and was able to focus outside myself.

The next most difficult part of my transition into a wheelchair was dealing with the way people began to treat me. This was by doing things "for me" instead of letting me proceed at my own slow pace. They rushed in to complete tasks I had begun, or started others before I had a chance. I felt like it wasn't acceptable for me to proceed my own way — that somehow I wasn't competent or whole any more. There was also a feeling of intrusion that I felt — that others were taking over what was mine. Over protection increased my already present feelings of inadequacy. Trying to cope with my frustration, I realized that there were certain things I did want help with, and others that I wanted to do alone. As it became clear to me that some help was beneficial I was more capable of making choices and stating my preferences assertively.

As a disabled person, a member of a minority, I am faced with a dilemma if I am to be psychologically healthy. Minorities are claimed to be inferior and assigned a label. Then the establishment proceeds to enforce those concepts by rules and behavior. These negative images must be refused if I am to value my personal identity and maintain self-esteem. The disabled are labeled weak, helpless and pitiful; are likened to children in that we need to be taken care of. Is it a coincidence that BART (Bay Area Rapid Transit) tickets for the handicapped are red — the same color assigned to children who are also considered helpless and incompetent? (Green is assigned for the elderly and blue for regular customers).

When I was first in a wheelchair I *felt* weak, helpless and sorry for myself. It was all too easy to accept society's stereotype. All my energy was spent on making necessary changes and none was left to dispute images of helplessness that seemed appropriate to me at the time. I had to regain my self-esteem before bucking negative images.

One problem the public has in relation to disability is the confusion about the "spread" of physical impairment to other competen-

cies. Recently a waitress asked my friend what *I* wanted to order —
an experience commonly shared by two blind people I know.

A stranger on the street asked my companion, not me, about my
wheelchair. Both times friends didn't know the answers, but for some
reason it was too threatening to ask me directly. I felt confused having
a stranger speak "through me". Didn't he know I was there? Did he
think I couldn't talk? I felt put down, at first, then annoyed. Something
was going on with this man. He had a problem. Perhaps he felt too
vulnerable about his own future. Old age, an accident or illness could
make him helpless. That's a scary thought, and the easiest way for him
to dismiss it was to distance himself from me. As an individual I can
model how I want to be treated, but there will be some who cannot
accept it.

Society's view of the disabled has changed, generally, for the better. Accessible buildings, sidewalk ramps and public buses with lifts
make my presence more visible. The message is I am active, mobile
and productive. Medical advances have increased the number of disabled people and seeing me cope helps others face their future. All of
society benefits as attitudinal barriers are broken down.

Last year I was present when a disabled woman applied for
attendant care. She seemed afraid to strike out on her own while needing
physical help in caring for herself. I was very touched by her. My first
response was apprehension and some pity. Then I realized she would
be okay and become stronger for it. While identifying with her and
her struggle, I felt glad to be a member of the disabled community.
We cope on a very basic level that gives us pride in our being. We confront issues of helplessness, autonomy and control daily and our struggle
helps us grow.

Ever since I moved to Walnut Creek six years ago I sought a support group to help me deal emotionally with being in a wheelchair.
Finally three years ago I joined one. What I discovered surprised me.
As others discussed their problems I realized my own attitudes had
changed. They no longer matched theirs although they had at one time.
I wasn't so frustrated any more. I was on the "other side" now, and
feeling comfortable about a lot of my adjustments. It was like suffering from a serious illness without noticing any improvement, then suddenly feeling okay and realizing that gradual changes had been going
on all the time without my notice. When other things pile up on me

and I am in a crisis, I still get very stressed. But I notice that I am not panicky any more and that my stressfulness is much less severe. Finding alternative ways of doing things and knowing that I can cope helps a lot.

Living With
A Hidden Disability

by anita l. pace

My illness is called agoraphobia. Some have named it the "Housewife's Syndrome," and some describe it as a fear of open spaces. Agoraphobia is neither confined to housewives, nor to the fear of open spaces; it is an illness which affects men and women, single and married, and manifests itself in different ways and to varying degrees.

For me, agoraphobia is an illness of anxiety. Unlike common nervousness, agoraphobia often produces unexplained anxiety attacks. Because anxiety symptoms come without apparent reason, one doesn't know when the next massive onslaught will occur. Thus one begins to avoid the scenes of previous attacks, which results in the paring down of places and situations which feel safe.

I was a nervous child even before experiencing my first anxiety attack. My upbringing was strict, religiously and culturally. Although my parents were born in the United States, their Italian heritage came through in their attitudes about right and wrong, how to dress, talk and feel. Between the Catholic Church and my parents, I felt I was very bad indeed. Yet, looking back, I was a rather pitiful, saintly child. I did my best to keep out of my parents' way, not to cause trouble, to cheer up my mother when she and my father fought, and to help with the cleaning, especially since my mother suffered with cancer and had been diagnosed "terminally ill" (she lived to prove otherwise). There were many holidays when my mother was in the hospital or my parents had a major fight. As a typical child I felt I was the cause of these maladies.

I wanted friends, but I didn't want them to come to the house and witness my fear during my parents' frequent arguments. I felt awkward in most places. I had an excuse-me-for-being-here feeling, a sense of being a burden and of doing things the "wrong" way. I was painfully lonely and didn't know it.

It was as if I was in training to be unable to handle stress. I was taught not to like myself ("conceit"), never to be satisfied with what I did, never to trust that I knew what I felt or wanted. I was taught to hold in laughter and to expect mocking if I cried ("go ahead, Anita, cry; it's good for you," my father would say). I believed sexuality was sinful, and I feared hell and punishment. I kept myself miserable to ward off misery, because I was taught to expect God's horrendous repercussions for any happiness I might experience.

With this background, at age thirteen my family and I moved and I began eighth grade in public school. The difference in values, language and clothing was overwhelming. I was laughed at every time I stood to answer a question, yet I felt it was disrespectful to speak from my seat. I was accustomed to uniforms of bobby socks and tee-shirts, not bras and stockings. My choices felt dichotomous: I could either fit in with my peers and feel guilty, bad, sinful, or I could do as my parents said and be a "good girl." For the most part, I opted for the latter and felt ostracized. Conflicts swarmed in me like bees, the humming of confusion twisting my thoughts.

A sense of panic arises. There is a strangenesss... something like nausea, but not quite. I am very hot and take off my sweater. I don't know what is happening to me. All my attention is focused on these very scary sensations. I watch the clock, hoping that I will make it through the class.

Another day. I cannot breathe. I feel unable to take in air and so I breathe even more, not knowing I am aggravating my system and perpetuating the vicious cycle. The more I breathe, the more I feel unable to breathe. Panic comes as I fear I will pass out in front of my classmates. I think I have epilepsy, or a brain tumor, or maybe even something yet undiscovered. I dare not leave the class.

For days, weeks and semesters, from eighth grade through four years of college, I sat through hundreds of classes in a panic. There were strange sensations, the impossibility of breathing normally, periods of stomach cramps and impending diarrhea. I'd sit in my chair and perspire from pain and fear — fear of pain and fear of discovery. I bore with it. I made it through college earning a Bachelor of Arts degree in Social Welfare with a 3.2 grade average, but I don't know how.

I didn't dare tell anyone about myself until college when I began therapy. Part of me sensed that the hell I was going through was of psychological origin, although I think I would have preferred a physical illness. My therapist told me I was experiencing anxiety and we delved into my life outside of these attacks. But I still didn't have a name for this strangeness. "Anxiety" seemed too simple to explain the horrible sensations I had.

The territory of illness expands. While driving I begin to experience lightheadedness, muscle tightness, difficult breathing. In the library I feel confused and unable to concentrate. I feel a tremendous desire to get out of that massive building.

Somehow I did manage to have relationships. At twenty-two I came out as a lesbian. I began a relationship, and discovered that, for me, the fear of being left was paramount. I could think of no better way to avoid abandonment than by being good, giving, understanding and never getting angry. Any other feeling was unacceptable and, therefore, repressed, except very rarely. My lover, Erin, noticed my nervousness, and I felt ashamed that my symptoms couldn't be covered up, and feared her disapproval.

Perhaps my anxiety problems would never have become so severe had I not been beaten by my next door neighbor after complaining about noise from his apartment. This man was often drunk and I could hear him abuse the woman he was with. The night of the assault, when he and his sister continued to beat Erin and I, even though we were not fighting back, I believed I was going to die. I felt myself shut down emotionally and reach a point of acceptance as I lay outside my door, already numbed to the pain of the blows. It wasn't until I realized I would live that the danger of the situation struck me. Erin and I moved immediately.

Neither of us was seriously injured physically, but the emotional impact of the assault was strong. At first I functioned very well, perhaps because Erin did not. She was extremely frightened for about six weeks and I took care of business, being the Rock of Gibraltar that I had always been. But as Erin became healthier, I sank into a state of severe, continual high anxiety.

Coffee shops and restaurants are more pain than pleasure. I can't seem to swallow when I want to. Instead, I swallow unexpectedly and choke. I am more afraid each time I eat, and I eat less and less around others. Standing in lines at the supermarket, bank and post office are becoming incredible ordeals for me, but I am forcing myself to go. Department stores, especially malls, are overwhelming stimuli and I go to such places as little as possible.

One day, Erin called me at work. She said that someone on a television talk show was talking about "what I have." The name of the mystery was finally made known to me, after nearly fourteen years of suffering. I had agoraphobia. Best of all, it was treatable.

A month later, I was diagnosed as "moderately agoraphobic," and within two months, I began a self-help process toward my recovery. Erin came to the meetings as my support person, just as the other fifteen or so came with spouses.

Once I began to learn about my illness, once I began to realize how hard I had been fighting all my life to "keep it together" when I felt I was falling apart, I began to feel anxiety on an ongoing basis to an extreme I had never experienced. Within two weeks after the group began, I couldn't drive one block. I rapidly became more and more dependent upon Erin and felt petrified by the loss of control and the sense of powerlessness I felt. Every sight, smell, sound and emotion became my enemy, a stimulus to a severe body reaction. I felt drained and scared continually, even in my phobia group.

I quickly became housebound and wasn't safe from anxiety there either. I had to go on disability. I couldn't stop the sensations, even by staying in my apartment. I became very low-functional. I soon felt unable to stand and began spending several hours of my day on the sofa, hyperventilating, gauging each breath, certain that if I didn't monitor myself I'd surely die.

I feared food poisoning, strange odors and medication. I finally consented to Valium, though I feared both dependency and an allergic reaction.

Most frightening was the feeling that there was no way out; no one had the key. I could barely stand up. A heaviness in my head, a tightness around it felt as if a belt of steel circled my forehead. I went to bed in the same clothes I had worn all day, day after day.

My relationship with Erin quickly deteriorated. Neither of us was getting enough of our needs met by the other and we both felt trapped: Erin by her feeling that she couldn't leave me in such a state, and I by my feeling of near total dependency on her. Our physical relationship was nearly totally defunct. Erin brought me flowers every Friday night, yet there was little affection and no sexual intimacy for months and sometimes for over a year at a time. At the same time I wanted affection and to be desired, I had little tolerance for intimacy of either a physical or emotional nature.

I had lived nearly thirty years believing that I could only be loved if I could meet another's needs. I was a person who had massive anxiety attacks from reading, showering, exercising or even walking down the block. Who could love me?

I began to make changes. I got up during commercials to wash dishes for two minutes at a time before lying down again. I began changing my clothes everyday. I learned some yoga and put it to practice by watching a daily television show. I took short walks halfway down the block when I could stand the anxiety, but more often, I practiced sitting in my car, then building up to driving around the block, and eventually to circling my neighborhood. I just kept doing it despite the anguish of my symptoms.

I started a journal, first recording what I had done each day, and eventually writing down feelings which had begun to emerge.

I knew I had to eat better. I hadn't eaten vegetables for years — the fiber seemed too easy to choke on. I bought baby food vegetables, and in a short time, I worked up to peas that I skinned individually. I ate hot cereal and struggled through chicken.

In time, I begin to tell people about my illness. Most don't understand. I feel hurt and angry when someone says, "Anita, everybody gets nervous. I get nervous. But you've got to keep working." Or, "Why should you feel nervous with me? We're friends."

Counseling interns are sent to my home. The pair that visits me tells me, "You must really enjoy staying inside. You don't have to go outside and have responsibilities." My blood boils, but the anger is foreign to me. I cannot touch my anger. I cannot say, "Fuck you! Do you think I'm having a goddamned good time hyperventilating in my apartment every goddamned waking moment of every goddamned day?"

I take a major leap and begin seeing a county social worker, driving a long four miles to reach her. Then, eleven miles to see a therapist. I begin my first assertiveness training session. The group situation is unbearable, but I can lessen my anxiety by sharing, and rediscover my long dormant sharp wit.

As I got better, I thought my relationship with Erin would improve. Instead, I had to face the reality that there was a great distance between us. By the time she moved out, I had gone through quite a bit of grieving. Nonetheless, it was difficult and scary. I didn't know what was worse, my loneliness or the fear of it. Living on my own, I was forced to be more independent and to make more changes. I stopped watching daytime television. I began drinking a mixture of milk and brewer's yeast. I took a disco class. I joined a lesbian organization that had a singles' support group.

But I needed people. I needed friends. And that need became stronger than my fear of anxiety. I began to see a Neo-Reichian therapist, during which time I learned to scream, express anger, and to let myself be touched. I even allowed myself to cry and be held, something I had only done a few times in my life. I began to feel emotions, loneliness, boredom, hopelessness, anger, sadness. It was the pain of one who had technically died and been revived.

I've made new friends and acquaintances, especially in the last year and a half. Besides my singles' group, I have begun acting lessons, paddle tennis, and have recently joined a softball team. I am still not working, but I occasionally clean someone's house, and in the past month, I began volunteer work at a cable television station, daring to learn new things.

I began using a new drug for agoraphobia, after having fought against such use on a regular basis. For me it has been helpful, but without all the other changes in my lifestyle, I believe the tranquilizer would only mask the source of my problem: lack of self-love.

I still have anxiety, but on the whole it's so much less. Some days I feel despair, but I still function. And some days, I feel rather well and happy. My disability has taught me compassion for others, but mostly for myself. I see that recovery doesn't mean days of bliss, the end of problems, sadness, loneliness, fear or hurt. Recovery means learning to accept myself and all the parts of myself. So, with the pain and fear in my life, there is also the excitement and self-love of being alive.

Disabled Women
In the Social Structure

by barbara mandell altman

*r*esearch in the past three years has uncovered the disadvantaged status of disabled women in our social structure (Altman, 1982; Barnartt, 1982; Fine and Asch, 1981). While the increased attention to our disabled population, particularly at government policy levels and among special interest groups, has benefited disabled workers and school aged disabled children, disabled women as a group have not improved their circumstances. This paper will examine disabled women's experiences within the social structure, especially their access to rehabilitation and their receipt of financial assistance. I will explore the specific demographic characteristics associated with women's disadvantaged status in an attempt to find some clues to the institutionalized patterns which appear to discriminate against disabled women.

As an example of the disadvantaged status of disabled women, Altman (1982) found that on all three common structural measures of social status, employment, occupational prestige and income, disabled women showed combination effects due to their gender and impairment. Disabled women had the lowest percentage employed compared to nondisabled women, disabled and nondisabled men. Of those who were employed, almost ⅓ had occupations in the very lowest rankings of the occupational prestige scale. Their mean income was 36% of nondisabled men's, 47% of disabled men's and 74% of nondisabled women's.

Disabled women's access to rehabilitation was also shown to be substantially less than disabled men's as was the public financial assistance which they received. What access there was to rehabilitation emphasized a medical model, concentrating on physical therapy. Disabled men participated in many more types of programs including job training and job counseling and received them from a much greater variety of organizations which emphasized a more utilitarian or reintegrative approach (Altman, 1982).

Rehabilitation and financial assistance are society's major answer to the problem of disability. Programs developed through workman's compensation legislation, veteran's legislation as well as through many private organizations seek to combat impairment or at least to alleviate its consequences. This is done either through payments of compensation for impairment or intervention programs aimed at restoring the disabled to their former functioning or adapting them to their handicap while legitimizing the disability role (Haber and Smith, 1972). Unfortunately the entre to these benefits most commonly is associated with the pre-disability occupational role which until recent years has created a strong barrier for disabled women because of their non-work force participation prior to disability.

Nationally only about 25% of the disabled receive rehabilitation benefits (Teitel, 1977); but since it is the only institutionalized means for the disabled to be reintegrated into society it is an important process to consider. There is good evidence in rehabilitation literature that disabled women are substantially disadvantaged in this area. Social Security statistics indicate 31% of disabled men receive some form of rehabilitation but only 20% of disabled women receive any rehabilitation (Teitel, 1977). In Nagi's study (1969), only 26% of those who applied for rehabilitation were women. The women in this sample, especially the white women, also had the highest rate of denial of services. In the final determination, 53.3% were denied compared to a denial rate of 37.8% for white men (Nagi, 1969).

Research shows that women who do receive access to a rehabilitation program are more likely to successfully complete that program than men. Better, et al (1979), found that the proportion of women who completed vocational rehabilitation programs was 10% greater than the men among those receiving Social Security benefits and even 4% greater among non-beneficiaries. Their sample was drawn from all 1975 closure records for general rehabilitation from vocational rehabilitation agencies nationwide.

Not only do women receive less rehabilitation services and benefits, they also receive less income support and maintenance benefits. William Johnson (1979) examining the "disability benefits system" of the United States is one of the few to compare the receipt of benefits between men and women. His work points up some large differences not only in amounts and proportions received, but also in sources of benefits. Using Social Security data, he found that while 49.5% of the men had impairments that effected their work 37% received any kind of transfer payments. However, though 50.5% of the women had impairments affecting their work, only 21.8% received any transfer payments. This sample consisted totally of individuals who had been employed prior to impairment thus eliminating the employment bias for women.

Johnson (1979) also found these discrepancies between men and women were greatest among the severely disabled. Fifty-seven percent of the severely disabled men received some transfer payments while only approximately 30% of the severely disabled women received any transfer payment. One possible reason for this great difference is the finding that women are much less likely to apply for any of the benefits available primarily because they consider themselves not eligible.

Sources of benefits for men and women were also demonstrated to be different by Johnson (1979). In both cases the greatest proportion of recipients received payment from the Social Security Administration (31.6% of the men and 26.1% of the women). However, higher proportions of men also received benefits from the Veteran's Administration (22.5%) and from government pensions (12.6%). Women, on the other hand, had a higher proportion receiving payments from APTD (Aid to the Permanently and Totally Disabled), a federally aided public assistance program.

The literature definitely shows that disabled women are disadvantaged in their receipt of social structural benefits such as rehabilitation and/or transfer payments. However, the reasons for this serious situation are not even considered. This study explored some possible explanatory factors including:

(1) Marital Status — concern is usually high if the male wage earner in the family becomes disabled and thereby jeopardizes the well-

being of an entire family. The problem is not seen as so serious if it is the spouse who stayed home anyway (or who could with less repercussions).

(2) Condition — specific conditions can be related to rehabilitation potential and/or availability. There are recognized programs for assisting the blind and the deaf but very little available to improve arthritis.

(3) Education — understanding the ramifications of a specific condition and familiarity with available resources plus the ability to navigate the application process could be very closely associated with an individual's education level.

(4) Age — the emphasis on age in our society values the young and thereby may favor the young in disability benefits in order to facilitate their resumption of normal role behavior.

This study was a secondary analysis of data collected and processed by the Bureau of the Census for the Social Security Administration. Of the 18,000 persons selected, 12,900 indicated they were disabled. Since the survey was large and very diverse in terms of disabling conditions, I limited this analysis to three prominent types of impairment conditions. These were life threatening, degenerative and communicative disorders. Those who indicated their primary health condition to be heart disease (987) represented the life threatening category; people with arthritis (1,248) were used as the degenerative group and the communicative disorders group combined those who were either deaf (197) or blind (191). The sample consisted of 1,395 men and 1,228 women who ranged in age from 20 to 66. Twelve percent of the sample was black.

The dependent variables focused on the individual's access to rehabilitation and their receipt of financial support. Rehabilitation was measured by a simple yes/no response to whether or not the individual had received rehabilitation services. Financial support was measured by summing all the dollar values from the various sources of transfer payments including Social Security, Veterans Administration, APTD, Government Pensions, Workman's Compensation, State Temporary Disability, and other public welfare sources.

The independent variables of concern included sociodemographic characteristics of the respondent such as education, race, sex and marital status. Other socioeconomic indicators such as occupation and income were unusable in this study because many of the women never worked and there was no question which ascertained their husband's income. In addition the respondent's medical condition, either heart disease, arthritis, deafness or blindness, was used as an independent indicator. In some instances deafness and blindness were combined into one category representing communicative disorders.

In the analysis I examined the differences in receipt of rehabilitation services and transfer payments between men and women and looked at these differences within each medical category. I also described the differences in the types of rehabilitation and the types of financial support that men and women received. Since my concern was with women's involvement in these disability system benefits, I assessed the relative importance of the independent variables in predicting receipt of these benefits. Once again men and women were examined separately.

In this particular sample men were more likely to receive rehabilitation (21.4% of the men compared to 15.3% of the women). Deaf or blind respondents were most likely to receive rehabilitation while people with heart disease were the least likely to receive it, particularly women. In examining the types of rehabilitation received, I found women were more likely to receive physical therapy while men had greater access to job counseling.

The data showed that a greater number of respondents received financial assistance. Once again, men were more likely to receive this assistance (41.5% compared to 38% of the women), and they were more likely to receive it from more than one source. Examining the sources of financial assistance revealed a somewhat surprising finding that a slightly higher proportion of women received social security benefits than men (24.6% compared to 23.2%). However, men received a much greater proportion of veterans benefits, workman's compensation and unemployment benefits. Women did receive more welfare type assistance than men but this accounted for only a small amount in the total financial assistance picture. The type of medical condition did not appear to be a factor in financial assistance as it was in rehabilitation.

Sociodemographic factors that influenced the receipt of rehabilitation services were similar for men and women. Age, education level and type of condition all were significantly associated with rehabilitation for both sexes, while race and marital status were not. Examining more closely, however, I found that the relative importance of these factors (age, education and condition) were different for men and women. Age was the most important factor for both groups, the younger the individual the more likely they received rehabilitation. However, education was second in importance for women, with higher levels of education associated with rehabilitation. For men this variable was less important than their specific condition.

Men and women did show differences in the effects of sociodemographic factors on financial assistance. Age and condition were the only two variables that are significant predictors of financial assistance for women, with older women and women with heart disease more likely to receive assistance than those who are deaf or blind.

Age was a similar predictor of financial assistance for men, but then the pattern changes. For men, *increased* education level led to increased financial assistance, whereas it was not a factor for women at all. Males with heart disease are also more likely than those with arthritis to receive such assistance and in greater amounts. Neither race nor marital status were important predictors for either men or women. Again, these variables only explained a little of the variation in financial assitance.

Probably one of the most surprising and disheartening results of this analysis is to note the very limited amount of assistance, either rehabilitation or financial, that was received by this disabled sample. It reinforces Johnson's findings that even among the most severely disabled the availability and/or use of the disability benefits system is limited.

The descriptive portion of the results also project another startling pattern. The experience of disability in our social structure is defined differently for men and women. In both rehabilitation and financial assistance areas the disabled male role is associated in one way or another with an active, work related nonstigmatizing philosophy. Rehabilitation for men includes job counseling and job placement. Financial assistance is associated with a past respectable, legitimate, normal male role and is earned via veterans' benefits, workman's compensation, unemployment, etc.

Women's disabled role on the other hand is a compounding of the dependent identity already associated with the female role. The rehabilitation model is a medical one, primarily physical therapy, as pointed out earlier by Altman (1982), that only obliquely addresses the resumption of independent functioning. Except for Social Security benefits, the financial assistance received by women is primarily in the form of welfare payments, once again a very dependent model without even the redeeming quality of "having been earned" that the male model provides. Thus disabled women experience more stigma.

Another important aspect of these results is that regardless of sex, age is an important factor in the receipt of benefits from the social structure. Younger patients are rehabilitated, while older patients are given financial assistance. Condition also appears to be a factor regardless of sex. Heart patients are less likely than the others to receive rehabilitation, but more likely to receive financial assistance.

Education has somewhat different effects for men and women. While increased education level was associated with rehabilitation for both, it was not a factor for women in predicting financial assistance while it was for men. Marital status showed no definite effects in association with rehabilitation or financial assistance for either sex but warrants further examination in light of the dependency model that appears to be associated with disabled women.

In all, the sociodemographic factors had very little association with either receipt of rehabilitation or financial assistance for men or women, yet the differences in receipt of disability benefits between the two groups is significant. This has been an exploratory study that demonstrates the need for further work in this area to explain these differences. Things to be considered in addition to marital status are pre-disability work experience, availability of rehabilitation for the impairment, attitudes of doctors and clients toward rehabilitation, eligibility requirements for financial assistance and whether they emphasize the individual or the family unit.

Note: This paper is part of a presentation made at the 26th annual meeting of the Western Social Science Association, April, 1984 in San Diego, California. For the entire paper, contact the author, Department of Sociology, University of Maryland, College Park, Maryland 20742. Funds for computer analysis supplied by the Computer Science Center, University of Maryland.

Bibliography

Altman, Barbara M. 1982. "Disabled women: doubly disadvantaged members of the social structure." Paper presented at the annual meeting of the American Sociological Association.

Barnartt, Sharon; 1982. "The socio-economic status of deaf women: are they doubly disadvantaged," in Christiansen and Egelston-Dodd (eds.) *Socioeconomic Status of the Deaf Population Conference: Sociology of Deafness*. Gallaudet College, Washington, D.C.

Brown, Julia and May E. Rawlinson; 1977. "Sex differences in sick role rejection and in work performance following cardiac surgery," *Journal of Health and Social Behavior*, 18:276-292.

Better, Sybil R., Phyllis R. Fine, Diane Simeson, Gordon H. Doss, Richard T. Walls, and Don E. McLaughlin; 1979. "Disability benefits as disincentives to rehabilitation," *Milbank Memorial Fund Quarterly/Health and Society*, 57: 412-427.

Berkowitz, Monroe, William G. Johnson and Edward H. Murphy; 1976. *Public Policy Toward Disability*. New York: Praeger.

Croog, S.H. and S. Levine; 1977. *The Heart Patient Recovers: Social and Psychological Aspects*. New York: Human Sciences Press.

Croog, Sydney and Sol Levine; 1982. *Life After a Heart Attack*. New York: Human Sciences Press.

Fine, Michelle and Adrienne Asch; 1981. "Disabled women: sexism without the pedestal," *Journal of Sociology and Social Welfare*, 233-248.

Finlayson, Angela and James McEwen; 1977. *Coronary Heart Disease and Patterns of Living*. New York: Prodist.

Haber, Lawrence and Richard T. Smith; 1971. "Disability and deviance: normative adaptations of role behavior," *American Sociological Review*, 36:87-97.

Johnson, William; 1979. "Disability, income support and social insurance," in Edward Berkowitz (ed.) *Disability Policies and Government Programs*. New York: Praeger.

Nagi, Saad; 1969. *Disability and Rehabilitation: Legal, Clinical and Self-Concepts and Measurement*. Columbus, Ohio: Ohio State University Press.

Smith, Richard T. and Lorraine Midanik; 1980. "The effects of social resources on recovery and perceived sense of control among the disabled," *Sociology of Health and Illness*, 2,1:48-63.

Teitel, Ralph; 1977. "Rehabilitation of disabled adults, 1972." Report No. 3. Disability Survey 1972. Disabled and Non-disabled Adults. DHEW Publication No. (SSA) 77-11717.

2.

Shout Out
— Using Our Anger —

Two stereotypes are frequently projected onto disabled women. One is the happy, humble woman who has "accepted her handicap" and is endlessly grateful for the help of others. Her counterpart is embittered, blames everyone else for her situation, and continually lashes out. Society approves of our complacency and discounts our anger. Either way, we are made invisible. It is comfortable to deny that anyone can become disabled at any time and gratifying to think that all that can be done for us is being done.

Disabled women have become a visible political force. We are angry and will not remain quietly locked away in our homes. Caught between two negative images, we have learned to use our anger as a political tool. We challenge society's perception of us and its discriminatory practices. Together, we are creating change.

Anger

by dai r. thompson

*a*nger is not a pretty emotion. And, in spite of a lot of rhetoric to the contrary, it is still not very well accepted even in women's communities, unless, perhaps, its source is rage against men. But anger is real, whatever its source. And it is strong. It can immobilize. It can twist a person's life into a warped mess completely out of touch with reality. It can turn inward, leading to severe depression and even suicide. On the other hand, anger can be a major force behind an individual's desire to accomplish. But even that productive aspect of anger can lead to serious burn-out problems. Anger is, then, a part of almost all of our lives. If it remains unacknowledged, it can rarely be successfully subliminated for any long period of time, and it can be disastrous to both the individual and those around her.

Anger felt by women because of our disabilities is rarely accepted in women's communities, or anywhere else for that matter. Disabled or not, most of us grew up with media images depicting pathetic little "crippled" children on various telethons or blind beggars with caps in hand ("handicap") or "brave" war heroes limping back to a home where they were promptly forgotten. Such individuals' anger was never seen, and still rarely is. Instead of acknowledging the basic humanity of our often-powerful emotions, able-bodied persons tend to view us either as helpless things to be pitied or as Super Crips, gallantly fighting to overcome insurmountable odds. Such attitudes display a bizarre two-tiered mindset: it is horrible beyond imagination to be disabled, but disabled people with guts can, if they only try hard enough, make themselves almost "normal". The absurdity of such all-or-nothing images is obvious. So, too, is the damage these images do to disabled people by robbing us of our sense of reality.

The reasoning behind such attitudes is certainly hard to understand. When able-bodied persons are temporarily sick or encumbered by a broken leg or a patched eye, it is understood they will be grouchy or out-of-sorts or childish. But if an individual happens to be disabled in any permanent or long-term way, the rules of the game suddenly switch. The permanent inability to perform a major life function, such as hearing or seeing or walking, seems to require silent endurance of often-excruciating pain, patience far beyond any normal human capacity, quiet acceptance of architectural and attitudinal barriers, and groveling gratitude for the pittances doled out by various welfare agencies. Unlike the temporarily ill, we who are permanently disabled are not supposed to be, do not in fact have the right to be, angry or even upset about all the things we can't or aren't allowed to do. Even non-disabled women willing to acknowledge our disabilities and even, perhaps, our right to be angry, caution us not to express our anger because most able-bodied persons just can't handle it. It's okay to be angry about rape or pornography or wife abuse or the KKK or the whole Nuke situation; it does not seem to be okay to get mad because your peers refuse to acknowledge the barriers they constantly help erect to shut out their disabled sisters.

It is not fun to be disabled. Being disabled is not a "challenge" we voluntarily undertake. Nor is it that we are merely "differently-abled." We are disabled; there are just some things that we can't do, at least not as quickly or easily as other people. Sure, the rehabilitation therapists and many disabled individuals have devised ingenious methods and gadgets for accomplishing all kinds of things our disabilities would not otherwise allow us to do. But being fluent in sign language or lip reading still does not give a person the ability to hear. Being able to use a prosthesis does not give someone back her lost leg. And certainly finally being deinstitutionalized does not automatically return to an individual her dignity or all the time she has lost behind bars. For probably all of us, at least at times, being disabled hurts. Even if the larger community would adopt totally fair and appropriate attitudes toward people with disabilities, this would still not eliminate the sense of loss, the frustration, and indeed the anger we feel just because we are disabled.

Non-acceptance of us and our needs, especially by the women's community, is destructive. We have trouble getting others to acknowledge even our most obvious problems such as the need for accessibility or interpretive services. How then can we make them deal with our emotional reality as well? How can we make others understand our anger, our frustrations, all those numerous bits and pieces of our lives that are different because we do happen to be disabled? Women's communities often refuse to give any credibility to our anger and may even trash us if we try to express it. Not surprisingly, such attitudes make us even more angry. And this, in turn, makes us even less acceptable to the able-bodied world.

Because we are disabled, many of us have pretty low self-esteem. Our physical appearance, for example, often does not fit any traditional standards: we fit neither "mother" nor "whore" images found in the straight world, and we are certainly often a far cry from the strong, tough dyke model. The very definition of being disabled means that we cannot do one or more basic life functions. This inability to do what others take for granted can also be extremely demoralizing. Added to our actual limitations are additional ones able-bodied persons frequently impose on us.

Women labelled mentally retarded are often considered to be incapable of ever working or living independently or even being sexual. Not fitting into the "American ideal" — having to put up with certain functional limitations, and having to cope with often-ludicrous stereotypes — can result in very depressed egos.

Self-image problems differ considerably, of course, depending on the type and origin of an individual's disability. Women disabled later in life may have fairly intact egos developed in disability-free childhoods. They do not, then, usually display the life-long self-esteem problems found in many women born with disabilities who grew up feeling isolated and rejected by almost everything and everyone around them, often including their own families.

But women disabled as adults do have to deal with a different set of problems that can often be just as anger provoking. Having experienced a life free of limitations for decades perhaps, most newly-disabled women cannot help but feel an often-overwhelming sense of loss and anger at all the things they cannot now do that they once used to. And their frustration often increases as those around them fail to understand the enormous changes they must make in even the simplest of daily tasks. In an effort to cheer up newly-disabled people, friends and relatives often try to point out the positive: even if you can't walk anymore, you can still use your hands; I know you can't read, but how 'bout all those wonderful recordings they make for the blind now; or — a real favorite — at least your mind is still intact. Positive thinking can, of course, be quite useful and is an important part of any successful rehabilitation program. But if a newly-disabled woman is constantly surrounded by only those spouting worn-out "it could be worse" cliches, she is likely to develop a very strong urge to strangle them all. Little Mary Sunshine types often mean well. But nothing they can say or do can make that disability disappear. It's there, and it's real, and it must be coped with.

Getting used to a new disability involves many things which vary, naturally, depending on the type and extent of the disability: getting through the initial diagnosis and rehabilitation period; making necessary adjustments in living space, modes of transportation, work possibilities, financial arrangements; trying to deal with numerous changes in personal, family, and sexual relationships. Most of these problems are, of course, a daily part of any disabled woman's life. But unlike those who have been trying to cope since early childhood, newly-disabled women often find their previously well-ordered lives have suddenly been turned upside down. They not only have to deal with their new limitations, but often also with the additional emotional losses caused by sudden and often drastic changes in self-image, feelings of independence, and their relationships with almost everyone around them.

Sometimes it's hard for birth-disabled women to understand the often out-of-control anger and frustration newly-disabled women feel. After all, they've had to deal with such limitations all their lives. At least previously able-bodied women had a chance at decent, unsegregated education. A chance to grow up with at least fairly healthy self-images, often a much easier chance to establish careers, develop financial security, meet potential lovers, have children. Of course, some women born with disabilities are lucky enough to enjoy these same experiences. But, even so, they probably had to fight a lot harder to get, as the saying goes, half as far. And so, the complexities of our anger grow.

Competing for who's got it worse is really not going to accomplish anything for anyone. It just feeds anger and division among all of us. But the desire to create a truly unified disabled community cannot negate the lack of understanding that does, indeed, foster this anger. And like the anger all disabled women feel, at times, towards this ignorant, inaccessible society, the anger felt by those disabled at different times in their lives is also quite real, and will not go away easily or automatically. And it must be acknowledged by all parties involved if any kind of solution is ever going to be found.

There is also a different kind of in-house dispute in the disabled community that can be equally frustrating and anger-provoking. This is based on a rarely-acknowledged but very real hierarchy that ranks people according to the "acceptability" of their disability. An individual's position in this hierarchy is generally determined by how well that person fits into society's "norm". In other words, the less disabled you look, the higher your rank. And this reasoning frequently applies in both the able-bodied and disabled communities.

Use of this hierarchy within the disabled community may well, of course, be just a reflection of able-bodied attitudes, similar to once-prevalent rankings in the Black community based on a preference for lighter-colored skin. The urge to "pass" is apparently fairly universal. But whether it's a reflection of able-bodied views or not, this hierarchy is often adopted by people with disabilities and it can thus become one more part of the anger cycle for those considered less acceptable.

The rungs on this ladder of conformity are not based just on type of disability. Rather they can vary considerably even within a single disability: the essential criteria depend on how closely an individual meets society's standards of appearance and behavior. For example, proponents of comprehensive learning programs for deaf children, which include sign, feel that strictly-oral curriculums unnecessarily limit children in order to try to force them to appear as non-disabled as possible. Lip readers seem to be high on the scale of acceptability; sign users are not. By the same reasoning, individuals with mobility problems often choose to suffer needless pain or to limit their lives needlessly rather than use any kind of mobility aid. Individuals with cerebral palsy can be seen all along the ladder, depending on how serious their communication and motor coordination problems are.

Probably the lowest on the general hierarchy of disability, set up by the able-bodied society and mirrored in the disabled community, are those individuals labelled mentally ill or mentally retarded. Both groups are still routinely referred to as incompetents, vegetables, basket cases, and, thanks to the media, dangerous threats to society. Frequently considered to be "better off" in institutions, we are often drugged up, locked away, shocked out of our minds, and totally rejected by both the able-bodied and otherwise-disabled communities.

Internalized attitudes about hierarchies are not the only things that help create barriers within the disabled community. Some factors which foster such feelings are very understandable and hence are even harder to overcome than mere prejudice. Once again, the whole issue comes from a vicious cycle of inaccurate labeling which causes anger which, in turn, leads to a strong desire to separate into distinct disability groups. The fact that individuals with mental disabilities are frequently shunned by those with physical or sensory ones is a prime example of this problem. People with learning disabilities, for example, are often labelled as mentally retarded because of the difficulties they have communicating. Naturally such individuals fight very hard to be recognized as the intelligent, competent people they are. To then develop alliances with mentally retarded people can, therefore, be enormously threatening. Likewise, those who begin to develop multiple sclerosis or other hard-to-diagnose disabilities frequently have their problems dismissed as purely psychiatric in nature. Fighting such dismissals and the denials of treatment and financial help because of them can often go on for years, building up enormous resentment. It is not surprising, then, that such people feel a strong desire to clearly separate themselves from those whose disabilities are, indeed, psychiatrically-based.

Issues like these are very complex and not easy to solve. But they are also very real and can be extremely anger-provoking when, for example, physically-disabled women refuse to even acknowledge their mentally-disabled sisters' existence.

The same kind of reasoning applies to barriers erected between disabled people because of their sex, race, religion, educational level, socio-economic background or current financial status. The latter can be particulary frustrating since it usually relates directly to the disability itself. Some disabled individuals, frequently those from more "acceptable" racial, religious and socio-economic backgrounds, are lucky enough to enjoy financial security thanks to decent jobs, substantial gains from lawsuits or insurance policies, or solid support from well-to-do families. Such individuals often display little understanding of their sisters who are dependent on the whims of government agencies for even their most basic needs. The demeaning and increasingly fruitless nature of the application and renewal process for Social Security and other entitlements can be one of the most anger-provoking barriers experienced by disabled individuals. And yet disabled people who have never had to go through such demoralizing procedures often seem to have no understanding of their sisters who must. So individuals on welfare find themselves doubly frustrated and angry at both the system itself and others who refuse to understand.

All these vicious cycles, then, tend to turn onward and inward, perpetuating and often deepening the anger felt by women with disabilities. Anger at being disabled at all, anger at being ostracized by society as a whole and by the women's community in particular, anger at the disabled community itself for judging individuals by their economic status or the type and origin of their disabilities. This anger grows strong as the cycles continue and it is not going to disappear either quickly or easily.

But slowly and surely, attempts can, and are, being made to dissipate this anger and so reduce its ability to further handicap women with disabilities. An absolutely essential beginning step in any such process is, of course, recognizing and giving credibility to the anger. Disabled women must learn to understand their own anger, and to accept that it is both reasonable and justified. It is lousy to be disabled and it is perfectly healthy and normal to feel that way, at least occasionally. The trick, however, is to learn how to control that anger so it does not become a liability in and of itself. Those with more acceptable disabilities, or those on a more sound economic footing, must examine the source of their prejudice against their sisters, recognize how harmful it can be, and then begin to discard their outmoded attitudes. On the other hand, those on the outs by hierarchy or finances must also try to understand why their prejudiced sisters feel and act the way they do. No one should be asked to accept discrimination from anyone. But recognizing its origin can make it a bit easier to deal with while the afflicted ones are getting their acts together.

And, of course, the able-bodied must begin tearing down the numerous physical, attitudinal and other barriers they have placed in front of people who happen to be disabled. Those of us who are disabled must learn to cope with the anger-provoking reality that all those many barriers are not going to come tumbling down all at once, as unjust, unfair and just plain infuriating as they are. It is not easy to constantly have to work our lives around the multitude of obstacles this society has put in our way. But it is also not very helpful, to ourselves or anyone else, to just sit around and scream at the injustice of it all. We need to find effective coping mechanisms to help us keep sane and strong. For some, political action may be useful. For others, a support group may help. There are numerous possibilities. The important thing is to find a way to survive.

All For Nothing

by mary anna ilves

This is for Marvin

As the curtain rises, we see a woman in a wheelchair talking on the telephone. Though the woman she is speaking to is offstage, we can hear her voice.

Woman in Wheelchair: Ms. Brewer, it's Jane Maxwell again. I was wondering if Dr. Hobson had received my message from earlier today.

Ms. Brewer *(offstage, very dignified)*: Jane we're having a difficult time locating Dr. Hobson. He's with a group of medical students right now and they're at another hospital.

Woman in Wheelchair *(somewhat upset)*: But I'm having alot of difficulty. I explained all this to you earlier.

Brewer: I know you did Jane, and I understand that you are concerned. Dr. Hobson will be informed of the situation and get back in touch with you.

Woman in Wheelchair *(exasperated)*: OK, thank you. Bye.

Brewer: You're very welcome. Goodbye.

Women in Wheelchair hangs up phone and begins nervously chewing on the side of her finger for a few seconds before she pulls out a phonebook from underneath the telephone, looks up a number and dials.

Woman in Wheelchair: May I have the SSI medi-cal worker?

Medi-cal man *(voice offstage)*: Can I help you?

Woman in Wheelchair: Yes, I've applied for SSI benefits and haven't begun receiving my medi-cal card through the mail. I was wondering if there was some way I could get it without having to come to the Oakland office. *(slight pause)* I live in Berkeley.

Medi-cal man: Nope, you've got to get a form from Social Security stating you haven't received a card for this month and bring it down to our office.

Woman in Wheelchair: But I'm very sick.

Medi-cal man: Lady, everybody who comes in here is sick. I've got a waiting room full of people right now who didn't receive their cards this month. People out there on oxygen tanks, on walkers, in wheelchairs.

Woman in Wheelchair *(small voice)*: I'm in a wheelchair.

Medi-cal man: If you don't come to the office you don't get the card.

Woman in Wheelchair *(getting upset and forceful)*: Can't someone come for a home visit?

Medi-cal man: Lady, they cut our funding so drastically we only have two SSI workers. We don't make home visits anymore.

Woman in Wheelchair: *(more upset)*: I'm really sick, and I have to take public transportation to your office. I don't know if I can do it.

Medi-cal man: Look Lady, all I can tell you is you can send the forms through the mail, but that'll take three weeks. If you want the card now, you've got to come in to the office.

Woman in Wheelchair *(voice faltering)*: Alright.

Hangs up and starts to cry.

Blackout

Lights come up on a Social Security office. There is a waiting area with rows of chairs and, in front of the waiting area, two desks side by side about 5 feet apart. The reception desk is downstage. Waiting to talk with the receptionist is the woman in the wheelchair. At the desk upstage is a man with a cane dressed in clothes that have seen better days. He politely holds his hat in his hands waiting for a Social Security worker to return to his desk. A partition partially conceals him from the waiting area, which is directly behind him.

Receptionist (male): Next please.

Woman in Wheelchair: I phoned yesterday and talked with Mrs. Smith about needing the form that verifies I haven't received this month's Medi-cal card. She said she would have it waiting for me at the reception desk.

Receptionist: Hmm, let me check. What's your name?

Woman in Wheelchair: Jane Maxwell.

Receptionist *(looking through papers)*: I don't seem to see it. Mrs. Smith isn't in today, if you'll just wait over there *(he points to waiting area)* I'll go check her desk so we can expedite this matter.

Woman in Wheelchair wheels over to the first row of seats in the waiting area. She can easily overhear conversation between Social Security worker (male) who has just returned, and the man with the cane. She reacts with widened eyes and heavy sighs to the conversation.

Man with Cane: Now they've gone and lost my October check too.

S.S. man *(cheerfully)*: Well, we'll just fill out a form for that one like we did for the September check.

Man with Cane: *(softly)*: I've used up the last of what little money I was able to save.

S.S. man *(indifferently)*: I'm very sorry, but we no longer have an emergency fund.

Man with Cane: Should I apply for foodstamps?

S.S. man: I don't think your application will be processed before your September check arrives. You should be getting it within the next two weeks.

Man with Cane *(upset and louder)*: But I don't have any money!

S.S. man: I'm very sorry sir, these things take time.

Blackout

A single spotlight on Social Security worker, obviously new to the job.

Novice: Sir, I overheard that conversation. Isn't there something we can do?

S.S. man: The most we can do for him and ourselves is process that claim efficiently and correctly.

Novice: But sir, maybe I could call around and see if there is some kind of county emergency money available.

S.S. man: Don't take all this so seriously, Gibbs. It can become insidious. Starts affecting your disposition, your sleep, your relationship with your wife. And all for nothing. We can't change the situation, we can't even change the system. It's here and we do our job.

Novice: Maybe there's more to the job than just processing papers. I mean isn't that why you became a social worker in the first place?

S.S. man: Gibbs, once I wanted to change the world too. Kept feeling responsible for the people who passed through these doors. Got myself so worked up over cases that I couldn't eat or sleep. It got to the point where I really believed if I didn't help these people some of them were going to starve, *(emphatically)* die! Do you know what believing that kind of stuff can do to your insides? These people manage, they always do. This man Brown, he'll go stay with some friends, or go stay at one of the churches where they'll feed him. I haven't heard one story yet of someone who was in here dying in the streets.

Novice: It just seems to me there should be something we could do.

S.S. man: There is, making sure the forms get processed efficiently and correctly. The only thing your kind of thinking is going to do is get you in trouble with yourself.

As the lights fade out a chorus of voices offstage chant in automaton fashion: "We only do exactly what we're told, we are the bureaucrats, we are the bureaucrats, we are the bureaucrats". Lights come up on Social Security office. Woman in Wheelchair is still waiting. She wheels over to receptionist.

Woman in Wheelchair: Excuse me, have you found out anything about the form I need?

Receptionist: I've tried to expedite this matter. I located the unsigned form on Mrs. Smith's desk and gave it to another worker to complete. Just a minute. *(He goes offstage for a moment only to return empty-handed.)* It appears she has gone for lunch, if you'll just wait over there *(points to waiting area),* she should return in 45 minutes.

Another Social Security worker (female) appears at the desk.

Receptionist II: I'll relieve you for lunch. *(Receptionist I exits; Receptionist II turns to Woman in Wheelchair:)* Can I help you?

Woman in Wheelchair *(becoming angry)*: Look, I've been here for an hour and a half waiting for a form that was supposed to have been completed yesterday. Now I'm told whoever is going to sign it has gone to lunch. I have to take public transportation to the Medi-Cal office before it closes today.

Receptionist II: Just a minute *(goes off stage. Woman in Wheelchair gives heavy sigh. Receptionist II returns with another woman.)* If you'll just explain your situation to Ms. Weber, our supervisor, I'm sure she can help you.

Woman in Wheelchair: I called yesterday... *(voice fades along with lights so that only Woman in Wheelchair is in the spotlight, alone with her thoughts).* What the hell goes on with these people? I swear I could wring Mr. Expedite's neck. *(with tired voice)* I don't know if I can go to Oakland, I need to lie down for awhile. I feel sick. *(frustrated and moaningly)* If I don't go I won't get the card and I've got to have those lab tests done. *(pause, then in a very tired voice)* Oh god, I just want to go to sleep.

Lights come back up and Weber is shaking her head negatively.

Weber: I'm very sorry, but you'll have to come back tomorrow.

Woman in Wheelchair *(almost yelling)*: Tomorrow? Why can't you just sign the form?

Weber: There seems to be a complication.

Woman in Wheelchair: Complication? I discussed this yesterday with Mrs. Smith, she didn't seem to think there was any complication.

Weber *(becoming distanced)*: I'm very sorry, but you'll just have to come back tomorrow. Now, if you'll excuse me I really am very busy.

Weber exits. Woman in Wheelchair exits.

BLACKOUT

Lights come up. It is nighttime. We see the closed sign on the Social Security office door. No person is in view, but we see an empty wheelchair strapped with dynamite careening through the front window. We hear glass shatter, then after a momentary pause we hear a loud explosion.

Disability, Sexism
And the Social Order

by debra connors

S oon after I began losing my vision, a friend asked if I would join her in a newly-forming support group of disabled women. My response was, "What do you mean *disabled? I'm* not disabled. I just can't *see,* that's all!" She agreed — the label was degrading and not at all how we felt about ourselves. Certainly it was better than *handicapped.* Residents of the state institution where I once worked and children on telethons were handicapped. Yet *disabled* was no consolation. It resounded with an all-encompassing, somehow too final thud in my ear.

A few years later, a classmate asked that I not refer to her as *disabled.* It offended her. She considered herself a person with a disability, she said, and would not be reduced to her deafness. A disability, she explained, is a physical or mental impairment. A handicap is a set of social conditions which impede our independence. Disabilities become handicaps only when we allow them to become insurmountable. We then become disabled; we become our disabilities.

Disabled, handicapped, differently-abled, physically or mentally different, physically challenged, women with disabilities — this is more than a mere discourse in semantics and a matter of personal preference. *Disabled women* is the term which most accurately characterizes our position in American society. Sexism and able-ism work in concert to disqualify us from vast areas of social life. Our unique set of barriers is further compounded by discrimination based on our race, age and sexual preference. Objectified as women and as medical, social work and charity cases, disabled women have been deeply invalidated as human beings. We have been disabled by our society. No euphemism will change this.

Disability is not a medical problem; nor is able-ism just a set of prejudicial ideas about disabled people. Disability is a societal institution which has developed alongside capitalism. Our societal position has been shaped by history and is inextricably woven into the fabric of American culture. There is no reason to assume that medical conditions are disabilities or that they should necessarily be stigmatizing. History reveals that policies, practices and ideas regarding disabled women have been socially constructed.

Disability first became institutionalized with the enactment of England's Elizabethan Poor Laws (1598-1601)[1]. As the old feudal order gave way to mercantile capitalism, unemployment emerged as a new social phenomenon. Serfs who had lost their birthrights to land as a result of the enclosure movement and old and sick people who had been ejected from their hospital and monastery shelters under the Protestant Acts of Dissolution flocked to market towns and cities which were unable to absorb them and ill prepared to cope with the problems they posed. With neither work nor relief available, life for most urban dwellers was characterized by suffering and protest. The Poor Laws were designed to squelch social unrest and control the vagabonds.

Prior to the Poor Laws, the Catholic Church had been the primary social service institution in medieval England. It provided a steady but slim trickle of alms to the poor. Travelers and old and sick people found shelter in the many hospitals (hospitality houses) under the governance of the monasteries. Pilgrims were charged a fee. Permanent residents of the hospitals were required to take vows of poverty and turn their few possessions over to the Church. Hospital life was severe and avoided by all who could manage to do so.[2] More generally, needy families received alms from the parish priests, if and when funds were available and depending on the political climate. Serfs expected charity and the Church sought to absolve itself as the major land and serf holder by redistributing to the poor a meager portion of the produce it had expropriated from them.

The Elizabethan Poor Laws differed from feudal custom in several important ways. They drew a distinction between those who were "deserving" and "not deserving" of charity. Poverty and unemployment came to be viewed as personal problems and defects of character. Receipt of charity became cause for humiliation. Newly defined as those who "could but would not work", able-bodied paupers were put to labor in workhouses. Children of poor families (orphans) were placed out as apprentices. Blind, old and lame people and others with "diverse maladies" were given licenses to beg. Those who were discovered begging without a license were publicly whipped. Overseers of the poor were appointed in each municipality to collect and establish poor taxes, remove vagabonds to their places of birth and charge their families responsible for the care of those deemed incapable of self-care.[3]. Almshouses were established for the care and incarceration of "invalids" and were administered by the overseers of poor people.

Persons who were ill or had physical impairments were legally defined as unemployable social dependents, incapable of self-care and in need of governance. Feudal paternalism had taken on a municipal guise. Those who were able to find employment or employ themselves were more directly taxed for the care of those who were destitute and were threatened with debtors' prison for failure to remit taxes to the overseer. This contributed to the opprobrium with which all "charity cases" were met. Poor relief was intended to restore social order, but it was never able to accomplish this. The social causes of poverty and unemployment were obscured in the Protestant work ethic and the working class began to be divided against itself.

The English Poor Laws were exported to the North American colonies and changed very little until 1935, when responsibility for and administration of poor people shifted from local, county and state to federal jurisdiction.[4] Like their historical antecedents, the Social Security Act and other New Deal measures were introduced in a period of high unemployment and social unrest. The federal government created some employment opportunities for able-bodied men and women. Disability continued to be defined as in inability to pursue an occupation because of physical impairment. Unemployment and disability have yet to be addressed as political and economic conditions endemic to capitalism.

The point to be made is, it hasn't always been the case that persons with medical or psychiatric disorders were categorically disabled — unemployed and unemployable. Indeed, the only persons free from labor in feudal Europe were the aristocrats. Some critically ill, contagious and dying persons were exempted from work in the hospitals, but most performed services in them.[5]. Bands of wandering minstrels who were blind, deaf and lame traveled from manor to manor, carrying messages and providing entertainment in exchange for food and shelter.[6] There is little record of the daily lives of serfs, as literacy was reserved for the ecclesiastical class, but it seems reasonable to conclude that everyone contributed to the manorial and family economies in whatever means they were able. Blind women, for example, spun yarn and wove cloth. There is no evidence to indicate that those who could not walk were not allowed to use their hands. Life was hard, scarcity tended to be the rule and labor was short during periods of plague. Survival depended on maximizing everyone's abilities.

Disabled people were denied passage to the American colonies, either as free persons or as indentured servants. But, many who began their journies in good health arrived quite ill and famished, as did enslaved Africans. Farm-centered family economies, plantation slavery and tenant farming predominated in America until the end of the nineteenth century. Women, men, children and elders, whether firm or infirm, contributed to family survival. Accidents and disease were common, but none could afford to be idle. Slaves harmed by brutality were not permitted respite. Disabled people have always existed and have always worked. Many no doubt labored beyond their capacities because there was no choice. They might have welcomed reprieve. But, in the urban-industrial cities, others found themselves in enforced idleness, unable to secure employment and ·with no means of support.

Disability became more fully institutionalized during the emergence of industrial capitalism. Industrialization had the potential to eliminate a substantial degree of disability, since machine power came to replace human power in many sectors of the economy. (The present computer revolution holds a similar promise.) Instead, more stamina was required of workers, industrial accidents caused more unemployability and efforts were made to eliminate disabled people. The industrial revolution, hailed as the epitome of human potential, often worked against the realization of that possibility.

Once time became money, workers who could not keep pace with the assembly line were systematically disabled from productive activity. Profit, after all, is created by paying workers less than the value of the work they have done.[7] It is less profitable to hire employees who work more slowly than young, able-bodied candidates. Since profit is the motive force of capitalism, workers with impaired profit generating abilities are regarded as useless — like broken machines.

Yet, less physical strength and dexterity are required to perform more tasks in today's work place than ever before.[8] Apparently disabled workers are no longer less profitable to employ. We, too, can be exploited at the maximal rate, at least until cost is considered. Workers who require adaptive equipment, a reader, sign language interpretation, a flexible work schedule, architectural reconstruction of the work place or a non-standard mode of work performance are unlikely to find work. Facilitation, accomodation, adaptive equipment and architectural redesign are expensive and avoidable, simply by hiring workers who do not need them.

One corporation, at least, would seem to disagree.[9] A recent study concluded that it is no more costly to hire disabled than non-disabled workers. Disabled workers were said to be as efficient and missed less work time than their co-workers. This superficially cheery picture soft-pedals the harsh truth that only those who can be fit into the corporate machine, as it exists, are ever hired. No report is given about the various physical attributes of these employees, which is obviously an important question. People with chronic progressive illnesses do miss more time from work, either due to fluctuating health or the fact that medical appointments are usually only available during business hours. Employers need not be aware of the added expenses involved in hiring a disabled person because either government subsidies or the employees pay the cost of our employability. We do not raise the cost of insurance plans because health insurance usually excludes pre-existing conditions. We should hardly be surprised to learn that these workers are satisfactory. They were no doubt carefully selected for their race, class, age, religion, appearance, gender — and of course — health.

What is tucked away, out of sight, by image-oriented approaches is that unemployment — and, thus, disability — is a necessary feature of a capitalist political economy. Business and industrial expansion *require* that a sector of the population be held in reserve — ready and willing to work for minimum wages. The conditions of unemployed and disabled workers serve as a constant reminder to even the most dissatisfied active worker that *any* job may be preferable to no job at all. The presence of readily available replacements effectively holds down wages and threatens unions. Fear and blame associated with unemployment mystifies its social origins and keeps workers in their place.[10]

Idealized notions of full employment do not include disabled people and old persons. Our unemployability is a given. We are not personally blamed for a dependence which is perceived to be beyond our control. We are pitied instead. Able-bodied people may lose their jobs, their lives may be falling apart, perhaps they've lost their partners or children, still a consoling friend will assure them, "at least you've got your health." Health offers hope for beginning anew, for taking personal control of a twist of fate. Illness and injury spell doom.

This pity — this doom writ large — has been called the common denominator of disabled people's oppression. We are said, by social scientists,[11] to suffer from the *opinions* others hold of us. We are viewed as "abnormal", "defectives", "deviants", partial persons who are not quite human. Our needs are a sign of our disgrace. Given our unemployable status and our reliance on family, friends and social services to cope with an inaccessible environment, it is not irrational that we are categorically defined as dependents in need of care. Able-ism is not only an oppressive idea; though, had anyone conspired against us, they coudn't have created a more effective institution.

It is unpardonable in an individualist society to fail to be "self-sufficient". Our society values a false sense of independence which results in pain and a sense of worthlessness for women and men whose capabilities have been ignored and whose potential has been uniformly underdeveloped. Yet, independence does not truly reflect anyone's reality. As a species, we are emphatically *interdependent*.[12] Disabled people cannot be independent, not because we are pitiable or helpless, but because we are human.

Americans are particularly unmindful of the many persons on

whom we daily depend for survival. A market economy — a cash nexus — obscures this fact. Moreover, class relations are hidden by the ideology of individualism. We firmly believe that if we are able to purchase the goods and services we are not able to produce for ourselves, we are free of dependence. Conversely, if we are not able to buy them, we suspect we do not deserve "charity". Those who are able to purchase a false sense of independence are revered and are a measure by which the working class evaluates its members. The fact that some grow rich at the expense of their employees is conveniently ignored, while people who are systematically disadvantaged are criticized for their dependence.

The stigma of dependence may be all but inescapable for disabled people. Society's resources are unavailable to us because we have been structurally defined as unemployable. It is considered a "special" privilege for us to be able to obtain an education, have a job or job skills, use public facilities or have access to medical care, sub-minimal social support and freedom of mobility. Without the financial resources to pay an attendant to enable us to negotiate an environment that was not designed for our participation, we are often isolated and may be led to prioritize our own needs — some as absolute and life-sustaining and others as "luxuries". Disability has become so institutionalized against a back-drop of Protestant individualism that we may question our own abilities and worthiness to live self-managed, interdependent lives.

Unequal distribution of wealth in feudal society was explained as divine will. Disease, famine and ill-fortune were a sign of having fallen from spiritual favor. Science has displaced religious authority since then and the oracular task of explanation has fallen to biological determinists. Religious appeals to a "calling" could not account for the immense fortunes of a few and the severe poverty of many. Social and medical scientists put forth theories of natural selection to legitimize the increasingly polarized class relations which evolved with the industrial revolution. Evolution, they argued, was in progress. The fit were thriving; the poor, who were by definition "unfit", had simly met the final outcome of their biological destinies. Policy makers were warned not to tamper with nature by providing for the welfare of destitute families.[13].

The myth of independence and theories of social evolution

essentially disguised and have continued to disguise the structural causes of virtually all social problems.[14] Biological determinism is the well-established idea that the personalities, capabilities and social positions of individuals are fundamentally and inevitably determined by their biological appearance or genetic characteristics. Science has justified and apologized for discrimination against women, third-world people, religious and ethnic groups, old people, lesbians and gay men and disabled people. While much of what was determined to be natural about social inequalities has been exposed as a conscious effort to manufacture myth, the legacy of these experiments retains a powerful strong-hold upon our imaginations and finds expression in our social policies and in our prejudiced attitudes.

Scientific able-ism is a specific instance of biological determinism. Based on our biological characteristics, medical science and legislature have worked in harmony to determine our membership. At various times throughout our history, attics, freak shows and circuses, hospitals, residential asylums, segregated schools and sheltered workshops have been established as our natural and proper environments. Myths concerning our feebleness, unnaturalness, beast-like sexuality or asexuality, ill-fittedness to parent, violent hostility and inherent evil prospered through time and have helped to keep us in our proper places.

Able-ist movements of the late-nineteenth and early twentieth centuries regarded disability as problematic for society, but not — once again — as a socially constructed problem. As with the earlier Poor Laws, solutions tended to be directed toward individuals. Past and current reform movements — whether liberal or conservative — try to fix the symptoms of what are structural problems, leaving the sources quite untouched. The eugenics and rehabilitation movements, for example, treated disability as a condition to be eliminated or corrected at an individual level. They were generally praised as humanitarian efforts.

The early eugenicists were medical scientists who essentially conducted an experiment in genocide. They sought to improve the quality of the human gene pool by preventing the births of disabled infants. Numerous studies were conducted in an attempt to document the hereditary nature of such diseases as diabetes, blindness and epilepsy, as well as deviant social behaviors as poverty, prostitution and criminality. Birth control literature, previously held in high disregard, suddenly found its way into the hands of poor women. Heredity counseling was advised for those with questionable genes in order to dissuade them from having children. State legislatures provided for the forced sterilization of mentally retarded women.

Despite the fact that evolution does not operate on an individual level and that most physical and emotional conditions are not inheritable, the search continues to this day for scientific documentation of genetically transmitted deviance. Recreational, automobile and industrial accidents, environmental pollution, iatrogenic disease, job-related stress and the impending threat of nuclear holocaust can safely be said to be among the major causes of physiological and psychological distress. Reproductive control of women's bodies continues, whether our genes or the genes of our partners are fallaciously considered problematic for society and our species. Twenty-seven states still provide for the sterilization of mentally retarded women. "Misdiagnosis" and coercion have lead blind, deaf, deaf-blind, third world and poor women to be sterilized against their will. Birth control chemicals are still rountinely dispensed to women in some institutions. Genetic counseling, available at most major medical centers, has found its way into popular opinion. (This is not to imply that information available through genetic counseling should not be made available to prospective parents but rather to point out the historical and frequent current misuse of genetic counseling.) Prenatal diagnosis, which the early eugenicists sought to discover, has been praised as a miracle of modern medicine, one which has made all too clear that only children who might some day permitted to be "productive" are welcomed into the world.

Common notions of disability continue to objectify us as patients. We are the failures of modern medicine, the "cases" whose births could not be foreseen and for whom there are no known cures. We testify against the omnipotence of medical science and represent a frightening truth. We are feared and hated and viewed as hopeless patients in all of our daily environments.

The consequences of viewing disabilities as irreparable impairments have been severe and far reaching. The investigatory nature and narrow conceptual scope of medical science — isolate the "defect", measure it, correct it, mask it and/or eliminate its recurrence — have often culminated in the abuse of disabled people.

Somehow, physicians often forget that we are whole people. Humanitarianism, the supposed god of the patient and the advancement of medical science are too often put forth as rationale for treating us as human rats, on the operating table and in the laboratories. The situation is rife with potential for personal violation and injustice.

Monopolized by the American Medical Association, medicine is produced and practiced for profit. Illness is a private problem for which individuals assume private responsibility. Because local, state and national health care programs are insufficient, because private insurance generally excludes pre-existing conditions and because disabled people are economically disadvantaged, we are generally unable to pursue needed health care — whether real or doctrinal — "independently". Our only choice may be to submit to experimentation. Personal, professional and societal messages about the virtue of health and the disgrace of disease render us a captive audience. If we are not willing to try every new experiment, no matter how slim the chance of cure or survival, we are blamed for wishing to remain impaired, either for opportunistic or masochistic reasons. Grateful for services we suspect we do not fully deserve and cannot justifiably refuse, we are unwittingly led to participate in our own abuse.

Women patients are more likely than men to be medically abused. Our physical and psychological concerns have been ignored, misdiagnosed and invalidated. Our physical symptoms have been treated as products of our imaginations. Psychotropic drugs are commonly prescribed as an all-purpose remedy to discount psychological distress. Vital information has been withheld and reserved for professionals. Disabled women have been medically controlled. Health, like disability, is politically defined by medical, insurance and governmental bureaucracies.

Our identities as patients have developed alongside the eugenics movement and the professionalization of medical science. In addition, education was becoming more specialized and more scientific during the late-nineteenth and early twentieth centuries. Both medical and educational reforms presumed what the English Poor Laws had decreed — that disabled people are unemployable and, therefore, in need of paternalistic care and governance. Rather than rehabilitating an able-ist society, medical science attempted to cure disabled people and educational reformers sought to correct them. Both of these individual solutions failed miserably, and not without harsh consequences.

The obvious solution is a fundamental restructuring of society. Instead, efforts remain focused on correcting *us*. Once medicine has failed, social workers, special educators and rehabilitators are called in to fix what are perceived to be our disabilities. Individual solutions merely mask fundamental causes, if they work at all. Structural impediments to our employability cannot be eradicated by teaching us to type, make brooms or run a computer. Rehabilitated workers remain largely disabled — underemployed or unemployed.

It would be absurd to deny the importance of literacy and the value of having marketable skills. For disabled people, quality education has long been non-existent, primarly because it was assumed we had no use for it. Educational resources and the efforts of teachers were thought to be wasted on us. The early efforts of doctors, teachers and philanthropists to solve disability by teaching disabled people to be "productive" demonstrated the futility of education as a solution.

Graduates of late-nineteenth century schools for blind, deaf and mentally retarded students found themselves without jobs and with no way to support themselves. Discouraged by this situation, the residential schools responded by establishing sheltered workshops, generally as an annex to the schools themselves. Broom factories, which employed blind workers, are a classic example. Sheltered workshops paid their employees less than subsistence wages, from which the cost of their room and board was then deducted. Frequently, these charges exceeded earnings and families were required to contribute to the support of workshop employees. When laws were enacted to ban prison workshops, only because of their unfair market competition, sheltered workshops for disabled people were exempted on the grounds that they were charitable institutions.[15] There is nothing charitable about exploiting workers and draining their resources such that many were never able to leave the institutions which profited from their labor. They were effectively enslaved. Those who controlled and incarcerated them argued that they were providing disabled workers with self-esteem and a sense of purpose.

State and private schools discovered teaching and communication methods for those who had previously been presumed uneducable. If some good came out of these schools, however, their results cannot possibly justify their inhumane means. Philanthropists became disillusioned when it was discovered that education did not necessarily facilitate employment or employability. Education was all but abandoned in most of the schools; they became warehouses for society's misfits.

Rehabilitation has recently been given new momentum and, again, has been hailed as the solution to our problems. Laws which seek to protect disabled people from educational and employment discrimination based on our physical or mental differences continue to presuppose our unemployability. Section 504 of the Rehabilitation Act, for example, applies principally to persons who are unable to work *because of a disability*.[16] This is a clear-cut case of biological determinism being used to reform institutionalized disability.

The dilemma of disabled women is especially poignant. Categorically, women have been significantly "disabled" from participating in skilled industrial, policy making and business spheres of society. Medical and/or psychiatric theories of biological inferiority, sexual dimorphism and hormonally induced "hysteria" have been sought to justify discrimination based on our sex. Domestic work and child rearing, whether we have worked outside of the home, have been determined to be our natural — instinctual — occupations. Disabled women have been disqualified from domestic and wage work, in a double bind of biological destination.

We experience institutionalized sexism in special education and rehabilitation programs. Vocational counselors, who have the authority to determine "appropriate" placements *for* us, often channel women into traditional "women's work". If we can type, sew and cook, we are considered rehabilitated. Inadequate education is likely to influence our scores on vocational aptitude tests, disqualifying us from training in non-traditional occupations. A lack of positive role models may influence our awareness of career possibilities for disabled women. Moreover, counselors often deny our own aspirations as impractical or inappropriate because we are women and disabled. Programs which may actually benefit some individual women more often control us.

On the other hand, the eugenics movement continues to shape the domestic life of disabled women. Victorian-era beliefs associating sex for women strictly with procreation have led to our being viewed as asexual. When we are sexual, our sexuality has been viewed as beast-like and in need of paternalistic control. Sex education is popularly thought to be misguided for disabled girls and women. Chastity belts seem to be in more appropriate order, especially since disabled women are regarded as unmarriageable and unfit to be mothers.

Popular notions of feminine beauty manufactured by cosmetic and fashion industries, myths of heredity and the private structure of the nuclear family have limited disabled women's potential for fulfilling traditional role prescriptions. Women who cannot perform an endless array of household and parenting responsibilities "independently" are considered unmarriageable and unfit mothers. Family wages are typically inadequate to hire someone to shop, transport children, cook, launder, clean or provide other consumer services. This privilege is reserved for the elite. If wages were enough to cover the cost of domestic accessibility, wage workers would have to be paid better. This arrangement would certainly be objectionable to employers, who refuse to be concerned with the "private" lives of employees. Disabled women are effectively disqualified to be housewives and mothers.

Current social welfare policies continue to place disabled women in a category of superfluous people. If we decide to marry, we may lose a substantial portion of our income. We are discriminated against in employment opportunities, even when it is no more costly and as profitable to employ us. When we are unable to find employment, we are forced to demonstrate to the bureaucracy that we are, in fact, unemployable. "Disincentives" to employment are built into the Social Security Act. Once our earned income has reached the poverty level, we are likely to be ineligible for any services at all.[17] This means that chronically ill women are asked, for example, to choose between having access to food or medical care. Our survival is thus threatened by employment. Able-ism has been built into the system; our poverty has been institutionalized. We cannot escape the clutches of bureaucratic control.

Our survival is also threatened when we do not comply with

the demands of law and our administrators. Welfare benefits are intentionally below the minimum wage in order to provide "incentive" to employment. We are relegated to dire poverty but are not expected to be able to subsist on such little income. Social workers know that we "cheat" the system by failing to report "under the table" employment and gifts of money from relatives; both of which would automatically be deducted from our welfare checks. They expect us to find additional means of support; yet, our very survival raises suspicions. Our survival is an act of resistance in a society which would just as soon eliminate us and is also a testament to our resourcefulness. Instead of encouraging our resourcefulness, we are interrogated no less than once a year. For this we are expected to be grateful.

In the wake of the women's liberation and independent living movements, disabled women have been thrown into a myriad of contradictions. Many of us have found satisyfing employment, live in accessible communities and homes and participate in reciprocal and rewarding relationships. Our resistance to sexism and able-ism has created better lives for many and increased opportunities for some individuals. Still, far too many of us remain in institutions. Poverty and isolation are far too prevalent in most of our lives. Our different abilities are not appreciated or acknowledged. Reforms in public services are in jeopardy. Funding has been cut and "special" programs have been eliminated. Able-ist oppression has been internalized and has divided us hierarchically against ourselves. We are experiencing a backlash against our collective protest and stand to lose much of what we've gained because we have not fully challenged the institutionalized nature of able-ism.

As we forge our way into new territories, disabled women have become more visible. Attitudes towards us are changing. Sensationalist television, for example, now features disabled women, but only disabled women who have "overcome their disabilities". We are praised for our "independence" and our refusal to be reduced to our disabilities. With little regard for the fact that we are legally defined as unemployable and that unemployment characterizes most of our lives, women who remain on social welfare programs are now criticized for continued dependence which is beginning to be perceived as a choice. Our collective resistance to systematically generated disability has been undermined. We must refuse to be co-opted by the idea that disabilities are personal shortcomings.

Disabled women have always resisted our no-win societal position. Indeed, the English Poor Laws, educational and medical reforms and recent welfare legislation have come about only because we have demanded them. We have refused to be incarcerated in "schools" and asylums. Able-ist notions that we are pitiable patients and charity cases have been exposed as efforts to keep us isolated, dependent, and discounted. Our history is rich with demonstrations, lobbying and petitions. But, these have been answered with reforms that disguise but continue the paternalistic suppression against which we have struggled. Our disabled status remains intact, as does the system which gave rise to it.

In essence, disabled women have demanded participation in a political economy which oppresses all workers. A small percent of the population owns most of the wealth and grows wealthier by exploiting employed and unemployed workers. Individualism mystifies the fact that our society is class structured. Ideals of equality and democracy mean that individuals are free to compete unequally for unequal rewards.[17] Disabled people are pitted against disabled people, women against women and political movements against one another as we compete for too few jobs, for piece meal gains and for validation of our cause. If we are to actualize our ideals of a true democracy and personal freedom, we must come together as disabled women and form alliances with other systematically disadvantaged groups in order to effect fundamental changes. Finding our own place within the system simply will not be enough.

Notes

1. Burn, Richard, H. Woodfall and W. Strahan; *The History of the Poor Laws,* London: Law Printers to the King's Most Highest Majesty, 1764.

2. Clay, Mary Rotha; *The Medieval Hospitals of England,* London: Frank Cass & Co. Ltd, 1909, Ch. I.

3. Heffernan, Joseph, *Introduction to Social Welfare: Power, Scarcity and Common Human Needs,* Itasca, IL: P.E. Peacock Publishers, 1981, p. 189.

4. ibid; pp. 188-206.

5. Clay, Mary Rotha, *The Medieval Hospitals of England,* London: Frank Cass & Co. Ltd, 1909, pp. 51-55.

6. French, Richard, *From Homer to Helen Keller: A Social and Educational History of the Blind,* New York: American Foundation for the Blind, 1932.

7. Marx, Karl, *Capital: A Critique of Political Economy, Vol, I,* New York: Vintage Books, 1977, Ch. 9 & 10, p. 346.

8. Braverman, Harry, *Labor and Monopoly Capital: The Degradation of Work in the Twenieth Century,* New York: Monthly Review Press, 1977, p. 83.

9. Ruffner, Robert, "DuPont Has the Answer", *Mainstream,* May, 1983.

10. Piven, Frances Fox and Richard Cloward, *Regulating the Poor: The Functions of Social Welfare,* New York: Vintage Books, 1976, pp. 3-38.

11. Goffman, Irving, *Stigma: Notes on the Management of Spoiled Identity,* Englewood Cliffs, NJ: Prentice-Hall, 1963, pp. 2-40.

12. Gould, Stephen Jay, *Ever Since Darwin: Reflections in Natural History,* New York: Norton, 1977, pp. 63-69.

13. Hofstadter, Richard, *Social Darwinism in American Thought,* Boston: Beacon Press, 1955.

14. Smith, Joan, *Social Issues and the Social Order: The Contradictions of Capitalism,* Cambridge, MA: Winthrop Publishers, 1981, pp. 6-11.

15. Koestler, Frances, *The Unseen Minority: A Social History of Blindness in the United States,* New York: David McKay Co. Inc., 1976, pp. 209-230.

16. _____ "Section 504 of the Rehabilitation Act of 1973: Briefing Guide", Washington, DC: Office for Civil Rights, 11/8/79.

17. Caulfield, Mina, "Equality, Sex and Mode of Production", in *Social Inequalities: Anthropological and Developmental Approaches,* edited by Gerald Berraman, New York: Academic Press, 1981, p. 203.

Catherine G. Nelson, Maria Stecenko, Deborah Lieberman and Carol Park have all provided me with greatly appreciated editorial assistance at various stages in the development of this essay. Deborah also typed several rather unwieldy versions of it, always on short notice. My dear friend, Carol, has been of tremendous support. Her warmth, advise and humor have made all the difference. I wish to thank each of you for your generosity, patience and encouragement.

Nicaragua: A Victory For Disabled Women

by joan tollifson

i am an amputee and a lesbian. I spent six weeks this past January and February living in Nicaragua, a recently liberated country in Central America, currently under U.S. attack. I went down as a student with the language school in Managua, where you live with a Nicaraguan family in a barrio and participate in community activities, as well as studying Spanish and learning about the revolution.

I was deeply moved by my experiences in this tiny country, whose people successfully expelled the U.S.-backed Somoza dictatorship four years ago. In that short period of time, despite *extremely* scarce resources and continuous military and economic attacks by the U.S.-backed Contras and the C.I.A., Nicaragua has made amazing changes. Unemployment has dropped from 60% to 16%. In a country where 80% of the population was illiterate four years ago, 87% can now read and write. The percentage of the national budget spent on healthcare has increased 600%. It is now illegal to use women's bodies in advertising.[1]

As a disabled woman, I was treated very differently than I am in the States. I was not looked at as an oddity because of my disability, and I felt more accepted as a full human being. I picked cotton and participated in all community activities without question. Children almost never stared at me or hassled me on the streets, which happens all the time here. I felt much less self-conscious. I don't mean to imply that the old ways are totally gone and that things are perfect, because they aren't. But there *is* a real difference.

[1]MADRE Fact Sheet, 853 Broadway, Rm 905, NY, NY 10003.

Women and disabled people fought in the revolution, and play an active role in the new Nicaragua. Disabled people can serve in the army, the militia, and the police force, which would be unheard of in our country. In the local militias, women and men, young and old, able-bodied and disabled all train and work together. You see people in wheelchairs in uniform, carrying rifles, and you see older women, with grey hair, in militia units. You see young teenage boys and older women working together and talking to each other with mutual respect, as equals, which would be a very uncommon sight here.

One of my neighbors in the barrio where I lived was a woman named Liduvina Gutierrez. She had lived in Estali during the war. One day a rocket tore through the side of her house, and she dove on top of her children to shield them with her body. She lost an arm and a leg, as well as part of her shoulder and other foot. Because of the National Guard, she couldn't leave the house for a day, and gangrene set in. Today she is a nurse and works at a rehabilitation center with other disabled people. She is a warm and energetic woman, full of tremendous spirit and love, and we had a great time talking to each other. I was deeply moved by her optimism, determination and generosity.

I was free to talk to anyone, and people expressed a wide range of political opinions openly and without fear. It was wonderful to live in a country that was *structured* around cooperation, social consciousness, and the welfare of the whole community, and *not* around material goods, consumerism, "rugged individualism," and personal gain at the expense of other people. I felt very safe there, despite the war, because people really cared about, and took care of each other. But perhaps the most striking thing for me was to be in a country where the government is actually *supporting* the struggles of disabled people, women, workers, and poor people, in contrast to our government which always *opposes* these movements and frequently attempts to destroy them.

I spent several days visiting with people at the Organization of Disabled Revolutionaries — Che Guevera (ORD), and the Center for Social and Vocational Rehabilitation — Gaspar Garcia Laviana (CRSV), the two main disability organizations. They are on the same street, next door to each other. ORD is a political organization that raises the issue of disability, struggling with society to see it as a problem of the *whole* society. ORD works to make the new Nicaragua accessible in all ways, and to gain full rights and participation for disabled people. They also have a wheelchair shop that builds and repairs chairs for all of Nicaragua. On the walls of ORD are photographs of people playing wheelchair basketball, militia members in wheelchairs with rifles, pictures of Che Guevera, posters about women's liberation, and a poster depicting a beggar in the streets and saying "we will never allow this to happen to our old people and our disabled people." ORD has had an on-going relationship with disabled organizations in the U.S. since its beginning.

Next door to ORD is the CRSV, named after Gaspar Garcia Laviana, a priest who died fighting with the Sandinistas in the revolution. They offer training programs in vocational skills. People live at the center while they are in the program, and learn a skill like weaving or TV repair.

At ORD they told me that their primary task and their biggest obstacle is ideological. All other problems grow out of this one. They told me that the economic situation is very hard, because of the poverty left over from many years of exploitation by the Somoza family, the wealthy minority, and U.S. corporations, as well as the war, and now the necessity of putting large amounts of their financial and human resources into the defense effort. As a result, it is not easy to create accessible transportation systems and buildings. Often the roads are unpaved and full of potholes and rubble. The buses are old and over-crowded. But their spirit is very high, the government is behind them, and they're doing everything they possibly can. This year the National University and one hospital have been made accessible. They are talking with the architecture students, to make them aware of the needs of disabled people. They are seeking equality in labor, education, legal rights, transportation, and all areas of life. The job of ORD is to do the political organizing to make that happen, to change the consciousness of society with respect to disability.

"We were born out of the revolution," Hector Segovia told me, the Director of ORD, a dark and beautiful man in a chair, with sharp, intelligent eyes. Before the revolution there was nothing for disabled people, except for some very bad, paternalistic religious charity programs. But now they have an open door to all the ministries of the government and the full support of the FSLN. In fact, many of them are members of the FSLN. Hector told me that the revolution is not paternalistic. "You don't sit back and receive benefits," he said, "you work very, very hard." And then he added: "Before we were outside of society , but now we are inside."

The disability movement and the women's movement in Nicaragua have a strong sense of themselves as part of the whole struggle. They have their own individual priorities and goals, but they never see themselves in isolation, as just single issues. They had tried peaceful and legal channels of struggle for many years, trying to reform the system and make it better from inside of it, but to no avail. They finally came to see that they would have to fight together to *take power,* and to create a *fundamentally different system,* a truly democratic society where workers, peasants, disabled people, and women had a significant voice. Now they have laid the groundwork for an on-going process of social change, a process that is encouraged and nurtured by the new government. I felt moved by the strength of the women and disabled people I met in Nicaragua. I think their strength came from the struggle they had waged and won, and from the process they were now part of, of building a whole new kind of society. To give you some idea of how it felt to be in such a place, imagine what it would be like if all the various progressive movements in this country got together and took over the government: people from the women's movement, the disability movement, the gay movement, the black liberation movement, the Native American movement, the peace movement, the ecology movement, and so forth. Imagine that people from all these different movements for social change would be running the government here instead of Reagan and his boys (or Mondale and his). Imagine that our whole country was structured around meeting people's real needs, and around people working together for the common good, instead of around profits for giant corporations and a small class of wealthy individuals. Obviously there would be plenty of problems, but at least we would be trying to live in harmony with the earth, and each other. We would be trying to create an alternative to the death culture of nuclear bombs and MX missiles, of the KKK and Jerry Falwell, of endless television programs about white male super-heroes rescuing physically perfect blonde women, of magazines like *Playboy,*

Hustler and *Glamour* that portray women as objects to be dressed and undressed or put through meat-grinders, and of "revolutionary" new dishwashing liquids instead of revolutionary social changes.

I gained a tremendous sense of hope for the future of the planet in Nicaragua. There I was in a small country which has little money and no weapons to speak of, and which is being attacked by the greatest military power on earth.* Yet the Nicaraguans seemed completely undaunted by this, and absolutely determined and sure of what they are doing. They are the first to admit that the revolution isn't perfect. But they're committed to making their best effort, so that things will be as good as possible for themselves and for the future generations. They have a deep sense of human community and wholeness. It felt *very* positive to live in that kind of atmosphere. I learned, not just intellectually, but in my heart, from my experience there, that it *is* possible to live another way and genuinely care about human life. I think it is this example that the U.S. government fears and is trying to destroy, because the idea that Nicaragua presents a military threat to the U.S. is ludicrous: the *entire* national budget of Nicaragua is *less* than the U.S. spends on the B-1 bomber program.[2]

I believe that the disability movement and the women's movement here in the U.S. can learn a great deal from our Nicaraguan counterparts. I think we can learn about unity, about the need for a strategy and vision that looks beyond single issues and begins to make connections with other oppressed groups, a strategy that begins to take on our system as a whole, at its roots. We *must* see beyond piecemeal reforms within a fundamentally unjust system, and move toward taking power into our own hands, so that we can begin to create the profound changes that will enable all of us to live as fully respected members of our society, and to share more equally its resources and its responsibilities.

Whenever I asked the people in Nicaragua what they wanted

*The U.S. is sending millions of dollars to the Contras, and the CIA has directed and financed the mining of Nicaraguan harbors, and attacks on key ports.

[2]Richard J. Barnet and Peter Kornbluh, "Contra/dictions in Nicaragua" *Sojourner Magazine,* May 1984.

from us here in the U.S., they would always tell me that they wanted us to stop the U.S. attacks and prevent a full-scale U.S. invasion. They told me that without the revolution, there is no hope for women or disabled people. If the Contras and the C.I.A. win, they will restore a system like the one that existed before, where women and disabled people are on the bottom, and the power rests with a small minority. They told me they are counting on us.

There is a process of transformation going on all over this planet. It is a very exciting, as well as terrifying, time to be alive. We feel that process here in the blossoming of many movements for social change. But too often, we fail to put it into an international perspective. We see ourselves and our struggles in isolation once again. But part of the importance of our struggles here in North America lies in the fact that we are *inside* the greatest military empire on earth. Our government is acting to perpetuate a world of madness, attacking Nicaragua, trying to destroy everything they have done there, and they are doing it with our tax dollars. Then they tell us that making America accessible or providing childcare for working mothers is "too expensive." There is a *direct link* between our oppression as disabled women and the attacks that our tax dollars are funding against the progressive government of Nicaragua. We are all part of one human community. We cannot afford to view what happens in Nicaragua as simply the affairs of a distant country, unrelated to our own lives and problems. Because in fact, their victory is our victory... and their defeat would be our own defeat.

My Last Legs

by suzanne beaucher

*t*hey came for me at 7:00 AM, two uniformed prison matrons whose grim expressions and stiff movements gave them all the personality of a pair of orthopedic shoes. My cell door was un-locked, by some unseen force, and the sunshine sisters entered. They stood on either side of me, as I sat on my cot scowling at nothing in particular. One handcuffed my hands behind my back and then they both yanked me to my feet. I teetered a little and hove to star-board while they deflected me between them like an oversized pinball.

When they were satisfied that I wasn't going to crash gracelessly to the floor (where they'd only have to pick me up) they handcuffed each of my arms to one of their own, wrinkling my freshly-ironed prison shirt. I'd had a prison dress at one time, but they took that away from me when they saw my legs, and gave me a coordinated shirt and slacks ensemble instead. The world of high-fashion followed me even to prison.

Dragging me between them, they began the solemn procession down the long narrow corridor. As I was being hauled along, I thought vaguely that the scene needed music, something inspira-tional like "You Light Up My Life". I knew, of course, that the priest wouldn't be there, for he'd called the night before to give me the "May God have mercy on your soul" which he uttered with the appropriate gasp of emotion. He apologized for not being able to make it in person but explained that he had to bless the Grand Open-ing of a used car lot.

At last, we approached the huge metal door at the end of the corridor and I was relieved, for even being dragged on a trip that far had exhausted me. One would think that Death Row would be more accessible. As the door swung silently open, I had a moment to reflect on my crime. What dark human passion had made me do it? How did I honestly feel, deep down inside, about what I had done?

I

I thought it singularly amusing that doctors would confer "an illness" on a patient and then administer enough tests and drugs to convince even the most stalwart patient that she did indeed have "an illness". The day my doctor awarded me my diagnosis, and we shook hands, he warned me that most people with my "illness" lead practically normal lives. I imagined myself caught up in a whirlwind of bridal showers and tupperware parties and developing a sudden compulsion to wear incredibly high heeled shoes that made important clacking sounds when I walked. I saw myself assuming my place in front of the crowded mirror in the "ladies" room and applying my eyeliner with the same air of frantic determination as everyone else. I confess I was more than a little frightened by it all.

The ceremony now over, I suddenly found myself on the sidewalk being swept along by a tide of corporate "up and comings". I felt myself in danger of being trampled until I pulled out a tattered copy of Dickens' *Bleakhouse* and began reading it. They regarded me nervously and then moved quickly away. Fear of the unknown, it gets them every time.

II

The first years of my life with an "illness" were the years I became the foremost American authority on floors. I used to pretend to trip over a stray paperclip or gumwrapper just so that I could get a closer look at the floor. During these years, I collected a total of $31.18 in carelessly dropped change and learned something of the mating rituals of carpenter ants.

Carpeted and linoleum floors were wonderfully comfortable, and of course I did achieve my crash and slide record of 8'6" on a linoleum no-wax óf imitation brick, but I've always been an outdoor-type and yearned for the challenge of pavement and cement. Broken glass was always exciting but I found that the snack foods were the real adventure. Melted ice cream bars and soggy french fries oozing ketchup made me feel like a real American but that was just a temporary high. It was the bubble gum that really stayed with you. I once spent two days with a wad of grape Bubbilicious stuck to my chin. I hated to give it up.

When winter came, I found that I lost some of my enthusiasm for groundwork; you see one snowbank, you've seen them all. The ice kept me very active of course, but I no longer wanted to devote the time to ground research. I was never one for winter sports, you see. I returned to my doctor and asked if there was a way he could help me spend more of my waking hours in an upright position. He regarded me suspiciously and then gave me a prescription slip upon which he scrawled the large letters MD. I thought he was probably flaunting his medical degree to intimidate the pharmacist.

I picked up the prescription on the way home and after an hour, finished reading all the warnings, which ended with DO NOT PASS GO, DO NOT COLLECT $200.00. That put me in a recreative mood so I loaded my syringe and thrust it into my thigh. It was no good, I was going to have to take off my jeans. I did so and repeated the action. This time the wonder drug was sucked right in. I waited a few minutes and tried to determine if I felt any different. I felt like a person with a hole in her leg.

When I stood up the metamorphosis began and, after one hour, was complete. I had turned into Moby Dick. Now it's not that I was unhappy being Moby Dick, I never dreamed I could become an American classic. It's just that none of my clothes fit.

I waddled happily around for about six months, losing most of my hair and telling people exactly what I thought of them. I seemed to have an incredible amount of energy, read two novels per day and even began writing one. I just couldn't seem to stop writing about this one-legged sea captain. I also developed a huge appetite which was never satisfied.

At the end of my six month term, my doctor advised me to stop taking the Moby Dick potion and see what happened. Gradually I returned to my normal size and, after about three months, regained most of my hair. I began carrying a cane to beat passers-by with. It was the only thing that cheered me up.

III.

One day as I stood on the edge of a curb bludgeoning a corporate "up and coming" with my cane, a strong gust of wind blew me off the sidewalk and into the traffic. As I rolled from side to side to avoid the cars, whose drivers were very annoyed that they had to swerve to avoid me, I pondered my situation. Thus far, my life with "an illness" had not been all glitter. I saw no point in returning to my doctor who could only give me more of the Moby Dick potion. He said he had a milder form which would only make me Orca the Killer Whale, but I just couldn't get excited about it. After all, as Gertrude Stein once said, "A whale is a whale is a whale." I needed an extremely different perspective, something... holistic. I rolled over onto my left side (that is my thinking side) and thought, Acupuncture! I'd once heard that some people who'd had my "illness" had been treated with acupuncture and had some good results. I struggled gracelessly to my feet and then smashed my cane triumphantly on the hood of an oversized Buick that was about to run me over. "Acupuncture!" I repeated. I lurched off into the sunset.

When I arrived at the Mellow Methods Health Center later that week, I found myself wandering about in a primeval cavern. The coat rack had been fashioned from a large oak tree on whose branches hung bark covered hangers decorated with clusters of acorns. When I hung my jacket on one of the hangers, a squirrel popped out of a hole, fixed its teeth on the collar of my jacket, and scurried off with it. It was an old jacket anyway. I was aware of the sound of running water and peered through some of the branches but found nothing. I took a step back and found my left foot ankle-deep in very cold water. Apparently, there was a small stream running through the center of the "room" and I noticed a body floating face down in this stream. I removed my foot and glanced nervously about. There were other people sitting around the stream on tree stumps reading magazines: *Planetary Oblivions, Awareness Through Tofu,* and *Meditating Your Way Through Nuclear Holocaust.* These people seemed unconcerned about the body so I decided to say nothing. I'm cool.

I caned my way over to a nearby pine tree and moved aside one of its low, over-hanging branches. I'd found the receptionist! She whispered dreamily into the telephone.

"It's like, no real problem to me, I don't even deal with the money thing myself, but, you know, M.M. says you owe us $400.00."

There was a pause before the receptionist continued.

"Yes, yes, I can relate to that. I see this image of you turning out your pockets and saying like 'Oh wow, there's nothing!' I can see that, it's a very clear image to me. But like... "

She turned her attention to me and smiled beatifically. She murmured something into the phone and laid it down on the moss-covered desk.

"Hi" she said soothingly.

"I have a 3:00 PM appointment with Elizabeth Rosenthal... " I began.

"Oh, with Liz, Liz is beautiful, a beautiful centered person."

"I'm happy for her," I responded.

"Please sit by the stream and read one of our relevant magazines, or you can just sit and, you know, be." She sighed with an awed kind of satisfaction.

I decided I'd just be, I thought I could handle that better than *Awareness Through Tofu.*

She spoke to the body in the stream gently. "Richard, your flotation period is over now."

The body responded by rising from the stream and walking in a dreamlike trance to the desk.

"Here's your wallet, Richard."

Richard took his wallet, extracted an American Express card, and handed it to the receptionist who deftly ran it through the machine, scribbled a few notations on the slip and then handed both back to him. He signed the slip, took his copy and his wallet and, wearing only a small hand towel walked floatingly out the door. The receptionist, seeing the puzzled look on my face, said, "Oh, it's his own towel."

I sat on a nearby stump to "be" until Elizabeth was ready for me.

When she finally arrived on the scene, I rose from my stump to shake her hand. She reached across the stream to take my outstretched hand and knocked one of the people reading a magazine off of her tree-stump and into the stream. The receptionist came over immediately and told the new occupant of the stream that it was $40.00 for the first ½ hour.

Elizabeth led me to a small room and helped to hoist me up onto the examination table. She chattered amiably as she pulled off my shoes and most of my clothing. I felt a momentary seizure of modesty but then overcame it. She arranged the needles in artistic patterns on my body and stood back to admire them.

I glanced out of the only window in the room, always careful to note all possible avenues of escape. Outside I saw a uniformed drum and bugle corps marching back and forth to the tune of "On The Street Where You Live". Meanwhile, Elizabeth thrust a needle into the tip of my nose.

She seemed to have seen some mark on my body, just above my navel, that intrigued her.

"Melvin should see this," she said excitedly. I tightened somewhat at the thought of this clinical show and tell but then relaxed when she remembered that he wasn't in this afternoon.

"Yes, he's out practicing with his drum and bugle group." She paused, "Hey, they're right out here." She flung open the window and bellowed with effortless projection, "Melvin, come here!"

Elizabeth had to be the kind of person whose commands are always obeyed. Melvin had to be the leader of the drum and bugle corps. The corps had to have been trained by a fanatical ex-marine who taught the group to follow their leader no matter what.

Within a matter of moments, there was a parade marching around me. I lay punctured with needles in all my semi-naked splendor. I hadn't noticed that Eyewitness News was also on the scene until the large TV cameras rolled into the room and zoomed in on the freckle that had been the cause of all the commotion. When I could endure no more, I plucked out the needles in handfuls and threw them at the camera crew. I rolled off of the table and onto the floor. For once, gravity was on my side. I scrambled into my clothes and staggered out of the room in an acupuncture stupor.

Elizabeth refused to treat me any further telling the receptionist that I was excessively modest and probably a Roman Catholic to boot. She'd treated child molesters, wife-beaters, even known Republicans but she just couldn't bring herself to treat a Catholic. She even hypothesized that my "illness" had been caused by my Catholicism. An exotic disease transmitted through rosary beads. This was a very popular theory in holistic circles.

I was ushered on to new Mellow Methods of Healing. Various therapists prescribed various vitamins and massive doses of sex. Apparently this was the only antidote to my Catholicism. I installed a machine outside my bedroom where the waiting personnel could take a number. This didn't last long though because I tired easily, often petering out after only number 151.

I tried the Miracle Eat Dirt Diet and was even coaxed into eating vegetables for a time. It was a beet that finally pushed me over the edge.

I was totally, thoroughly and completely exhausted one evening and wanted to finish my carrot juice and vegetable super-salad and drag myself on my forearm crutches off to bed. I just had to finish this salad, maybe I'd survive without the carrot juice, others had. Just get through the salad. I took a deep breath and hoisted a mouthful up towards my mouth. No good, I overshot it and it went off into space. I'd clean it up sometime when I had the energy, maybe next year. I took another mouthful and dropped my head into the salad to shorten the distance between fork and mouth. I could use the rest. I got down most of it and it tasted as horrible as ever. Finally, all that remained was one pickled beet slice.

I was going to do it. I stabbed the beet slice and brought my mouth down to it. I tried to thrust it in but it was too wide for my ever-delicate little mouth. I would have to cut it. I groped for the fork and it dropped under the table. I bent painfully at the waist and felt for it on the floor. My floor skills were not what they once were and I couldn't find it.

I finally found the fork lodged under my foot. I pulled but I couldn't dislodge it. But I was going to do it. I tried foolishly to move my foot but at this hour my feet and legs were dead to the world.

They usually knock off at about 2:30 PM, but I was going to do it. I decided I'd try to break it in half with my bare hands, if I had that much strength left. I was going to do it.

I grabbed the beet slice with my right hand and it squirmed out of my grasp. I cornered it with both hands and pressed hard when it shot out of my hands and into the living room. I could have abandoned the fight right then and there but I had said I was going to do it and I was going to do it.

Somehow, I managed to heave myself to my feet on my crutches and drag myself almost three feet before I collapsed on the floor. I'd never get up now, I knew it, but I was going to get that beet and eat it. I was going to do it somehow, someway. I crawled, groaning in my best Barbara Stanwyck style, and saw the beet in the distance. When I was as close as I thought I could get, I stretched out my right arm and the fingers of my right hand and just touched it with my middle fingernail. One more millimeter. I virtually dislocated my shoulder with stretching but got the millimeter I needed.

IV

When I woke up the next morning, still lying on the living room floor, I felt an odd change in my psyche and in the state of the world. Today had something to do with Fate, I could feel it. I showered, dressed and went out to work as I had for the past seven years, unaware of what had transpired late last night, in an abandoned orthopedic shoe factory.

My doctor, all of my former therapists, and attending physicians had formed a secret alliance to destroy me. They called it the Society Against Sally, which was most interesting since that was not my name. Clever of them to leave no clues linking their society to me. They even wore team jackets in orange, yellow, and aqua, my three least favorite colors.

Their reasons for wanting me destroyed varied. For some, it was a mercy killing, for others it was to save face, since their treatments hadn't worked on me, but for most it was a reaction against the fear that they all lived with, that I'd make another appointment and come back!

As I crutched my way towards the building in which I worked, I noticed a black car pull stealthily in toward the curb, blocking the ramp for the disabled. I felt myself becoming angry. The battle with the beet the night before had unhinged me a bit. It was just one battle in a seven-year-long war but every woman has her breaking point and that had been mine. I felt myself losing control. I crutched over to the car and stared angrily in through the open window. There was no one inside. I began trembling and turning purple, angry adrenaline pumping through my body. Finally I let loose a savage growl, threw my crutches to the ground, and overturned the car. It was still blocking the ramp but I felt better seeing it balanced on its roof.

Within minutes the local and state police were on the scene accompanied by two federal agencies and the National Guard. Since I knew the penalty in Massachusetts was death for any offence other than littering and driving on the Southeast Expressway with intent to kill, I knew I had been framed. These therapists had known exactly when my breaking point would come and had hired the beet to insure that I was partially unhinged by the next morning. So, it had been a stunt-beet.

And so I was arrested, tried and sentenced to death, and shipped off to prison. Here, I spent my final days reading back issues of TV Guide and weaving a long chain of cigarette butts, which I intended to use as a tool in my escape. The chain was only nine inches long the morning they came for me.

The matrons dragged me into the room and swung the heavy door shut. They removed my handcuffs and led me to a large metal chair. So this was "the chair". They strapped me in securely and put a stainless steel mixing bowl on my head. They asked if I had any last requests and I told them I didn't like the bowl on my head and could I see something in a Stetson.

They never cracked a smile as they moved toward "the switches". How nice to spend my final moments with such a rollicking pair of cut-ups. Each threw her respective switch and I felt the electricity surge through my body, curling my toes. Suddenly, inexplicably, and unbelievably, I stood up, breaking the straps. I was completely better (except for my toes which were still curled). I jumped up and down in joyful leaps and then began tap-dancing like Ruby Keeler. I grabbed one of the matrons and began waltzing. She wasn't a bad dancer but was still not much of a conversationalist.

I offered to trade my striped prison outift for her own. She refused. I threatened to foxtrot her to death if she did not swap and she still refused. It wasn't until I told her that stripes were in this year that she agreed.

The exchange complete, I grabbed the other matron and tangoed back down Death Row. The Head Prison Matron took me aside at the end of the corridor and asked me how everything went. I said "Fine." She asked me how I was feeling, I said "Fine." Then she said that maybe I should go home. I said "Fine" and tap-danced out of the gates, leaving my seven-year imprisonment behind me.

Abuse of Women With Disabilities

by rebecca s. grothaus

are disabled women victims of physical, sexual, and/or psychological abuse? If you answer the question based on what you read about the problem, you must say "No", or at least, "They don't seem to be."

But, if your knowledge of disabled women in general is based on what you read, or hear, or see on television or in the movies, you wouldn't be sure there are any disabled women. You know that there are disabled girls; you see us on posters and on cans in convenience stores being hugged by Jerry Lewis. What happens to us when we're too old to be Jerry's kids?

We grow up, we go to college, we try to get jobs, we fall in love, we have children of our own, and, despite the lack of information on the subject, we can be the victims of sexual assault, battery, and psychological abuse.

Violence against women was a real, but unrecognized, problem long before the feminist movement made it an issue. It was, and largely still is, a shameful secret, a situation women blamed ourselves for causing. Whether rape victim, battered wife or sexually abused child, women always felt ourselves to be at fault.

Friends, neighbors, teachers, the police and the courts all conspired to keep the violence against women a personal problem. Violence against women is many things in America: an expression of contempt for females, a way for men to assert power over women, a mental illness, "fun" for a group of college students on a Saturday night drunk, a source of humor, a way to sell records or clothes, a multi-million dollar pornography industry; but it is more than a personal problem.

It is a political problem and it requires a political solution. Political solutions are being sought and found. More and more women and girls are reporting their victimization. Laws are changing. More shelters and underground railroads exist to help women escape batterers. All these changes impact the situation of disabled women who are victims of abuse.

Disabled women, no matter the subject being explored, are an invisible population. We are often lumped together with senior citizens in statistical reports, and in the thinking of public policy makers, so that our unique concerns, and even our numbers, are lost.

The Government, in funding programs for victims of violence, does not even follow its own non-discrimination regulations. Shelters for battered women are not always required to be physically accessible. This means that women with mobility impairments cannot get up the stairs or in the door to seek shelter. No special funding is available for the programs to provide ramps or other necessities like sign-language interpreters for the deaf. No government-funded studies have been done on the extent of violence against disabled women, or, if they have, they have not been publicized.

The disability civil rights movement does not recognize the unique concerns of disabled women. Most women working in this movement perceive our disabilities as the only cause of our problems. It requires a considerable leap to recognize sex-based discrimination and identify with feminist issues like volence against women, even if we are the victims of such violence.

In actuality, disabled women have two threats to our civil rights, if not to our bodies: discrimination based on disability and discrimination based on sex.

Often, shelters are not accessible to disabled women. Few self-defense classes are designed for women with disabilities. Rape and battery hotlines usually do not have tele-communications devices for deaf women. When a battered women's shelter is accessible, the staff may be afraid to take in a battered disabled woman. They fear she won't fit in, that she can't do her share of the work, or that other women find her depressing.

If all the programs, shelters and hot-lines were fully accessible, some disabled women would still not seek help. All of the factors that keep non-disabled women from reporting rape or battery are present for disabled women. The feeling that it is somehow her own fault, fear of public knowledge of her shameful secret, of the courts, of retaliation by the accused batterer or rapist all occur in a disabled victim of violence, but there are additional considerations for disabled women.

A severely disabled women who has finally achieved independence from institutions, doctors and parents and is living alone may not report a rape because she knows the reaction will be to put her somewhere ''safe''. She may fear re-institutionalization in a board and care facility, or in her parents' home, more than she fears rape.

A severely disabled woman in an abusive relationship may be unable to leave, due to limited job opportunities, lack of adequate transportation, or low self-esteem. As medical bills mount, she may feel that it is somehow ''right'' for her to be beaten or punished for the financial and social tensions her disability brings to a relationship.

Her companion may be sexually stimulated by a perception that she is powerless. If so, she may tolerate the physical or psychological abuse, reasoning that if she cannot offer physical beauty or ''normalcy,'' she must somehow make up for that lack.

Women with severe disabilities are not expected to have relationships. We are perceived as asexual, as not desiring love or sex or committed involvement. When a disabled woman does have a relationship, she may feel validated as a woman and as a sexual being. It may be very hard for her to reject that role of lover/wife that she never expected to have in the first place.

The problem of abuse of disabled women exists, but several factors prevent the finding of solutions. They are the general lack of information and awareness of the concerns of women with disabilities, non-enforcement of accessibility requirements in publicly funded programs and shelters and the failure of the feminist movement to include the nearly 20 percent of women with disabilities when action is taken on such issues as rape and battery.

The following recommendations present a starting point for discussion and action to find solutions:

1. Increased attention by policy makers to determine the extent of

the problem of abuse of disabled women in their jurisdiction. Studies should be funded and widely publicized.

2. Increased enforcement of disability non-discrimination laws in all publicly funded programs that deal with violence against women.

3. Increased funding for programs to make themselves accessible through structural changes like ramps and through the purchase of telecommunications devices for deaf women and providing sign language interpreters. Line items for accessibility provisions should be included in budgets and paid for by the funding source.

4. Education by disabled persons of workers in all violence-oriented programs to reduce their fear of disabilities and their ignorance of the abilities of women who may need their help. Programs should seek out such in-service training.

5. Development of resource lists in programs that provide specialized assistance such as disabled peer counseling or interpreters for deaf women.

6. Better education of staff in medical facilities which treat victims of violence as to the requirements for adequate handling of severely disabled women. For example, a woman with osteogenesis imperfecta could receive further damage to her brittle bones by the injudicious handling by medical staff. It is not enough to rely on the woman's ability to communicate warnings to the staff. Victims of violence who need emergency medical attention are usually distraught, to say the least, and at times incoherent.

7. Provision of adequate equipment in medical facilities so that severely disabled women can be examined safely and with dignity, for example, the provision of Hoyer lifts to get a woman from her wheelchair onto the examining table.

8. Recognition by the disability civil rights movement that women with disabilities face double discrimination. Following recognition should come action to bring disabled women's issues onto the agendas of organized groups. Feminists should be invited to speak at disability group meetings. Support should be given

to feminist causes by disabled persons, with bodies at protest rallies and by speaking out.

9. Recognition by the feminist movement that disabled women are being excluded by inaccessible meeting places and by ignorance. Following this recognition should also come action to include disabled women. Outreach programs should be targeted to disabled women. Speakers from disability groups should be invited to educate the members. Feminists should lend support to disability causes; women are the majority of disabled persons and any effort to secure the rights of disabled people helps women.

10. Agitation by disabled women to demand that their concerns be considered and that their needs be met. Disabled women must organize themselves and take on the systems that have ignored them and now claim that they don't exist. Women with disabilities have legal and civil rights, among them the right to be safe in our homes and on the streets and to have access to help when we are victimized. Disabled women must demand our rights, because waiting for someone else to do it hasn't worked yet.

3.

Growing Up In Our Families

Growing up in our families has laid the foundation for our self perceptions, all our future interactions and how we deal with our disabilities. For those of us disabled as children, our disabilities have profoundly affected those early life experiences.

We have been influenced by the valued myth that our families should be self sufficient in raising children. In reality parents often act as coordinators of their children's participation in education, medical and recreational resources provided outside the nuclear family. When there is a disabled child and services are not accessible, the responsibility for attending to the child's basic needs reverts back to the family. With so few people trying to meet the needs, the family system can quickly become overwhelmed and exhausted.

Since childrearing is viewed as a family affair, and family matters are private, parents may struggle in intense isolation to provide for their disabled children. Without the necessary resources, they may be forced to deny the existence or seriousness of the disability. When disabilities are acknowledged, parents may experience great shame and guilt, believing they are responsible for having created a disabled child. Although most disabilities are not inherited, placing cause within the family serves the purpose of diverting responsibility away from industries that manufacture toxins and contaminate our air, water and food supplies.

Caring for a disability may be so time consuming that there is little energy left for caring for the child. As disabled children, we often become the scapegoats for an already exhausted and strained family system, bearing the burdens of the family's frustrations and resentments. Parents and siblings may see us as the problem, and we may come to believe that we are guilty for being disabled and for causing the family trouble.

Because there are so few community resources available to encourage the full development of disabled children and so few role models of disabled adults, parents naturally have few images of how their children could grow up to be functioning adults in society's mainstream. It may seem best to protect us from the outside world and teach us to be dependent on the family. But meeting all the child's needs is an impossible task for even the most caring and loving family. Institutionalizing the disabled child may be the only available alternative to relieve some of the family's burden.

Disabled children deserve to grow up in families supported by the same community resources available to others. For instance, all families, including those with disabled children, would benefit from adequate, accessible childcare. We need the same opportunity to learn to love and respect ourselves and to function in the world as adults. For us this may mean learning to work with attendants to get our physical needs met in a way that leaves us feeling mature, respected, and whole.

We also deserve the opportunity to associate with other disabled children and adults in atmospheres that foster our individual growth and the incorporation of our disabilities into positive self-concepts. Our parents deserve access to adequate services including support groups for parents raising disabled children.

Inheritance

by pennyota ahladas

h e was somebody who didn't hear, somebody I hardly knew. I wondered what his world was like. I tried sometimes to see what it was like. I walked the house with my hands over my ears. It never lasted long; I was afraid my brother might sneak up behind me. It was so lonely to cover my ears. I could hear only hollow empty sounds like the sea on a quiet day.

I never stopped talking to him. He never spoke back. Maybe he didn't like me, and was only pretending not to hear. Sometimes he used to sit in the big armchair by the piano. I wanted to play for him but I was afraid he would get angry to see me striking at the keys when he didn't know the sound that I was making.

One Saturday afternoon, I was sitting on the couch playing my guitar. I had saved for a year to buy it, because I would have never asked him for the money. He flared up in a rage, tore the guitar from me, and threw it against the wall. The twanging strings of the cracked instrument pulsed in my head as I ran frightened and confused into my room. I cried with my face in my pillow, not understanding what I had done. One week later, I understood.

He took me to see a doctor. It was the first time that we ever went anywhere serious together. There were lots of tests that different people did to me, shuffling me from room to room. When they were done, they sat me in the doctor's office. After too long a time, the doctor came into the room. "Your father has a disease," he said, "you too have that disease. Someday, you too will not be able to hear. There is nothing I can do to help you." Inside me, I was flooded with tears. They poured and poured. I felt my eyes swell with water, though I let none roll down my cheek. I didn't want my father to see that I even minded, that I was afraid, that I was mad at him, that I felt all alone, that I could still hear the rain pounding on the roof.

Now, I can't hear the rain pounding on the roof. I write him a letter, "Dad, I can no longer hear the rain pounding on the roof. I don't know when the telephone rings." He answers, "It's in your head, the hearing loss is in your head. You have created it in your mind."

My father's father was deaf, my father's aunts and uncles were deaf, and my father refuses to admit my own deafness. My father does not read lips, he will not learn sign. My father, a deaf man, lives alone in a silent house, lives alone in a silent world. A life like his I will not live.

Waiting Again

by frances lynn

before I tell you about Frances Lynn today, I want to plead with all the Kentucky readers of this piece to work on attendant care for all of us, because if we don't get a program I may not last much longer. I'm tired of how I am living now and I don't see any answer for me other than moving away from home and to freedom!

Let me explain. For those of you who know me, I never did get to go to college. Right after Christmas, my grandfather died. He and my grandmother had lived all their lives in a small town in the southern part of the state. They own a grocery store a few blocks from their home. I used to love to visit when I was little because Mom would push me to the store and I would sit behind the counter and pretend to help my grandparents. I learned how to make change, even though I couldn't hold the coins very well, and since my wheelchair was a child's size, I couldn't reach the cash register. Still, Grandma said I did help her out a lot.

Everybody worried about Grandma after Grandpa died. She had never been alone from the day they had married. Af first, my Uncle Bob went home to Grandma's and stayed, but he is an Army man and he had gotten his orders for overseas before Christmas so we all realized it was only a temporary solution.

One of the best things about my family is the way we all take care of each other. Uncle Jake, remember, took my mom and dad and me in when we needed him, and we lived with him for years. But that is also a bad thing about my family.

When I try to talk about attendant care, my mom says, "Honey, you have a family to take care of you. Why would you want a stranger? You don't need to get involved with that as long as you have an aunt, or cousin, or whatever. Someone from the family will always be here to look after you."

Well, Uncle Bob had to leave early last year and since Pop had been laid off again, my parents decided that the best solution for Grandma was for us to move down there with her, and Mom and Pop could help out with the store. That decision did not bother me 'cause I did not see how it would affect my plans to go away and live in the dorm at college.

But Mom could not see how I could go.

"Honey, you can go to that school anytime. Grandma needs us and I can't be down there trying to help her over Grandpa's death and run that store and worry about you in that strange town, in college with some young kid taking care of you." I reminded her that the student I would share my room with had worked as an attendant for two years already.

"But what if you get sick?" She shouted at me. "I won't be there. I'll worry to death. NO! You can't make all this harder for me. You're just being selfish. You *must* move to Grandma's with us, and that's final!"

Mom seldom shouts. She was really upset. So what could I do? I was being selfish, but don't you *have* to be selfish sometimes?

Mom made me feel much worse when she got over being upset and came into my room and took my hand and said, "Besides, I need you. Grandma is taking this all very hard. She loves you very much, and you have to help me take care of her and that big house. We will buy you that electric wheelchair with the money Grandpa's leaving us. And we will talk about college next year, OK?"

What could I say? If I knew what I was about to get into I might have done something drastic — like gone to court to get my independence. Don't teenagers get to do that? I guess I'm being silly, but there must be *some* way I can be in charge of my own life. There must be.

We all moved to Grandma's in late January last year. I told my social worker that I really loved my grandma and that I could not be happy at college knowing she needed me. Mom went with me to my social worker's office and told me later how proud she was of me and what I had said.

I don't mean to ramble on but this is the first time I have told anyone what I am going through.

Mom took me to a drive-in restaurant after the meeting with my social worker to get a malt. I always used to get to do that after I had been to the doctor's if I had been good and didn't cry. I did cry that night after Mom put me to bed and turned out my light.

Making plans to go to college had been hard. Coping with the changes, calling strangers there and interviewing an attendant, figuring out all the finances for college had all been hard. I had been scared to death to leave home but I had made a decision and I was going to do it even if it did actually scare me to death!

Now all that was gone. No more fear of moving away from my family. I cried. I felt I would never be free. I would never be free. I would never get to make my own decisions, decisions for the good of no one but me. And I became *really* afraid.

We have been here at Grandma's a little over a year. I *do* have more responsibility here. Shortly after we moved here Grandma had a stroke. She is not able to get out of bed most of the time. Since there is only one decent room on the first floor of Grandma's house, and neither of us can get up the stairs, we made it into a big bedroom and she and I share it.

Whenever Mom works at the store I get in my electric wheelchair (at least I did get *that*), so I can reach the phone in case Grandma needs attention. Also Mom leaves food and drinks where I can reach them. I serve lunch for Grandma, sort of. If you had told me a year ago that I would be an attendant myself, I would have called the nut wagon for you.

This house has steps off the porch so only once in a while do I get out in my electric wheelchair. But once out, I do ride around ALONE. This town is so small that there is not much traffic — or many sidewalks. During this time alone I think and plan and psych myself up for my next chance at freedom. I am going to work hard for an attendant care program. I *do* love my family but someone else will have to take care of them. I want to take care of myself for a change.

"Ask Mummy"

by elb

*i*n the locked-off days of my childhood when my parents were bringing me up in careful isolation in the country, I remember how, on one of those useless sunny afternoons that inevitably come one's way in the teen years, I had gone out into the garden at the front of my parents' village house. My mother was out there, industriously picking a generous supply of apples. I hung around wondering whether I should avail her of my help, knowing full well that she hardly needed it anyway. On the other hand, there was nothing else in the world to do on that lengthy afternoon. The strange immature boy with whom I had grown up also came listlessly around the corner. It felt like the two of us.

At that moment the gate opened and a new neighbor who lived at the other side of the village came into the garden. My mother, who did not usually care for neighbors, was quite happy to see her because she and my father were interested to call her and her husband their friends as they were apparently doing well in the buying-homes-for-people business. My mother was also interested in their eldest son as a prospect on my behalf. However it was the first time that this neighbor had the opportunity to meet my brother and me. What she did, apart from giving me a cursory look-over, was to turn to my brother and to start talking about what a lovely boy he was, very natural in manners, but why quite like that? My mother explained that he was backward; the neighbor was apparently not satisfied with that explanation and wanted to know more; why he was backward.

My mother said — "The reason he is backward is as a result of a nervous breakdown suffered when small, due to worry and concern over his sister going deaf." That I would say is how the sun sinks down in the afternoons of one's middle teenage.

Letters From the Moon

by kathleen m. white

The Hospital
December 29, 1965

Dear Daddy:

If I tried to put down all my thoughts and feelings in the journal Dick got for me, my poor non-focusing eyes would probably turn inside out and my writing would look like upside down Arabic. So Mom has agreed to take on the chore of recording my momentous observations in a letter to you.

The strangest thing is that the accident itself still doesn't seem credible to me. I was half asleep when it happened and unconscious or only semi-conscious for a week thereafter, so it has no reality for me. I've learned some of the details so I can reply intelligently when people ask me about it, but it is mostly just a story to me. Of course I believe it happened, mainly because it's an explanation of why I'm here. It's like asking, "Why do the tides come in and out" and being told, "It's the moon." As an explanation, it's acceptable but somehow remote.

When I first became fully conscious I simply felt that I had a new situation to deal with. All of a sudden I found myself in a hospital bed with two strange and numb legs attached to my body. I felt very, very weak and very helpless. Mummy was with me as well as Dick, so I was aware that something was out of the ordinary. Even as I became informed of the details of the accident and my injury, I couldn't really become depressed because I just felt like me in a new situation. I've been in lots of new situations in my life and have come to feel the best way to handle them is to keep laughing and shoot high. I don't feel any different now...

Dear Bestest Friends:

Goldwater country is probably the last place you ever expected to see postmarked on a letter to you. Just before Christmas Dick and I started impulsively east, cat and dog in tow; we planned to call you as a big surprise when we had gotten close to home. Unfortunately, someone must have let it out of the bag that we were good liberal Democrats because we weren't able to make it through this state. In the midst of a snowstorm our poor little "Baby Cadillac" and a great big tough old Republican car went skidding into each other. Virtue failed to win out and the poor Democratic Volkswagen got demolished and I got pretty banged up myself.

Dick and Lurch and Mopsy proved too tough for injury, but I guess I had everyone pretty worried for awhile. My mother and father came out from Boston to help Dick, and Mummy is still here, keeping me company. As soon as I'm strong enough the doctor will put me in a body cast and send me back to Boston. It's been kind of a long trip but I still can't wait to get home.

Dick reluctantly went back to Berkeley to finish his semester, then he'll be back in Massachusetts, too. The doctor expects to get me out of here in three weeks. I can't wait to begin some real therapy — there are two legs in bed with me, but no real indication that they're mine. Since I'm determined to be swimming, sailing, horseback riding and wrestling with Dick by next summer, I am naturally very anxious to get started on my progress.

Lunch just came, and since eating is supposed to help me strengthen fast, I'll sign off to you now. While I eat, Mom is going to fill in some of the events between December 23, when I was still unconscious, and today, when I'm obviously my outspoken old self. I am very anxious for mail, so please take time to write to me here. Love to you all...

Dear Friends of Kathie:

When Kathie's father and I arrived in Arizona, she was still unconscious, but by December 23, she was having periods of hazy consciousness. On Christmas Eve, I asked the doctor, "she will be able to read and write again, won't she?"

His dubious look as he replied, "I don't know, it's a little early to tell yet," filled me with dread, but Kathie herself settled the matter the next day when she unwrapped a present I had given her.

"*The I Hate to Housekeep Book* by Peg Bracken," she murmured, gazing at the cover while Dick and I exchanged relieved glances.

"If it's loose, pick it up;" she added drowsily, "if it isn't, dust it; if it moves, feed it."

Dick took the book from her hand and his brow cleared as he read the fine print blurb above the title. "That's what it says, all right."

I know you'll be glad to hear that our Christmas wasn't as miserable an occasion as you might think. Dick had bought a huge red stocking which he filled with little surprises and hung on the curtain railing above Kathie's bed. Her favorite presents were a stuffed poodle which looked like Moppet and a perky red reindeer.

Dick and I were invited for Christmas dinner by a Williams couple who had learned of our situation, but as much as we appreciated this kind-hearted gesture, neither of us felt up to accepting. When it was suggested by a member of the hospital staff that we have dinner in Kathie's room, this we gratefully did, taking turns feeding her what little she would eat from her plate of turkey and "all the fixings." It must be difficult for her to eat and drink lying flat on her back, but at least she is doing well enough so she no longer needs to be fed intravenously.

On Tuesday the 21st, the day Ed returned to Boston, Kathie was still semi-delirious. She doesn't remember saying, "Hello, Daddy, I love you." Nor does she recall saying to Dick, when he gently placed a damp cloth on her hot forehead: "You're a good husband. I don't know if you're *my* husband, but you're a good husband."

"Would you like to see your mother?"

"I want to see you the most."

"I'll be here, too — your mother will just be an added attraction."

"Hi, Mummy. There's something I want you both to know. I think you both did a wonderful job bringing me up and now you're going to take care of me and watch over me all my life, aren't you, and never let me get hurt or lost or abandoned... "

On Christmas day she talked on the telephone to Dick's family. I heard her say, "I'm grateful to be alive."

By Monday, the 27th, ten days after the accident, Kathie was thinking very clearly indeed. "I have been mentally composing a projectory to present to the doctor," she informed Dick and me, "giving him various reasons why I feel I should be put in a cast as soon as possible, my arguments being based on the pre-med courses I took when I was thinking of being a nurse."

Obviously charmed by Kathie's intelligence and wit, Dr. Burns nevertheless refuses to be rushed. He explains that she will have to be given an anesthetic when the cast is put on, and in her weakened condition the use of an anesthetic could be dangerous. We will just have to be patient and hope her strength returns in the near future.

You asked about pain. I would say Kathie had two days when she was aware of pain and discomfort, despite the medications which were supposed to help her.

But even under these circumstances she was able to wisecrack.

Nurse: "Is your pain any better, Kathie?"

Kathie, wryly: "Is my pain better? How can pain be *better?* Pain is pain!"

Monday afternoon, she demanded, "Where is that sexpot doctor? I want him front and center immediately!"

Nurse: "I don't believe he'll be back today. He's gone to his office in Flagstaff."

"Is he arranging my plane reservations so I can fly home tomorrow? I get so tired of just lying here all the time. I want to be sitted up."

(Laughter from Dick, myself, and nurse.)

Nurse: "The doctor said he might let you be propped up a bit toward the end of the week."

"What's today?"

Nurse: "Monday."

"Is tomorrow the end of the week?"

She told us she wants so much to be home "where I can be near the people I know. I'd even like to see the idiot-people. I'd much rather see old idiot-people than new idiot-people."

As Kathie mentioned, Dick returned to Berkeley on Sunday to finish the three weeks remaining in the first semester so he will have salvaged at least that much of his senior year. I am so proud of Kathie for insisting that he go... and proud of him, too. It will be hard for him to return alone to their memory-filled apartment, furnished with so many things they made or refinished with their own hands. Do call him if he doesn't call you. I'm sure he'll appreciate seeing you.

January 5, 1966

Dear Favorite Principal Boss:

You can't imagine how much your call meant to me. Every card, every letter reminds me that I belong in a non-hospital world, too — not that the hospital routine is dull... as a matter of fact every day begins with a Battle Royale! I am forced to fight fiercely for my beauty sleep against a hoard of uncooperative nurses. At 6:00 a.m. (imagine!) the first wake-up nurse crashes into my room, hooks open my door, and turns on two lights. At 6:15 the next bright-eyed wake-up nurse comes bounding in to get my water pitcher. She doesn't refill it, mind you, she puts it on a cart with all the other water pitchers and clanks the cart up and down the hall a few times until she is sure everyone is wide awake.

Six-thirty is pill time. A sweet, friendly looking old nurse who looks like somebody's grandmother brings me about eighty pills and stands over me until every one of them has gone down the hatch. At 6:45 come the cruelest of all blows — some unidentified nurse wakes up every baby in the nursery and urges each to howl his loudest. I would like to think that the cold, wet washcloth which is brought in at 7:00 is intended to sooth our brows after fifteen minutes of listening to baby squalls; however, judging from the nurse's expression when she hands me the wet cloth and says, "Get ready for breakfast, dear," I doubt if this is her motive. Apparently she is not satisfied with eyes that are only half open and expects me to undergo a form of medieval water torture to complete the journey to wakefulness.

Breakfast provides additional fun and novelty. The nurses optimistically drape a king-sized towel under my chin, but in my groggy state, I still manage to feed at least half of my oatmeal to the sheet, blanket, and pillow case, as well as amply nourishing my neck, throat, and shoulder-blades.

Most of the morning passes quite pleasantly because my mother is with me to read and write letters. This is so out of keeping with the usual scheme of things that she is shooed out from time to time by nurses zealously devoted to restoring hospital normalcy. The customary excuse is that my bedsores need treatment. Who would have thought that one could develop sores just from lying in a soft, clean, comfortable bed! The treatment is unique: the nurses prop me up on my side with a few pillows and then direct a bright lamp on the trouble spots. Never in my wildest nightmares did I ever picture myself with that particular part of my anatomy in the spotlight.

Despite the obvious zest in hospital living, I appreciate my Manzanita mail more than I can say. I expect to be in Arizona for another two or three weeks and hope the mail bag will continue to be full. Thereafter I will be at Massachusetts General Hospital. I miss Manzanita and hope to be back there before too long. Make sure my substitute is giving my kiddies enough loving...

January 6, 1966

Dear Gram:

A steady stream of letters from home have helped to brighten every day. Reminders and memories help the hospital routine pass more easily, not that the routine is very complicated — they feed me, wash me, roll me around and rub my back, somehow change the bed with me in it, massage my legs, give me different pills forty times a day and regularly take my temperature, pulse, and blood pressure.

The hardest part isn't the external hospital routine, it's getting used to me. Like there's a strange pair of legs in my bed. I have a vague feeling of a numb pair of bent legs attached to my body, but every time I look, there is very clearly a pair of *flat* legs lying here. I can't feel a thing though the nurses prod them and rub them and move them, but Mom tells me originally I couldn't feel anything below my neck, so I figure by next week I should have feeling to the knees, and another week I should even be able to wiggle my toes.

There's been a lot of progress, anyway. Instead of lying flat in bed like a pancake, I am wound up to a sitting position, trusted to wash my own face and hands, and I'm even allowed to feed myself. I wonder if my kiddies would mind a teacher with egg all over her face.

The doctor was a little worried about the injury to my head, but obviously I'm as quick and clever as ever. I think the plan of action is to get me well enough to go back to Boston for therapy. I'll keep you in touch and meanwhile would appreciate as much news as possible. Please write again...

January 11, 1966

Dear Ted:

It was wonderful to hear from my favorite older brother. Writing an answer isn't as easy as you might think. I still have a problem of quadruple, over-lapping, intermingling, and thoroughly confusing vision. I can't even read what I'm writing when I attempt to be my own secretary, unless I keep one eye closed in one-eyed pirate fashion.

Other than my skewed vision, my progress continues to be very good. I had a problem of a squeaky ear, but that was only because of a low pressure area at our high altitude. The doctor's carefully weighed and well-considered prescription for this malady was a wad of bubble-gum, which was intended to equalize the unbalanced pressures between my ear and Eustachian tube. I've applied myself so steadfastly to this cure that I can now down my hourly pills without so much as breaking rhythm in my chewing. Lucky my children can't see me chomping away; they'd probably think I should stay after school.

One of the most exciting signs of progress is that I'm beginning to have some sensation in my legs. Now that I'm becoming convinced they are really mine, I have stopped requesting that the nurses return them to their proper owner. I can't move them yet, but expect that with the proper concentration I should be able to waggle my toes in a week or two... You'll be interested to hear that Daddy has thoughtfully arranged that I go to General (so I can be near the Union Boat Club). Dr. Burns hasn't been at all cooperative about my getting exercise. When I requested that a jungle-gym be installed over my bed so I could do chin-ups and pull-ups to restore the bod-beautiful, he merely suggested that knitting would be a more appropriate occupation and hurried on to his next patient. Realizing that planning ahead can solve many problems, I have my scheme all worked out for Boston: whenever you and Dad plan to play squash, come to the hospital to see me first, then you take my place in bed and I'll go play squash with Daddy. See you at the hospital...

January 20, 1966

Dear Daddy:

The last few days have been particularly exciting. Tuesday morning they wheeled my bed down to the operating room.
I was pleased to be getting my cast at last but had no idea it would so closely resemble a corset. They began by wrapping me in felt, pulling it tighter and tighter, despite my protests that I needed room to get my figure back. They assured me there would be room for my tummy to expand but I couldn't convince them that this was not the only area where I intended to do some growing.

During my badinage with the nurses I noticed a mild-looking young man leaning in the corner and laughing at our conversation. My glances toward him changed from coy to alarmed when he wheeled over a tall pole from which dangled a jar of fluid and a long tube terminating in a menacing looking needle. In confirmation of my fears, it took the anesthetist three jabs before he could find a vein. I was about to protest loudly when, without so much as a goodbye, the doctor, two nurses, and the anesthetist all disappeared.

The next thing I knew Mummy was saying, "How do you feel, hon?" I probably shouldn't tell you this, but she must have been drinking because she was so blurry I could hardly see her, and her vision was so confused, the room looked spinny even to me. I was about to chastise her for her moral lassitude when the doctor came in. I began to have doubts about him, too, when he walked up to my bed and cheerfully thumped me on the chest. I should have realized that the hollow thump my chest gave in response wasn't my heart, but I still reacted with modest defensiveness when he swept back the covers to my waist. To my amazement, there before my eyes rose a much larger bust than I ever expected to see attached to this body. As my delighted eyes began to focus more clearly on this unexpected development, I noted that it was white, nubbly, crisscrossed with tape and all in all not the texture you'd find in a Reubens painting.

"Is it comfortable?" Dr. Burns asked, drumming thoughtfully on my chest.

I was forced to admit I suspected his creation was designed solely as a punishment for all my flippancies of the past few weeks. I had expected rough spots in the plaster, but not sandpaper, bottle caps, and old coat hangers.

As a reward for not resorting to physical violence to defend myself, I was placed in a wheelchair for the first time and taken on a Cook's Tour of the hospital. Everything looked a little blurry because I had been in a supine position for so long, but I was as thrilled as if I were seeing the whole world for the first time.

General Hospital
Thursday, January 27, 1966

Dear Favorite Principal:

Whatever you do, don't write and tell me about California weather! Snow is not confined to Arizona — the drifts were six feet high when we arrived in Boston. I tried to fill my thoughts of California with billowing smog, but the warm sun and crisp air of February insist on coloring my memories.

Although the trip to Boston was cold and wintry, I enjoyed every minute of it. The air was fresh and without a trace of ether, rubbing alcohol or antiseptic. Instead of four walls there were mountains, lakes, clouds, and whole cities in miniature to see from my Pullman-type berth on the plane. When the stewardess suggested that I might close my curtains for privacy as the other passengers were boarding, I insisted that it would be a pleasure to see people who weren't dressed in hospital garb.

No one tapped me on the shoulder every hour and said, "Pill time!" Best of all, I had a nice big tenderloin steak for dinner.

We arrived in Boston about 10:30 p.m.; I was wheeled all over the hospital before they finally found a bed for me. The details of my first night are too grim to be recounted, but now that I'm established in the rehabilitation ward, I feel as comfortable and at home as anyone could be in a hospital.

My therapist has just come to put my body through some paces, so I must close. It's nice to be rehabilitating instead of just recuperating. I feel as if I've started a whole new chapter of my life. I can't wait for the next chapter, which should be one of returning to normal life. Love to everyone...

Dear Nanci

*by pam herbert**

Sept. 1983 — July, 1984

Dear Nanci,

There are so many things I want to share with you. I don't know
where to start. I hope you won't mind too much, me running on
about the things I have experienced in my life, but I have never really
had anyone I could talk to. When I got your letter, I thought to
myself, maybe I can do somebody some good. I want to tell you about
my family.

My daddy is a bread man; he works for Rainbow Bread. He's
been in the bread business for about 33 years. He is about 6' tall,
overweight, has arthritis in his knees and off and on he's had
problems with his heart. He's 57 years old. He's been great to us
kids all along the way, through bad times and good times.

My mom is a housewife; always has been and probably always
will be. She babysits for two of her grandsons and three other kids.
She also does quilting for a lot of people. Some people bring their
quilt tops from as far as Texas just to have my mom quilt them. She's
about 5' tall, average weight, 55 years old and has done alot for us
kids. The main thing she does for me and Mark is cook for us and
do our wash. We buy the food and laundry soap, but she does the
rest. My mom is a very special lady, because she's had to live with
three handicapped kids, which has taken a great deal of patience.

My older sister Anne is 34. She's married and has two boys.
James is seven and Troy is four. She got a job at one of the power
companies here in Hays. Her husband's name is Steve. He is part
owner of a furniture store. They have been married almost ten years.

* *Pam typed this letter using her tongue to operate a computer.*

My older brother Michael is 32. He is also married and has two boys; Elmer is four and James is four months. His wife's name is Kay. Michael and Kay have a job working together. They train slow learners to take care of physically handicapped people. Kay is the coordinator of the program. Michael is the actual trainer. The trainees learn to cook, do the laundry, and how to transfer, feed and dress people. Michael and Kay have been doing this program about three years. They seem to enjoy it. Michael and Kay live in Wichita. By the way, Michael also has muscular dystrophy.

My little sister Mish is 21. She has a job at a local department store. Mish is about 6' tall and very pretty. She has her own car and a little black dog called Tish. She likes photography; she bought a movie camera and a VCR (video cassette recorder). She once tried living on her own, but it didn't work out, so she's living at home again.

Now we come to the baby of the family, only he isn't a baby anymore. His name is Francis. He is 19 and a graduate of Hays High School. He, too, has muscular dystrophy, so he had tutors come to the house, but he did go to one or two classes at school. Francis also likes to write, and he is real good at making up stories. He has won quite a few ribbons for creative writing.

Francis is the weakest of the three of us. So when he gets sick, he has a pretty hard time getting over it. He has his good days and his bad days. My mom is about the only one that can get him situated comfortably in his bed or his wheelchair. Francis has a hard time sitting up for long periods, so he spends most of his time in bed. If Francis could stand up he'd be about 6' tall. He is all skin and bones.

As for me, I'm the third oldest in the family. I weigh about 130 pounds; I'm about four feet tall. It's pretty hard to get an accurate measurement on me because both of my knees are permanently bent and my spine is curved, so 4' is an estimate. I wear size two tennis shoes and strong glasses; my hair is dishwater blonde and shoulder length. My hair used to be down to the middle of my back before I was married and now Mark wants it that way again, so I'm letting it grow out. I was born right here in Hays, Kansas on October 27, 1956. I appeared normal at first, but when it came time for me to crawl and sit up and walk, I didn't do it, so that's when Mom and Dad figured out that something was wrong. They had already been through all this stuff with Michael, the doctors, the tests, the hospitals, the braces, the "I don't know what it is" and, of course, the tears. So they weren't going to go through that again with me. I don't remember when I got my first wheelchair, but I do remember sitting on Michael's lap most of the time. I must have been about four years old when I got my chair. I started school when I was about five and the tutor came to my house. I learned pretty quickly how to read and spell. I loved my teacher; she was really great!

When I was seven, I went to a boarding school in Topeka, the Capper Foundation for Crippled Children. Michael had already been there about five years, so he knew the ropes, but for me it was a whole new scary experience. I was always shy, afraid to talk. Michael brought me out of that stage in my life. So now, when I want to say something, I either say it or tell Mark or my aide and they interpret it; but I don't keep quiet anymore. I learned a long time ago that if you want to say something, you have to make up your mind and say it, otherwise people can walk all over you.

Now back to Capper's. It was a school and a boarding home. They were beside each other. At the time, there was only one living unit. Now there are three. We did our regular school work plus we had physical therapy and occupational therapy. We also had scouts (I was a Brownie), dances, and basketball games (one time, the Harlem Globe Trotters even came), and many other activities like that. We got up at six every morning, went to school, came home, ate supper at four thirty, and we little kids had to go to bed at six. Older ones got to stay up til seven. It was a real treat when something special was going on, because we got to stay up later. At the home we had house parents, usually a couple, and aides that would come in at certain times. There was one very special aide named Debbie. She's quite a lady. She is what I call dedicated. I don't say that about too many people, but Debbie is one of them. Whenever I had to go to the bathroom, all I had to do was cross my legs and she'd come running. Debbie was married and had a little boy. She loved kids. She could hardly stand to leave us at night. We were always calling Debbie instead of anybody else. Even the house mother couldn't do much with us.

A few years later, Debbie and her husband became the house parents. Then Debbie got very sick and lost all feeling below the waist, but she could still walk around and do her job. About a year ago, Debbie got bit by a spider on her leg and didn't know it until she saw a terrible rash. She was in the hospital about a month. When she got back, she could walk around the living unit OK, but she had to use a wheelchair to go over to the school, because her doctor said it was too far to walk. She only had to go to the school for conferences held *once a month*. Her boss saw her in the wheelchair and said that it *looked bad* to have a house parent in a wheelchair. He said she should quit. She said, "You'll have to fire me." So, he eventually fired her. Since then, that place has had three sets of house parents. Debbie had been there twenty years. It hurt me deeply to find out she was fired, because I know how much the kids love and need someone who is dedicated like Debbie.

I was there at Cappers only two years. I left because Michael's hip was out of place and needed surgery, and Mom and Dad decided they didn't want me to be alone there, so they brought us both home. When I came home it seemed like I had never been there before. There was a whole new routine that we all had to adjust to, especially my mom. Once again there were three of us to take care of instead of one. Michael and I had a tutor. She taught both of us, one at a time, every day. We didn't like her very much.

About two years after we came home, Mom hurt her back lifting the three of us all the time. It was decided to let Michael and me go to the nursing home. It was called Hillcrest Manor at the time. We were in the same room together, so that made it a little bit easier for me. The people that worked there were very nice. Some of them even became good friends. The administrator would come to see us. He was really sweet to us. He even bought Michael a beer for his eighteenth birthday. He was the best they ever had, even to this day.

There was some kind of law that wouldn't allow me to stay there because of my age. So about a year later I had to move to St. Anthony's Hospital. That was quite an experience for me because I didn't have my brother Michael around to tell them what I wanted. I was totally on my own. Of course my family did come over to see me, but it just wasn't the same thing. I was only about twelve then. I got to meet a lot of interesting people: doctors, nurses, visitors, pink ladies and other patients.

I got to know one of the pink ladies very well. Her name is

Barbara. She's one of the wealthiest people in Hays. Barb always used to come and take me for walks. We would walk to the nursing home where Michael lived. While we were walking we went by a school that I always admired. I told Barb my dream of going to a regular school, so when I was sixteen I got to go to that school. We did all kinds of things together, like painting and going out for ice cream. She's still a very special friend.

From St. Anthony's Hospital, I went to a little town named Lacrosse. I lived in the long term care unit of a hospital. I lived there about one year. While I was there I had a number of interesting experiences.

I had two tutors, one named Lisa, the other named Polly. Lisa was my first teacher. She was really sweet. That summer she took me to a Girl Scout day camp. It was a five day session. Lisa always used to come get me early in the morning and take me back again. We did a lot of neat things — crafts, songs, and cooking. It was really great to be with all those kids.

Polly was also a very good teacher. She and her husband, Tim, did a lot for me. They took me quite a few places. One example of this is when a film crew started filming a movie called "Paper Moon," starring Ryan O'Neal, who I was dearly in love with at the time. Anyway, Tim and Polly knew how much I liked Ryan, so one day they surprised me by talking me to one of the sets nearby. We had to wait about an hour before he came over to the car, but when he did come, it was like a dream. All I could do was stare at the poor guy. I think I said a few things, but mostly I just stared at him. We asked if we could take a picture. He said "OK." I got a really nice color 8 x 10 that I will always treasure.

This happened on October 7, 1972. My birthday was the 27th of October, so I thought, "Hey, this is a really fantastic birthday gift," but I was in for another big surprise. I didn't know it at the time, but Barbara was planning to surprise me with another visit to the set. She came and got me on my birthday. My whole family was there: Mom, Dad, Anne, Michael, Mish and Francis. Anyway, they were shooting when we got there, so we had to wait a little while. Finally, guess who walks out the door, the one and only Ryan O'Neal. He came over to my wheelchair and kissed me right on the cheek, and said, "Happy birthday." Right then I thought I was going to die. But that wasn't all. To top it off, they had their own cook bake a cake with sixteen candles on it. You see, I was "sweet sixteen and had never been kissed". It was quite an exciting day for me.

All the way home all I could do was cry. I think I was in shock. I never dreamed that I would get to see my favorite movie star, but I did, and I will always remember it as long as I live.

There's another day in my life that I will never forget. It was to be a commitment of a lifetime. It was two days after my birthday that I met the man of my dreams.

It was a Sunday, and it was raining a cold October drizzle. Mom and Dad usually visited me on Sundays, but this time they called and said they wouldn't make it. Then, at suppertime, while I was waiting for someone to feed me, guess who walks in the door: my brother Michael and three of his friends.

The friends that brought Michael over to see me were Ward Herbert and his two boys, Mark and Loren. Ward was at that time administrator for the nursing home where Michael was staying. They got to be good friends, so Michael had asked them if they would take him over to see me. Anyway, they all came in the door that night, and all I could do was stare at Mark. He was so good looking. He had long dark hair, greenish brown eyes, and a nice looking body. You see, this was about the first time I had had contact with a guy, other than a few friends, so I was a little nervous, but happy. The one thing I remember most about that night is that Mark fed me a piece of my birthday cake, and this was to mean something five years later, on our wedding day.

The next five years had their ups and downs. I remember Christmas time, 1972. Mark was running around with Michael quite a bit, doing this and that, and I was falling more and more in love with him. I felt like he didn't give a damn about me, until one night I was listening to Donny Osmond singing "Puppy Love" and I was crying. Michael and Mark came in. Michael said, "What's wrong?" so I told him. He said, "Hey, look you two, you're in love with each other, so why not show it?" Mark came over and kissed and hugged me. He said, "I love you Pam." I couldn't believe it, somebody actually loved me, a quad who couldn't do much of anything.

1973 started off great, but gradually got worse. One night Mark and I went over to his house. We were there for a little while and then my daddy came storming in and said, "What the hell are you doing over here?" All I could do was stare at him. Then he said, "I don't ever want you to see my daughter again." By this time I was in tears. He took me back to the nursing home and I cried and cried. I just couldn't believe my daddy could get so mad, but he did.

I will never forget that night as long as I live. The only thing was I never did know why my daddy was so mad. I guess he didn't want his little girl to get hurt. From that night in January until sometime in June I wasn't supposed to see Mark at all, but we would sneak around anyway. We would write letters back and forth, he would write amost everyday and I wrote about once a week. We also talked through my bedroom window. So when I knew Mark was coming over to see Michael, I would have the aides open the window so we could talk. During this time I had two speech teachers that would come twice a week. They were the ones who helped me write my letters to Mark.

In August I started going to school at Marian High. It was a girl's Catholic high school. We had to wear uniforms. They were a pretty blue color. The other girls wore a vest and a skirt with a white blouse, but they let me wear slacks instead of a skirt. I thought it was kind of nice not having to worry about what you are going to wear every day, but most of the girls didn't like wearing uniforms. It didn't bother me because I didn't have that many nice clothes to wear. I met a lot of people, some even became my friends. Most of the girls had their own groups and I never did quite fit in with the crowd. Sometimes it hurt my feelings, but I usually tried not to let it bother me too much. My grades were about a C average. I took as many classes as I could take at Marian, plus I had two tutors to teach me what I couldn't take in school like Math, English, and Government.

My teachers were very good to me. My math teacher's name was Mrs. Barris. Even though she couldn't always understand me, we would get along great. My other teacher's name was Mrs. Ross. She was the main one that helped get all of my credits, so I would be able to graduate with my class and all my friends. I didn't think I would make it in four years, but I did, thanks to Mrs. Ross. She and I became very close, and I will always remember what she did for me.

1973 was coming to an end, and I was falling more and more in love with Mark. I was seeing him almost everyday. He got fired from the nursing home in the spring of '74. The nursing supervisor said that his hands weren't clean enough for them, because he was usually working on cars before he went to work. But I didn't think that was the real reason they fired him. I think they just didn't approve of us going together, of course nobody did.

Earlier that year Kay came into my brother Michael's life. She was a student nurse and was working at the nursing home. Michael started going out with her and fell in love. Michael moved out of the nursing home. Michael and Kay got married. Later that summer, the four of us took a trip to attend my cousin's wedding. We headed home the day after the wedding. We got a little ways out of Topeka and the rear end went out on our car, so we hitched a ride back to Topeka. We called a few people trying to get some money to get back home. Finally, we got a hold of some relatives and asked if we could borrow $100.00 to get an airplane ticket home. They said yes. So off we went in the air with two dogs, two quads, two able bodied people and a whole lot of luggage.

It was Christmas time once again, and I was full of anticipation of officially getting engaged. My Mom and Dad were still a little bit leery of Mark's love for me, and to tell you the truth, I was still a little scared myself, but deep down inside I knew he was the right man for me. Mark took me to his house. They all welcomed me as if I was already part of the family. This made me feel so good. We talked for quite awhile then it was time for the big moment. Opening presents. Mark brought mine over to me and started opening them. Finally, he got to the most important present of the evening, my engagement ring. When he opened that tiny little box and took out the ring and showed it to me, all I could do was cry. He put the ring on my finger and I cried some more. The evening was coming to an end and I said my goodbyes to the family. Mark took me back to the nursing home. Of course, everyone knew what was going on. Most of the aides were happy for me, and a few weren't. I didn't show my Mom right away, I guess I was scared to. I avoided showing her for a couple of weeks. When I did show her, she didn't say much. But despite all this, I was still on Cloud Nine for a very long time.

1977 was the biggest year of my life. Two great events happened. My graduation and my wedding. Graduation night was quite a night for me. Like I said before, I didn't think I would make it in four years, but I did. I actually got all my credits. Finally they started passing the diplomas. They got to my name and everybody started standing up and clapping their hands. It made me feel so good that all I could do was cry and then we started singing. Saying goodbye wasn't easy for me and still isn't. After graduation a lot of people came and brought presents and cards. When I think of that night, it still brings tears to my eyes, even though I was never a part of the crowd, I still feel very much a part of that school.

Well, the big day was getting closer and closer. The biggest day of my life, my wedding day, October 29, 1977. My sister Mish was my bridesmaid and my brother Michael was the best man. My wedding wasn't quite like I wanted, but at least I got married. I couldn't sleep the night before, I was too excited and happy. Anyway, the girls at the nursing home started getting me dressed about 12:00 that day, makeup and everything. They were all very excited and happy. My Mom and Dad came and got me about 3:00 and took me to the church. At 4:00 it was time to walk down the aisle. Mish pushed Michael down the aisle, and both our parents walked us down the aisle. The ceremony was very beautiful, but the guy we hired to sing wasn't the greatest. Finally, the preacher said, ''Pam, do you take this man to be your husband,'' etc. All I could do was sort of squeal out the words, ''I do.''

''I now pronounce you Husband and Wife,'' said the preacher. We turned around and the whole church was jam packed with people. Of course, they were all crying. I was OK until we started down the aisle, then I cried. I just couldn't believe I was married. It was like a dream come true. Anyway, everyone came to congratulate us and I still was crying. I couldn't help it I was so happy. Finally, I calmed down enough to take some pictures. We couldn't afford a professional photographer, so my sister Anne volunteered to take pictures for us. She took about 100 pictures in all. After we were done with that, we had dinner reservations at the Ramada Inn. It was a very good dinner. Every one seemed to have a very good time.

After the dinner we stopped by my parents' house so I could go to the bathroom. But I couldn't go because I was too nervous and uptight to go, so we went on to our wedding dance, which was at the National Guard Armory. We had a polka band play, but I would have rather had a rock and roll band, but as usual couldn't afford it. The band was pretty anyway. A lot of people came and everybody had a very good time. Mark and I danced and he danced with other people too. About midnight, I started getting tired, so I told Mark and we got ready to leave. Earlier that evening Mark's brother-in-law gave us a 20 dollar bill and told us to go get a motel room for the night, so that's exactly what we did.

We went to the Holiday Inn and got a room. The 20 dollars barely covered the room, but Mark told them that we just got married, so they let us have a lower rate. We got to our room and Mark laid me down on the bed because I was so tired from sitting all day. Anyway, I hadn't gone to the bathroom all day so Mark had to catheterize me. I had been having trouble going to the bathroom for many years, so it was nothing new to Mark, he had done it lots of times before.

It was time now for the biggest moment of my life, making love. Of course, I was a little nervous and scared. Mark was very gentle with me. He started undressing me and kissing me. We tried making love in the normal fashion with Mark on top and me on the bottom. Well, that position didn't work at all, so then we tried laying on our sides coming in from behind. This was a little better. Anyway, we went to sleep that night a little discouraged because we didn't have a very good lovemaking session. You would have thought that it would be great, but sometimes things don't always go the way we want them to. We didn't get the hang of making love for about two months. It hurt for a long time. The next day was Sunday and we had to get up early and get ready for church.

After church, we went to my parents' house to open all our wedding presents. We got a lot of nice things, and quite a bit of money. After we were done opening our presents, we went home to our little 10 by 55 foot mobile home. Talk about inaccessibility, try going through a very narrow hallway just to get to your bedroom. Let me tell you, it's hell. Mark had to carry me up and down the hallway three or four times a day. It got to be very tiring. Anyway, Mark took a week off from work so we could get settled in our new home. He had to quit his job as a roofer because they usually stayed out of town all week and that wouldn't have worked for us because there was no one to take care of me while he would be gone. So he got a job as an attendant at a gas station.

It wasn't the greatest job in the world, but at least we had an income. What happened to me while Mark was at work? Well, there was a girl who lived across the alley from us that babysat for kids, so Mark asked her if she would watch me. She said yes. Mark thought it would be great, but it was hell. All she ever cooked for lunch was frozen pizza and canned spaghetti. I wasn't happy at all. I came home crying almost every night. Finally, Mark talked to the administrator at the nursing home to see if I could stay there during the day. He said OK but it would cost five dollars a day. We thought that wouldn't be too bad as long as we stayed caught up with it, but we didn't. We got so far behind that they were going to kick me out until my cousin's Dad came to our rescue and paid the $1200 debt for us. Can you believe someone doing that for us? I still can't.

We did this for about two years. Then, finally, in the fall of 1980 the SRS Office got their act together and started paying for an aide to take care of me in our home. It took them about two years to get all their paperwork done. Can you believe it, two years? Well, my first aide was pretty nice in the beginning, but after a few months she couldn't get along with Mark. He would ask her to do something and she would say, "Oh, I can't do that, that's not my job." At that time, my aides were getting $4.50 an hour, 40 hours a week. I felt if they were going to get that kind of money they should do just about anything that we wanted within reason, of course. She quit. My next aide was a college girl, and we didn't get along at all. She was too picky. My third could barely read and write, so I taught her how. Before she became my aide, she helped me with school. We were neighbors at the time and got to be good friends. We got along great until she got hurt and then things went downhill. We finally had to let her go. Next was Mark's sister. She was already working at the nursing home as an aide, but she needed the money really bad because she was supporting three kids by herself. She stayed with us for about one year. Then she decided to take a medications aide course so she could get a little more pay. We got along great, but after she left our aide situation went downhill. They would come and go like hotcakes for the next five months. Then we thought we had finally found someone who would cooperate with us. We hired a guy and he was very sweet for about the first month, then he got just like all the rest of my aides. He was always getting into it with Mark.

Mark was getting home late from work and he didn't like that because he was too dedicated to school. Anyway, Mark had a change in his work schedule, so he quit. Then an old buddy of mine tried work for about a month. He couldn't handle it, so he quit. Now I have a girl with CP. She is really sweet and we get along great. She can do every thing but get me up and down, so we have another girl to do the lifting. It's working out really good now. I really like my girls. They are doing a really good job for me, and I hope it stays this way a little while. That is how it has been going for four years now and I don't think it's going to get any easier for us because there aren't enough people willing to take care of the handicapped. This is only what I have experienced with aides, maybe you have had better luck, if so, I sure would like to know how you did it.

Between 1977 and 1984, we moved six times for one reason or another. We moved out of the trailer because there were so many roaches in it that I couldn't stand it anymore. One night, I had one crawl across me, I told Mark that's it, we are moving, so we did. Another reason was because it was awful scary in tornado season. It could have blown us up very easily.

We moved to a ground floor apartment. It was very nice. It had two bedrooms. We were only there for four months. The owner sold it. The new owner wanted to remodel the whole apartment building, so that meant that the rent was going to be sky high, so we had to move again. We found another place pretty fast. This time it was a basement apartment. We had to build a very steep ramp. It was in the worst part of town, the flood area. We got flooded out a couple of times while living there, and we lived there for about two years. It also had roaches. The landlord was OK, but he had a heart condition and he was a teacher at the college, so he didn't have much time to fix up the apartment building. Anyway we got pretty fed up with the whole thing and decided it was time to move again, so we started looking for another place to live. We found another ground floor apartment. It was a two car garage turned into an apartment. It was attached to a bigger house. It had two bedrooms, a small kitchen and living room and bathroom. We really liked this apartment but then we decided to apply for a rent subsidy, so we talked to the landlords about it. They said they didn't want anything to do with the government, so they gave us 30 days notice to get out. Here we go again, apartment hunting. We found one pretty fast. It was another basement apartment. We looked at it once before and didn't take it because it didn't have a tub, only a shower. But this time we decided to take it and work out the bath problem later. I would go to my Mom's once a week and take a bath there. Anyway, the apartment was OK. It had two bedrooms, etc. The landlord was a lady, and she was very sweet and cooperative. But the lady who lived upstairs wasn't so nice. Everytime we made the least little sound, she would have fits. That summer, we decided to put out a garden. Everything was growing so good. Then she got all upset about something and ripped up the tomato plants, and they were still growing. We were getting tired of her complaining all the time, so we thought about moving again. Then we met this old lady who lived across the street from us, and she was looking for someone to rent her apartment. We would always go by her house and say hi. She begged us to move in her apartment. We thought about it for awhile and decided anything had to be better than living with a grumpy person, so we moved again.

This time it was a small one bedroom apartment. The lady lived in the big part of the house, and we lived at one end of it. We called her grandma. We got along pretty good, but her son was a different story. They were hard headed as hell. You can't talk to people like that. They won't listen to reason at all. We lived there about a year, then we brought a friend of ours to stay with us for awhile, so he could look for a job. He had long hair and a beard and Grandma was scared he was going to kill her or something. Anyway, her son got all upset because we brought him here. There was a big fight and he said either he leaves or you all leave, so we left.

Now we live in a small two bedroom house. The hallway is so narrow that I can't even get back in the bedrooms, so we have our bed in the living room.

Well, I guess I had better end this letter. Thank you for giving me a chance to be in your book. It really means alot to me.

Like I said before, I hope to meet you someday. I am also hoping to write a book of my own someday. Thank you again, I love you.

A See-By-Logic Life

by naomi woronov

*i*f you ask the experts how people as blind as James Joyce or
James Thurber managed to get through school, they'll tell you it
was by a process of cognitive interpretation and subsequent conceptual integration of environmental stimuli.

I call it the "common-sense-sight" or "see-by-logic" system.

Today, of course, school is much easier for partially-sighted
youngsters because of technological innovations, psychological insights
and even new terminology (e.g., "partially-sighted" for "half-blind").
Nonetheless, common-sense-sight remains the dominant mode of
operation for people like me, and I hope that this account of my own
education will help uncover the mystery of how it works.

Perhaps the first thing to realize is that see-by-logic doesn't always
work.

I was with a friend in New York's Washington Square Park on
a warm, breezy holiday afternoon just before a mayoral election. The
place was mobbed. Election speeches blared from sound trucks and
fused into background noise. A man in a blue shirt stood high above
the crowd of several hundred people milling around and in the large,
dry fountain. He was orating energetically, anxiously turning here and
there that his message might reach all those people — people who
seemed a good deal more interested in gawking at local guitarists than
in listening to him.

I turned to my friend. "I wonder who's that man in the blue shirt
preaching at all these people?"

My friend replied, "He's a blue balloon."

But see-by-logic does work well enough for Joyce and Thurber
and my sister and brother and me and several million people like us
to wend our ways through school (and life) — if only others will let

us do what we can, help us do what we cannot, and make the effort required to distinguish between them.*

For his three "cockeyed" children, it was the luckiest as well as most ironic of coincidences that my father was an optometrist. My parents could in good conscience ignore the opinions of eye doctors and educators who counselled them to send us to schools for the blind, or at least to sight-saving classes. (Remember them?) Furthermore, the notes my father sent to school on his professional stationery undoubtedly carried more weight that they otherwise might, and probably, at least in the early years, saved us much grief.

As far as I can determine, my pre-school sensory adjustment to the physical world was hardly any different from that of any child. I established conceptual relationships with the objects around me as any child does. As a child learns, empirically, that a little hand won't hold a large glass of milk, so I learned, empirically, that if I reached for a glass of milk where it appeared to me to be, I'd knock it over.

Perhaps an illustration of a consciously arranged adjustment in later years will clarify this normally unconscious process.

I was not the best-of-all possible tennis players. Nor was I brilliant at baseball. But I was superb at archery. The target was stationary, and so was I. At the beginning of each session I carefully aimed at that round blur of colors out there, and let fly. I heard the arrow go, but saw nothing. A companion informed me that I had hit the top

---

*"Legal blindness" (in most states and by federal definition for tax purposes) is visual acuity that cannot be corrected to better than 20/200 in both eyes. A person with 20/200 vision receives basically the same impression at 20 feet that a normally-sighted person (20/20) has at 200 feet.

My own vision is 20/200 in the left eye, 20/400 in the right. This disparity in focal ranges, together with an astigmatism (a structural defect that prevents light rays from an object from meeting in a single focal point so that indistinct images are formed) creates what I imagine are blurred images to other people; since my condition is congenital and incorrectable, however, I have only a vague notion of what such words as "sharp" and "blurred" mean to others. As a nystagmus (uncontrollable rapid eye movement) is the only observable aspect of the condition, I appear perfectly normal.

My sister and brother have almost precisely the same condition I have, even to the disparity between left and right eyes. My parents have fine vision as had all of our relatives as far back as anyone can trace. I have five nieces and nephews and a grand-niece and two grandnephews, all of whom have excellent eyesight.

branches of a tree way to the left of my target. Okay. Now I carefully aimed at a farmhouse way to the right of the target. Much better. This time, I was told, I hit halfway between the top of the trees and the top of the target, and just a bit to the left of it.

I believe that this game of narrowing the field was as much fun for my friends as it was for me, though the camp was none too happy about all the lost arrows. We played it until I determined that by aiming at a huge rock nowhere near the vicinity of the target I could consistently hit the bull's eye.

Thus my earliest adjustments to physical phenomenon were as natural as those of any child, and nearly as complete, with the exception of such objects as glasses of water, which are essentially invisible and which, to this day, I knock over on floors and laps. I had trouble, too, with stairs, and was thus a very colorful child, i.e., black and blue. I was not permitted to ride a bike (I was well over thirty when I achieved that feat, and take immense pleasure in it today), but since we lived on the top of a very steep hill I saw nothing strange in that. There was little difference between my activities and those of my playmates. I had little idea of any physical limitations — certainly no one at home breathed a word.

This conceptual reasoning process saw me without major incident through nursery school and kindergarten. In the first grade, I encountered my first vision-related problem.

It was apparently requisite for a first grade teacher to train her pupils to hold reading matter at a "proper" distance. I brought old Dick and Jane within my own focal range, which was not, of course, the "proper" distance. The teacher straightened my arm and admonished me not to move it. So I brought my head down to my hand.

This sort of nonsense went on for several days. I still find it difficult to imagine a teacher so insensitive, but in those days (the 40s) teachers were as ignorant about sight and hearing disabilities as most teachers still are about such problems as dyslexia. So it was a difficult and confusing time for a child too "stubborn" to follow instructions, and already uncomfortable about talking things out at home.

But Mother and Dad realized that something was amiss, and the first of that long line of notes was issued on my father's stationery. After all, they had been through this before: my sister is eleven years older than I, my brother seven years older. Yet not a scrap of information, not a shred of experience (good or bad), not a tinge of support or comfort was ever shared in our household.

I have no doubt that this refusal to admit the existence of a handicap is preferable to over protection, yet how sad it is that we each reinvented our own problem-solving wheel. As we grew older and faced serious constraints and sometimes anguish, it was as impossible to offer one another the aid or empathy that should have flowed naturally as it was for us to discuss sex.

As I moved from grade to grade in elementary school, book print became smaller and I simply brought the books closer to my eyes. Italicized passages began to appear in my texts; I couldn't read them, so I just skipped over them. I sought ways of getting light between my nose and my books. If the print was too difficult to read, I turned it sideways and read letter by letter. I did what I had to do; there was no one to instruct me how to manage better, but there were also no naysayers, no one to tell me what someone with my eyesight was supposed to be unable to do. As an adult, for example, I have been told by social workers and administrators in agencies for the blind that someone with my vision cannot read newspapers. But they don't appreciate the see-by-logic system. I can and do read newspapers.

It's difficult to conjecture what I might or might not have tried to do had I been trained in schools for the blind. I cannot help but think of a college student I know who does very badly with print, but sight-reads Braille beautifully.

I read for about fifteen minutes at a time, then rest my eyes for a like period. I didn't plan this procedure, it *happened* to me through an unconscious process of trial and error (error = headaches). I read very slowly, for the closer a book is held to the eyes, the narrower the field that can be focused on. This precludes the reading of groups of lines, whole lines, or even groups of words, depending on typeface and size and on focal range. This necessarily limits reading speed. On a battery of tests I took when I entered college, I disturbed psychologists by breaking the bottom of the curve on speed and the top of the curve on comprehension. But the issue of speed never concerned me — for that matter never occurred to me — until college, when the amount of required reading multiplied substantially.

When I read aloud to my classes now, I sometimes misread words, though it's hard to say which errors are visual and which Freudian.

I have difficulty distinguishing certain letters, especially vertical ones, which are easily fused or mistaken. But one doesn't normally need to distinguish the letters of her native language. The amount of cognitive interpretation (or see-by-logic) one regularly does in reading becomes apparent only in studying a foreign language. I can't say to what extent this "educated guess" or *gestalt* process accounts for my miserable handwriting or for my abominable spelling — a shocking fault in an English teacher.

Recently I was assigned to observe the class of a junior colleague. I sat in the front row and noticed with a sudden panicky feeling that I could not read the blackboard. Of course I had never been able to read a blackboard, but until the blossoming self-consciousness of my high school years, it rarely crossed my mind that anyone else could.

Most teachers use blackboards to emphasize remarks or to summarize. What is written normally coincides rather closely with what is said. Add to this the teacher's tone as well as the number, length, and "look" of words (e.g., capitals, crossed and dotted letters which you can watch the teacher make even if you cannot see the finished product). With all these data, the human mind is likely to come up with relatively accurate surmises, more accurate the better skilled one becomes at the see-by-logic game. It's something like playing Pac-man a lot.

Furthermore, in grade school at least, I was not at all shy and never hesitated to ask questions. If an exam was written on a blackboard, for example, I would simply walk up to the board and across the room and write down the questions. I had been with most of my classmates for a few years by then; they were involved in their own work. Teachers often caught on quickly and provided me with their own handwritten copies of the tests.

The memory of one grade school exam, however, still stings. My favorite teacher, Patrick Le Patre, taught geography. I had already taken several history and current affairs courses with him, and he was well acquainted with what I could and couldn't see. But geography! The maps hanging around the room were big globs of pretty colors. I could rarely participate in class. I had never been so forcefully aware that other people could see what I could not. At home, in the cell of myself, I poured over book maps with the highest-powered magnifying glass I could find, but to no avail.

I missed the first geography exam. Mr. Le Patre gave me a make-up. He sat me in a room with a blank map and question sheet. When he returned, I was sitting, chin in hand, staring off into space — space which happened to be occupied by a large map of the world. He was furious. He ripped up my paper. What was the matter with me? I had been acting peculiar all semester, and now this! He had trusted me not to cheat; how could I disappoint him? I was too distresed to tell him what I saw on the walls: great colonies of ants crawling around undefined red, orange, blue, green and yellow smears.

When I couldn't get away with playing sick any longer, I returned to a teacher awaiting me with open arms and apologies. It was hard, he explained, for others to remember that someone who looked and functioned just like anyone else couldn't see like everyone else. Why hadn't I said anything? Teachers would certainly try to help me if I asked for help, but I must try to understand and help them too. But I was like a tourist in a foreign capital who needs to pretend he knows the city's surfaces and secrets as well as a native — asking was absolutely last resort.

But push can come to shove. It was graduation year and all the little girls sat in sewing class. Day one: thread the needle. Day two: sew together two tiny pieces of cloth. Day three: begin work on an apron. I was still on day one, trying to explain that if the teacher would only thread the needle for me, I was certain I could sew together two pieces of cloth. I was the only child who graduated in a store-bought dress.

For all that, however, eyesight problems in grade school were few and minor. Classes were relatively small, and almost all teachers found ways of helping me without physically or psychologically isolating me from my classmates. I can recall no incident in which a child taunted me for peering at things or rubbing my nose in a book. (I cannot say the same about adults.) Thus no one and nothing in grade school prepared me to cope with the problems — my own and others' — that I was to encounter in high school. I continued to use the common-sense-sight methods I'd devised, but they no longer covered all contingencies. I adopted my parents' implied attitude: If you can't see it, ignore it.

My elementary education was excellent. I had been taught to read, to write clear English, and to reason mathematically. I even had a sound, fundamental knowledge of French. My first year in high school should have been easy, but Mother, well-meaning no doubt, contrived to make it difficult.

"You already studied French," she told me. "Why waste time in beginning classes?" So I was tested and placed in French IV. I was a freshman amongst juniors and seniors. My methods of deciphering blackboard writing in classes conducted in English did not work here, for my French-thinking mind did not compute fast enough to make logical assumptions. And I was now a teenager, too self-conscious to ask a lot of obvious questions and prance about the classroom and up to the board. I squeaked through the exam on previously-acquired knowledge, but French V had more students and a teacher who chattered away at a furious pace, whitewashing blackboards all around the room as she did so. I failed. Havoc at home.

I tried to explain, but was accused of fabricating visual excuses to cover an unwillingness to study. That had just enough grains of truth in it to make me feel guilty. After many stormy scenes, we compromised on a tutor. As a result of the feelings that flowed during this fight, however, I never again admitted in my house to having trouble seeing anything, and I was unwilling to seek help from anyone in school lest my parents learn of it. Minor vision-related problems swelled into traumatic experiences. Every moment in the library, for example, was excruciating: I could rarely copy call numbers accurately, and was humiliated by the consequent confusion; I could not read a book title above nose level, and was embarassed at having to take down one book after another to find what I needed; I often could not manage without a magnifying glass, and was mortified as other youngsters tried not to notice. But God forbid I should ask for help!

And then there was geometry class. I had done exceptionally well in algebra. The teacher, seeing me with my nose pressed against my book concluded that I had trouble seeing and asked how she could help me with blackboard and other work. Math was fun. Then came geometry, and Miss Begrunt.

Miss Begrunt insisted on maintaining alphabetical seating order. "Woronov" didn't show up in the front row. I explained that I could see neither the board nor her from where I sat, and she, in turn, explained that if I was too vain to wear glasses I would simply have to suffer. All semester she called on me in class, asked me to rise, state my name, and determine the area of "this" trapezoid or the volume of "that" sphere. Each time I asked its dimensions, and each time she replied that "vanity is stupidity." I wasn't an entirely satisfactory victim: since I couldn't really see her, I could stare her down.

I somehow managed to scrape through the finals. I suppose I had absorbed something from the text, that I was too afraid of my parents to fail, that it was a great way of getting even.

The rest of my high school career followed the same pattern: reasonable and unreasonable, sympathetic and apathetic teachers, courses such as biology in which I would have done better had I been able to see more, and courses such as chemistry which I might or might not have mastered.

But if it was a difficult and lonely time for me, it was a worse period for my brother Marvin who had recently graduated from college. If I was embarrassed on dates because I was so clumsy, had to sit near the front row at the movies, and felt a social outcast because thought a snob — I would pass friends only a few feet away and not recognize them — and if I struggled alone through all the vicissitudes of a half-blind female adolescence, it was in many ways also difficult for a boy.

Marvin had been in college during the war, and continually had to explain why he wasn't in the Army. He was a male who could not drive. And what about a career? The purpose of my education was to get me culturally gussied up for sale to a proper marriage partner. (My sister was already married to a doctor.) But a boy had to have a proper middle-class career. Sitting at the top of the stairs in our house one night, I listened as my parents told my brother that he was too blind to do anything but go into their business.

I had never before heard that word uttered in our household. I was staggered: Mother and Dad simultaneously and firmly embraced both horns: (a) there is absolutely no problem, and (b) there is a severe handicap. I myself have bled on those two points ever since, for even in writing this article for this anthology I have asked myself (a) if I have the right to contribute at all (I am not, afer all, "disabled"), and (b) if I have glossed over the physical, psychological, educational, financial and social difficulties which did then and now confront a partially sighted person — me.

Today I see it this way: My parents were unconsciously angry with us for making their lives difficult, for were they not constantly explaining to friends, neighbors, teachers and even strangers that we were "incorrectably nearsighted," that they had not neglected to take us to eye doctors or to buy us glasses? They must have felt guilty, for had they not produced not one, not two, but three half-blind children? They were ignorant, believing that any mention of or attempt to help us with problems was mollycoddling, which would make us soft, dependent.

They were also superstitious. Theirs was a world of knocking on wood and throwing salt over shoulders. Thus there had never been and could never be the slightest expression of admiration for what any of us had achieved without a lot of assistance. Harriette had a B.A. in psychology. Marvin had one in business. I had published many articles in the high school paper, was vice-president of the New York City High School Press Council and liaison between that group and the High School UNESCO Council. But to compliment any of us was to call down the wrath of their strange and mighty libra God who, hearing of success, would surely balance the scales with some great misery.

The other side of "no compliments" is "no complaints." If I expressed so much as annoyance over some physical or emotional matter, Mother would tell me the story of the man who complained so bitterly that he had no shoes, until he saw a man with no feet. Frankly, that concept never made my feet any warmer.

By the middle of my third year in high school, I was flunking chemistry, floundering in French — again — and doing poorly in subjects I'd previously enjoyed. Arguing that I was bored and unchallenged, my parents asked the school authorities to give me the appropriate four-year Regents exams and let me graduate. They refused. To my great relief, I was shipped off to a boarding school, thus skirting all the failures I had anticipated in June. This was a school for girls who couldn't make it elsewhere academically, so by default, as it were, I got superb grades and graduated in August after three years of high school. In September, at the age of sixteen, I went off to Syracuse University where, ironically, the defenses that prevented me from requesting needed help also insulated me against most of the well-meaning naysayers.

The first of these was Dr. Joy. Student Health, apparently unimpressed with my father's and doctors' reports, sent me to a local optholmologist. Dr. Joy scrutinized my eyes with every testing device known to science — or at least to him — for three solid hours. He was a nice old man, a sympathetic soul. I felt sorry for him as he advised me to pack my bags and go home because no one with my eyesight could make it through college.

How many professors and doctors have since assured me that I could not make it through a bachelor's degree, a master's degree, a doctoral degree or as an English teacher. When applying to graduate school I was told by certain department chairmen (and they were all men, then) that their programs were second only to Harvard — how dare I think could compete? Another brief trauma was created by a nervous neurologist I visited years later in graduate school because I had migraines. He lectured me at length on how to deal with the fact that no man would ever want to marry me.

"Why?" I whispered, thinking of my mother's perpetual warning that nobody loves a fat girl.

"Why, because of your handicap," he answered, as though it was the most obvious thing in the world.

I was genuinely mystified, for I had never thought of myself as having a "handicap."

But in many ways, except for the proliferation of reading requirements, college was easier than high school. I sat where I would, asked questions at will and found the old see-by-logic system adequate for blackboard work — except, of course, in French, which I had guaranteed my mother I would take.

I had a one-year science requirement. Remembering Thurber's experience in biology lab, I chose geology, the only non-microscope science. And, indeed, there was no microscope work; instead you had to scratch at little rocks and read topographic maps. My "D" in geology must have been a gift, for the Dean of Students called me in before the end of the semester.

"Taking geology, are you?"

"Yes, sir."

"Not doing well, are you?"

"No, sir."

"Don't see too well, do you?"

"No, sir."

"Well, finish up the term and we'll waive the rest of your science requirement."

"Thank you, sir."

Syracuse had some fifteen thousand students at the time. I was and am still astonished that the Dean of Students bothered to seek me out on such a matter.

I avoided courses known to be book heavy. What I did read, I read as was my custom, completely and thoroughly, about a quarter of the work in most courses. For some reason the idea of skimming books, even for research papers, never occurred to me. I think I thought it was cheating. I passed many an exam on books I hadn't read by studying the tables of contents and indexes, and by skillfuly synthesizing the little information I did have into coherent English.

I had chosen Syracuse University because of its journalism school, and I was deeply disappointed when I was rejected on the grounds that I didn't have enough eyesight to get through such required courses as Printing I and Printing II. It seemed silly to me even then. Today I'm convinced that the rejection had a great deal more to do with my sex than with my vision.

I wandered in and out of radio-TV, speech and drama departments. I worked as a waitress in an off-campus restaurant (talk about jobs that someone like me really *shouldn't* do), and wandered through various groups of people. When I finally settled down I found myself in the English Department, and among people who did a lot of painting and sculpting, composing and writing, a lot of talking and a lot of reading. I had read very little, but I had a passion for language, and now I began to develop a complementary passion for ideas. Every book now sent my mind reeling, and led to dozens of others equally important and exciting. I was hooked, and I grew increasingly frustrated at my visual limitations. Oh, the urge to kill when my roommate came back from the library to yawn that she had read *only* 150 pages today.

I began to read for longer periods of time and then to develop such severe headaches I couldn't read for days. My class notes were interspersed with the word "headache" etched in endless varieties of print and script. The school doctor suggested the headaches were psychological, and as I had never seriously taxed my vision (or mind) before, I had no way of distinguishing eye strain from mind strain.

I made Dean's List in my last four semesters. By then I was deeply immersed in other people's theories of literature, and was beginning to develop some of my own. I *had* to go to graduate school. But the headaches increased in number and intensity; how could I possibly manage the reading? I wondered, somewhat vaguely at first, how blind people get through school. It finally came to me: Braille, of course. I, who had so long ignored what I could not see, took myself to the Special Education Center at the University and expressed a desire to learn Braille.

"Why Braille?" the counselor asked. If I were legally blind, I could have a talking book machine which would serve my purposes much better than Braille. Me? Legally blind? I was twenty years old, had been through three and a half years of college. I was incorrectably near-sighted. I couldn't possibly be *legally blind*.

But I was. I reasoned with myself that I could see no less today than I saw yesterday because it had a name attached to it. This was an intellectually convincing argument; emotionally, it didn't suffice. The idea frightened me, the words horrified me.

I didn't write to my parents until I had confirmation of a full-tuition scholarship to graduate school from the New York State Commission for the Blind, and had been accepted by the University of Chicago. As casually as I could, I wrote home about my discovery, my scholarship and my plans. By return mail I got a frantic letter: "Don't tell anybody. If you don't tell anybody, no one will ever know." No one, of course, referred to eligible men. I spent the next two years imperiling my graduate and teaching careers (and social life) by slipping my newly acquired label into the tiniest pinhole in any conversation.

I went off to Chicago with enough funds to cover tuition, fees, books and supplies, and six dollars a week living expenses. I had to find jobs which required little or no eyesight to supplement my income, and I was no better equipped to deal with my reading problem than I had been the day I decided to learn Braille, for I had been given a tape recorder instead of a talking book machine, and offered no guidance on what use to make of it in my studies. Naturally, I didn't ask.*

*Talking book machines play recorded books at very slow speeds; a 400-page book comes on 16-18 sides of eight feather-weight disks or four, four-track cassettes — but it takes 18 hours to listen to it. The Library of Congress produces hundreds each year, and provides them free to all legally blind, and now all homebound, persons. Since I learned about this service, years after I left Chicago, I have listened to many dozens of excellent novels, stories and non-ficton works I would never otherwise have had access to.

I did get my M.A. at Chicago and I did become a teacher. But I never did get a job where my credentials arrived before I did, for my scholarship from the Commission for the Blind became a stigma and, unbeknownst to me, one of my professors wrote a "recommendation" stating that I was a sweet, bright young thing, but too blind to be a teacher. So I got the jobs that had been vacated in late September, and had been an effective classroom teacher for months before my dossier arrived. Today, I would file suits against the people who refused to hire me or tried to fire me on the grounds my eyesight constituted an insurance risk for them, but in the late 60s, few of us knew about legal recourse, and the laws were worse anyway.

Like so many of us trained as literature teachers, I ended up teaching freshmen composition — take what you can where you can get it. Grading papers was, quite literally, a pain for me, but I managed by spreading the work out over many more hours than other teachers might. Since the New York City budget cuts of the mid-70s, however, the student load has become so overwhelming that I now share my salary with someone who helps me plow through the papers.

But while the education system crumbles, science advances; new glasses invented by the Retina Institute in Boston have lengthened my reading time, improved my ability to distinguish letters instead of "guess" reading, and reduced my headaches. I now have about three hours a day of reading time; but if I try to use too much of it at one sitting or to push beyond that limit, I can and do put myself out of commission for two or three days.

In the classroom there is no problem. It takes students about a week to get used to this nut with her nose in the book — a student recently suggested I am the only teacher in the school who knows what paper smells like.

But in the "real" world are real problems. The supermarket: there I am trying to decipher the blood-blurred price on a raw rump roast when the store manager approaches: "Lady," he says, "don't eat the meat here. Take it home and cook it first."

Or I find myself explaining to the nice policeman that I thought I was hailing a taxicab.

And then there's the business of distinguishing between the ladies' and the mens' rooms.

I mean to make neither light nor heavy of all this. Yes, we are lucky to have feet, but there's no reason those feet have to be so damn cold. My experience says that parents and educators need to carefully assess each child's strengths and weaknesses, and to understand that:

• aid in the conscious development of methods of confronting or skirting a handicap does not promote dependence, but rather more fruitful, creative independence;

• praise is essential to feelings of strength and worth as is encouragement not to brag, but to take pleasure in accomplishment in the context of limitation;

• a correlative to learning to do for oneself is learning to ask for help when needed, and to do so without shame;

• the need for children *and* parents to talk is crucial, to share information, techniques, ideas, experiences, and to express pleasure. pain, joy and anger, comfort and fear, satisfaction and frustration and even (gasp!) to admit to sometimes feeling sorry for yourself.

It hasn't been and isn't and won't be easy for the likes of me, and I am frankly proud of how well I've done. But it should and could have been easier and better; the time and energy wasted on doubt, confusion and anguish were neither useful nor necessary. This, I hope, is the lesson of my upbringing and my education, of the story of a see-by-logic life.

4.

Invisible and
On Center Stage
— Who Do We Think
We Are, Anyway? —

We are each made up of a myriad of identities forged through our interactions with other people. Disabled women experience a lack of role models, especially positive ones through which to form our own identities. We are apt to be invisible to others or seen only as our disabilities.

We develop strategies for maintaining positive self concepts when vital parts of our selves are unacceptable to those around us. Withdrawal, passing and disclosing our identities are all ways we work to be ourselves and be O.K. with ourselves. Sometimes it is safer to withdraw from interaction with others than disclose our vulnerabilities to a hostile audience. At other times we may choose to interact, but pass ourselves off as able-bodied. Those of us with invisible disabilities can do this to the extreme, whereas visibly disabled women may have no choice about sharing some aspects of our disabilities. On rare and special occasions we feel safe and are totally open and sharing about our issues.

We may bounce back and forth among these ways of presenting ourselves. There are costs and rewards involved in using each. Withdrawal, while protecting us from negativity also insulates us from all that is positive and life sustaining in relating to other people. In a vacuum, we may feel very alone and isolated and may never come to know who we really are. We may internalize negative attitudes about ourselves and feel ashamed and embarassed about being disabled. Passing as able-bodied may allow us to avoid being seen as only our disabilities, and feel, if for only a short time "normal", a part of a world designed for the able-bodied. But the risks are heavy. We may come to dislike ourselves for being less than honest about who we are. We may endanger our physical health rather than admit we need the cooperation of others to meet our disability needs. By acting as if we have no needs, we may perpetuate a ''super-crip'' image — disabled people can do anything we want if we only try hard enough. We may exhaust ourselves trying and come to believe that we are better than other disabled people who have not accomplished as much. This can separate us from a very important resource in developing whole self concepts, other disabled women. As disabled women, we may also fit the social expectation for disabled women by appearing dependent, compliant and pitiful.

Sharing our disabilities with others makes it clear where we can and where we cannot get the support we need. Some people refuse to discuss our disabilities, or blame us for our condition. They have a hard time believing we are really disabled. We can choose to associate with people who acknowledge and accept all of who we are. Through this process, we begin to incorporate our disabilities into realistic and positive conceptions of ourselves. Holding onto our positive self images is a more difficult task if we are also old, lesbian, or women of color. Each of these identities needs nourishment to grow.

Our bodies and our abilities are an integral part of our identities. We need visible, available role models of other disabled women who can share with us realistic pictures of their lives. We need a shift in societal values, so that these genuine pictures are allowed to be seen instead of only images that offer false reassurance to able-bodied and disabled people alike. Our disabilities need not dominate our lives and identities if the individual differences of all people are valued and accommodated.

Like the Hully-Gully But Not So Slow

by anne finger

they have this rule here at the library that we innocent young things under the age of sixteen aren't allowed in the Adult Room. I guess they're afraid we'll pick up a copy of *Lolita* or *The Carpetbaggers* and see something raunchy and our minds will be permanently warped. So if you want to read something besides *Sue Barton at Nursing School, Beanie Goes to College,* or *The Wonderful World of Electricity* — the books that they have in the Young Adult section — then you've got to fill out this Book Request Slip for the librarian and she goes and fetches whatever it is you want. That way, there's no chance that your eyes will alight on anything forbidden.

I pass my slip to the librarian.

"Aren't you old enough to — "

"I'm eleven."

"Eleven?" she asks. She gives me a cool long once-over, down and then up, with her gaze finally coming to rest on my breasts.

I hunch my shoulders, suck in my chest. "Eleven," I say, in a digusted tone of voice, to show her that I don't like it one bit better than she does. People are always acting like it's my *fault,* for Christ's sake. "Precocious puberty," that's what the doctor said. "Nothing to be alarmed about." Easy for him to say: he wasn't five feet tall at the age of eight; sprouting breasts and hair in strange places. Bleeding. "Too bad you're not a dairy cow." That's what my father said. "You'd be worth something then." He's a stupid bastard, which is not just my individual opinion. It happens to be a fact. F-A-C-T. Ask anyone.

The librarian returns with her arms full of books. "Do you really think you're going to be able to understand these?"

I shove my library card across the counter; give her one of my well-practiced glares.

She offers me a smile as a peace token, asks: "How did you break your leg?"

I lean slightly across the counter. "I was born this way," I hiss.

My parents' house is really pretty classy. It's this big old Victorian job, three stories, twelve rooms. The only reason we can afford it is that it's on the wrong side of Hope Street — *i.e.,* too close to where the Negroes live. I mean, I really can't believe that grown adults would not want to buy a house because Negroes live two blocks away, but that's the way the way the world is. I'm not complaining. We've got this nice house because of it.

Guess I'm the first one home: the mail is still lying on the floor under the mail slot. I dump my bookbag and crutches in the corner of the hall, go back and pick it up. There's a letter from some guy named Dr. Fishbein — I don't know who the hell he is, just that my father's always getting bills from him. Yesterday's *New York Times, The Proceedings of the American Academy of Philology* — my parents' dull stuff. They have such boring lives — sometimes I don't know how they manage to stay awake through them.

I go up the backstairs, which were made for the servants to use. My mother's old green bookbag from college is slung over my shoulder: it slops from side to side banging against my crutches as I climb the stairs. My room's on the third floor, in the front of the house. It's kind of a lookout — I can keep an eye on who's coming and going. Usually, I'm looking out the window around six o'clock when my father comes home from work. I try to figure out from the way he pulls his VW into the driveway what kind of mood he's in. Sometimes he's furious, racing headlong for the end of the drive and you think he's not going to stop, just keep going, smash into the chain link fence that separates our property from the Patinsky's and keep hurtling on — and then, at the last second, he slams on the brakes and the car lurches to a halt. Other days, it's a sad, slow creep.

God, I hate these braces. I have to get up fifteen minutes earlier than everybody else and start strapping and buckling myself into them. I'm supposed to leave them on until I go to bed at night, but forget it.

I sit down at my desk; stack my library books next to me. People

are always asking me: "What kind of scientist are you going to be?"
I shrug my shoulders and say, "I don't know." But the truth of it is
that I don't want to limit myself to just one thing — I want to know
everything there is to know. Everything about astronomy, zoology,
electrical engineering, chemistry — organic and inorganic,
microbiology. Everything.

Even when I can't understand all the books I read, I love the
sounds of the words: quantum, lambda, muon, strangeness is not conserved, klystron, well-collimated beam.

"Do you believe it?"

"I would never... "

"I'd just want to *di-ie* if... "

Giggle, giggle, giggle. That's my sister, Suzanne, and her best
friend, Doreen. That's D as in dopey, O as in obnoxious, R as in ran-
cid, E as in — never mind.

Suzanne is my older sister. She's fourteen. Frankly, I've known
two-year-olds who were more mature. She and Doreen are probably
going to spend the afternoon practicing their giggles. Or maybe they'll
discuss eyebrow plucking. Talk about whether they'd rather have an
XKE or a Sting Ray. Did you hear about the new French teacher?
I think Howie Abott's a creep.

"Listen," Suzanne is saying as they go into her bedroom and
shut the door, "Did you know she made out with... "

"Euuuuuuhhh," Doreen says. "Gross me out."

"Turn up the radio a little bit, would you? I don't want my stupid
sister," she's practically shouting, "EAVESDROPPING."

Doreen starts fiddling with the radio dial, "Coming at you live
from Providence, Rhode... " a bleep of sound, another bleep, "WJ...
kind of like the monkey, kind of like the fish... "

"I love this song."

"*Pretend you're in the water and* — I was just so pissed off at her, she's
such an — *like the hully-gully but not so slow...* "

My door yanks open: "Would you fucking stop listening?"

"I'm not — "

"Sure. You're just sitting there. With your ear practically to the
wall."

"I'm *thinking.*"

"What are you *thinking* about?"

"The human condition," I say.

"The human condition," Suzanne snorts. "God. You're such an asshole. I wish you weren't my sister. I was sitting in algebra class during fourth period and you walked down the hall. Everyone heard you. Clunk. Squeak. Clunk. Squeak. Why don't you ever oil yourself?" and she slams the door shut.

Screw you. Just for that, I'm not ever going to oil my crutches again. I'm going to let them get so bad that the whole school will be able to hear me coming when I walk down the empty hallways; I'll creak and the walls will echo back, "Creak; CREAK."

I pull my notebook out from under my pillow, cross off "1758;" next to it I write, "1757." Only those thousand seven hundred and fifty-seven days of this crap left. Then I will be sixteen years old. Sixteen. I will walk into the principal's office and say: "Mr. Dolan. I am withdrawing from school." "Excuse me?" He'll think he heard wrong. "Today's my sixteenth birthday. I am withdrawing from school. Quitting."

Then I'll go to Paris — free myself from the straitjacket of this provincial town. Like Madame Curie, I'll go to the Sorbonne, starve in an attic, live on black bread and tea. I will waste. I suck in my cheeks, anchoring them between my teeth, to get an idea of how I will feel when my dedication to science has burned away all but my flesh. I have $143 — babysitting money — saved up now. At the current rate of exchange, that is 623 French francs.

"Dinner!" my mother hollers up the stairs. "Re-bec-ca! Suzanne! Ka-ate! Jim-my! Din-ner!"

Our dining room furniture is old, made of mahogany, hand-carved. My parents got it second-hand from this crackpot professor emeritus, or however the hell you pronounce it, who was about to be carted off to a nursing home for doddering intellectuals.

My father sits at the head of the table in a chair with arms that are carved into great curlicues, ending in the heads of animals — dogs, maybe; or lions — with teeth bared. My mother sits at the foot of the table. Her chair has arms too, but plain ones.

I sit between my mother and Rebecca. A place of great safety: flanked on my left side by my mother's gentleness, on the right by Rebecca's coldness.

My father stands, the carving knife in one hand, the sharpening steel in the other. With a long clean motion he slices the knife against the sharpener. We are all studying his face, watching for a sign of his mood.

He sets a slice of beef on the first plate, passes it to Rebecca, who passes it to me. I hand it to my mother. She dollops instant mashed potatoes and canned peas onto it and returns it to me.

"Well," my mother says when we have all been served; we bend over our plates. But my father is sitting, hands folded in front of him on the table, not eating.

"Josh?" my mother ventures.

"I taught the most fascinating class today. Sometimes I think, gee whiz, Josh, you sure are a boring old windbag. Do you ever have those days? When you look out at your students and they're sitting there with chins resting in their hands, two kids in the back row are playing footsie, and you think, 'What the hell am I doing here?' You ever have those days?"

"Sometimes," my mother says hesitantly.

He stands up. "Today," he says, holding his open hands, slightly cupped, in front of him, "Today I taught the most marvelous class." He brings his fingers to his thumbs, a gesture of appreciation. "Different theories on the nature and creation of the universe. This is fascinating," he says, and we obediently all set our knives and forks down on our plates and turn our heads towards him. He is leaning across the table now, hands clutching the edge, eyes glistening. "There are two main theories, Steady State and Big Bang. Steady State posits that the universe has always existed in its present form and always will. Big Bang says that the universe was created about eighteen billion years ago... primordial fireball... of course, the universe is expanding..."

He sketches out our possible futures: a steady universe in which the stars and galaxies drift slowly apart, growing colder and colder, floating away from each other into the nothingness of space. I don't like that idea much. Or a universe expanding until like a rubber band it snaps back, atoms imploding, worlds destroyed.

"Some say the world will end in fire," my mother quotes, "some say — "

The telephone rings.

And rings again. Each burr lashes across the room like lightening.

"I don't want to hear that goddamn telephone," he shouts.

Suzanne pushes back her chair and dashes for it. "Fine," she whispers. "Listen, I can't talk to you now. You know. My father."

I squish my peas into my mashed potatoes with my fork. The green oozes into the white: squish. I sneak a glance at my father. His eyes are on Suzanne, cold and fierce.

"Hang that goddamn thing up!" he shouts.

"There he goes," Suzanne whispers.

"Hang it up!" His hands are shaking. "Sit down." His upper lip is pointed, like the beak of a hawk.

"I don't want to hear that telephone ring one more time tonight."

"Mommy," Suzanne pleads as she takes her seat.

"Shut up," he says.

In the back of the *New York Times Magazine* every Sunday there's an advertisement that says, "Your Thoughts Have Wings." Underneath, there is a drawing of a man with a mystical look on his face and winged orbs flying from his head: his thoughts with wings. Underneath it explains how, through studious concentration, you can beam your thoughts into the minds of others. (There's a coupon underneath which you can mail to the Rosicrucians, who will send you more information. But of course, I don't dare... suppose I didn't get to the mail first.)

I am sending a thought throughout the city of Providence: "Don't call Suzanne tonight. Don't call her. She'll get in trouble with her father. Don't call." I send my winged orb flying down Lancaster Street: it makes a left turn onto Hope Street, floats up Doyle Avenue, slowly oozing its way out over the whole East Side: a fog of "Don't call. Don't call Suzanne Evans. Don't call."

I don't have to worry about the phone ringing and it being for me — the last time anybody called me was three weeks ago. It was Charlotte Rodriguez, who sits next to me in homeroom. She said, "We just got a telephone. I'm calling everybody I know."

"Oh," I said.

"So how you doing?"

"Pretty good," I said. I moved my jaw up and down as if I were chewing a piece of gum. These were the things I was supposed to do: chew gum, talk on the telephone. "Pretty good," I said again.

"Yeah?"

"Yeah. How about you?"

"All right."

"That's good." I tried to make my voice sound drawn out and tough, like Suzanne's.

A door slammed shut on her end. "That's my father," Charlotte said. "He just got off work."

"Oh." Then: "My father's still at work."

"Oh."

"So — uh — how's school?"

"It sucks," Charlotte said.

"Really?"

"Sucks." There was the very faint sound of static on the line. "Listen," she said, "I better get going. My father doesn't like me talking on the phone too much."

The telephone rings again. My thoughts have not been traveling quickly enough: I am making them fly now, not just floating them gently through the air. Quick, quick, hang up the phone, hang it up, just — whoever you are, just —

My father strides to the telephone. "Suzanne is eating her dinner," he shouts and slams the receiver down into its cradle.

"What was that?" Suzanne asks.

"One of your punk boyfriends."

"Who?"

"How the hell should I know? You're running around with half the creeps in this town."

"Josh," my mother says.

"Don't you Josh me." He draws his breath in sharp and long, so long I think he will suck all the air out of this room.

"Daddy," Suzanne says, "I'm not running around with — "

"Don't tell me what you're doing. I know what you're doing. I know what you are."

"I'm not."

"I know what you are."

"You're crazy," Suzanne says.

My throat is so tight that my food cannot get down. I lift my napkin to my lips and spit a half-chewed piece of meat into it. "I don't feel — " I say, shoving my napkin under my plate and standing. "May

I be excused... "

I swing myself up the stairs, two at a time. At the top, I hear his footsteps coming after me.

In my room, I scurry under the blankets, pulling them up over my head. The air inside this tent of flannel is musty and good.

"You — " he says. "Look at me." He shuts the door. "You know better than to act that way."

"I didn't feel well. I — "

"Shut up," he says. He sits down on the bed next to me. "Your old man tries. He's not such a bad guy," and his rough hand strokes my face. I shudder away from him.

"Goddamn you," he says. He crouches over me, fixes his hands around my throat.

"No. Let... " I try to say, but my words are lost, unable to pass the grip of his hands. I am falling, swirling downwards although still on the bed. Cannot stop and. In one thousand seven hundred and. Sixteen years. The strangeness is not conserved. In one.

He lets up the pressure for a second. "Mommy!" I scream.

The door opens. She is here. The light from the hallway is bright; I am safe. In one thousand seven hundred and fifty seven days I will be sixteen years old.

"What did you do that for?" he shouts. "This has nothing to do with her."

"Mommy," I cry.

Her arms are folded across her chest. All I can ask is that she rescue me. I cannot ask her for comfort. "Kate," she says. "You shouldn't upset your father... "

Monday morning, I get down to the kitchen before anybody else. My mother's mixing orange juice. Very casually, I ask her: "Who's Doctor Fishbein?"

She doesn't say anything.

"He sends bills to Daddy."

"You know better than to read other people's mail."

I snort. "I knew you weren't supposed to read the *inside*. I didn't know it was a crime to read the outside."

She walks over to the clothes dryer in the corner of the kitchen, picks up a stack of folded clothes, and walks out of the room. I swear to God if my mother ever found out that the Russians were about to drop the Bomb, she'd start putting my father's shorts away in his drawer. Really.

"What're you doing here?" Charlotte says to me when I get to homeroom.

"Huh?"

"Aren't you Jewish?"

"No."

"Ooohh," she says, "I didn't know you were Catholic."

"I'm not."

"What are you?"

"Nothing," I say.

"*Nothing?* You've got to be something."

"We don't go to church," I say.

"But you've got to *be* something."

I shrug.

First period is English class. There are thirty desks in this classroom, in rows six across and five deep. Twenty-nine of them are empty. It's Yom Kippur. I'm in the smart class. All the other smart kids are Jewish.

"Your mother wouldn't let you bunk today, huh?" Mr. Dolan says.

"No, sir."

"You know, if you weren't here I could go down to the teacher's room and smoke a cigarette."

"Oh."

When I get home from school, there's another bill from Dr. Fishbein. And no one else is home — my parents are both at work; Suzanne's out — she's always out; Rebecca's wracking up her extracurricular activities that she can list on her college applications; Jimmy's playing hockey in the muddy vacant lot two blocks away.

I put the kettle on the stove to boil. I learned this trick on *Love of Life* — my favorite of all the soap operas I watched last summer when I was in the hospital.

When it boils, I hold Dr. Fishbein's bill in the jet of steam. My hands turn red and sting from the heat. The paper wrinkles, growing damp. Should I try to pull it open now? Suppose I do and it's not ready, the paper rips? I could always throw it away, in the bottom of the wastebasket. My father would think it had gotten lost in the mail.

Gently, I edge my finger under the flap. It gives way easily, almost miraculously.

I am holding the piece of paper in my hand, unfolding it: "Office visits: October 2, 9, 16, 23, 30 @ $35 $175." I fold the paper up quickly, stick it back in the envelope, press down the flap. I thought it would say what it was for. $175, in one month. Where does he get that much money? Something must be really wrong with him. Maybe a brain tumor, like in *Death Be Not Proud*. Maybe cancer.

I've made a resolution. I've decided to stop being such a klutz and always getting flack from everyone because I'm not clean enough, because I don't smell the right way, because my braces clunk, because I don't have any friends. Not that I'm planning to give up anything — get a Ph.D. in giggling or anything like that — just that I'm going to start being more normal.

So this morning, I went down to the drugstore and bought a copy of *Young Teen* magazine. Suzanne says that the only people who read magazines written for teenagers are the real losers and she would not be "caught dead" — her exact words — reading them. But then, she doesn't need to — she already knows everything you're supposed to do and not supposed to do, and how to dress and have friends.

The first thing I turn to is the Fashion Hints column — I figure I need help in that department. In the Fashion Hints column you write a letter and tell them what your particular fashion problem is and they answer it for you. The first letter is from someone with short legs who wants to know what kind of clothing would be "most flattering." The Fashion Editor tells her that she's in luck — the new empire dresses that flair out from beneath the bustline are just perfect for girls with short legs.

"Dear Fashion Editor," I could write, "my problem is that I wear braces on both my legs and walk with crutches. When I get dressed up nicely, I look like a robot in a party dress. Any fashion suggestions?"

You're in luck. The fashion shows in Paris this year featured the metal look. It hasn't hit these shores yet, but within a year the other girls at school will be dressing themselves up in aluminum foil and carrying purses made of steel girders — and casting jealous eyes at your high-grade aluminum and anodized steel. So just hold on for a little bit more and you'll be right in the swing of things!

Or maybe:

Might we suggest a tent? It's not nearly as uncomfortable as it sounds — you just cut a hole for your head in the top and leave out the stakes and poles. Step inside, zip it up, and all your problems will be discreetly hidden. And don't think that just because you have to wear a tent you'll be stuck in drab browns and khakis — L.L. Bean has a great new line that comes in fashionable reds, yellows, and blues!

I know what I'd really get. True beauty shines from within. Wear a pleasant smile and clothes that are wrinkle free. Avoid loud prints. Take part in a lot of afterschool activities.

And then, I see this announcement: "Just published: *Young Teen*'s informative new booklet, "Facts About Love and Sex for Teens..." I don't need to read anymore: I put my fifty cents in an envelope and send away for it.

The kids are asleep. Dave and Trina (who absolutely won't *allow* you to call them "Mr. & Mrs. Sandersen," perish the thought) have gone out with my parents.

Dave is a pretty sad case, if you ask me. He has this moustache. One time I got here a few minutes early, and as I'm coming up the walk I see him sitting in the living room with this stupid little brush in his hand, combing his moustache. He sees me and dips it into his pocket, real quick. Uh-oh, the babysitter caught me brushing my moustache. Come on.

You really get to know people when you babysit for them. Not that I go snooping in people's drawers or anything like that. I've only done that a couple of times. Dave is a real pseud. He has this copy of *Playboy* magazine sitting on his coffee table. I just know that when people see it there he says, "Oh, I just bought that because I wanted to read the interview with Thelonious Monk." Sure you did, Dave.

Plus, downstairs he has all these books that sound dirty but aren't. He's got this one called *Eros and Civilization* which I thought was going to be pretty hot. I picked it up and got treated to:

At the same time, however, the sexual relations themselves became more closely assimilated with social relations; sexual liberty is harmonized with profitable conformity.

I'm not kidding. The whole book was like that.

But upstairs, Dave has all his real dirty books. Upstairs, where his hot-shot lawyer and architect and doctor friends won't see them. Even then, he never goes out and buys the real honest raunch-o stuff like they have behind the counter at Izzie's. Oh, no. He's got these books that have introductions by some guy with a Ph.D. in psychology that says how this book is full of redeeming social value because it points out how awful it is to be a loose woman. Or else they have the woman do all this wild stuff and then in the last chapter she becomes a nun or a missionary to Africa or something. The only problem with these books is that you never find out what people actually do. You know what I mean. Everyone pants and moans but they never actually describe the whole thing.

Dave and Trina and my folks come rolling in around midnight. Trina's laughing: they must have stopped off at a club — *i.e.,* a bar.

"Stay and have another drink," Trina's saying to my folks. I'm putting on my jacket, hoping that they're not so drunk they'll forget to pay me. My father picks up *Playboy.*

"There's a good article in there about — " Dave says.

"I don't want to read any article," my father says. "I just want to look at the tits."

"Josh," my mother says.

I flop myself down across my bed, pick up my copy of *Young Teen.* Here's an article on how to shop for your new fall fashion wardrobe — I can skip that. The way I shop for my new fall fashion wardrobe is that I go into Suzanne's room and she goes through her closet and says, "I hate this," and throws the offending garment on the bed; "I *never* wear this," and that gets tossed onto the heap. *Voila,* my fall wardrobe.

"Moddess Because... " and underneath there's a picture of this beautiful girl in her prom gown. "Problem Fingernails?" "Invite the whole crowd over for a big autumn bash!" And there's a two-page color spread of all these moronically happy young teens dancing, laughing, talking, snacking. (I could invite my whole crowd over for a big bash and still have plenty of room left over for the Rhode Island Philharmonic Orchestra.)

In the back there's this column called "Problems of Young Living." It begins with this letter from a thirteen year old who's having problems getting along with her parents; lives on a farm and has to get up at 4 a.m. to do chores, they're so strict and blah, blah, blah. The Problems of Young Living Editor suggests that she talk to her doctor or minister. Then there's one from some poor dork who's just moved to a new town and doesn't have any friends. The answer lady says: "You say no one ever invites you *anyplace*. Have you tried inviting *them?* Strike up a conversation with someone interesting and say: 'How about a game of tennis this afternoon?' "

I come downstairs a little before dinner time. My mother is pouring frozen peas into boiling water. Thin strips of bacon are frying in the skillet. This is the food we eat when my father is not coming home for dinner: bacon, eggs, leftovers. Tuesday night, when he has a late class and eats at school, is "clean out the refrigerator night." My mother sets in front of us leftover broccoli and wilted salad, an odd lamb chop or two congealed in its pale fat, barely warmed white rice. But this is not Tuesday. And my mother's eyes are rimmed with red.

"What's wrong?"

"Nothing's wrong," she says. "Everything's fine. Fine. Dinner. Call your sisters and brother."

"Where's Daddy?" Jimmy asks when we are all seated around the kitchen table.

"He's not going to be here for dinner tonight," my mother says.

"How come?" Jimmy asks.

"I'm going to do a project for the science fair," I say. "I think something about the Sargasso Sea."

" 'Your mind and you are our Sargasso Sea... ' " my mother says, tilting her head into the air the way she always does when she's delivering a quote.

"Where's Daddy?" Suzanne asks.

My mother lays her knife and fork down. She opens her mouth to speak; a tear runs down her cheek. "Your father," she says, and then rises, walking to the corner of the counter where the kleenexes are kept, pulling out one and then another, "Your father's been under a lot of pressure lately. He — he's gone away for a rest."

"Where?" Suzanne asks.

"Well," my mother says, clearing her throat. "It's not exactly a hospital."

"Exactly what is it?" Suzanne asks.

"It's a place where people can go and rest for awhile, get away from their problems."

I imagine a resort somewhere, the South Seas, perhaps, a ramshackle hotel in the background, like the one on *Adventures in Paradise* where tired men lie all day in hammocks, eased by tropical breezes, drinking sweet cocktails from the hollowed-out shells of pineapples.

"Butler?" Suzanne asks.

"Yes," my mother says softly. "Butler."

Butler? That is the nut house, the funny farm, the looney bin.

"The Sargasso Sea is actually a marine desert," I say. "Isn't that — "

Suzanne glares at me: "Would you shut up?"

After I take a shower and wash my hair, I wrap my head in a towel. I look at myself in the mirror — with my hair wrapped up in this turban I look very old — seventeen, or maybe even twenty. I hold an imaginary cigarette at a jaunty angle. I am sitting in the Deux Maggots, talking with my good friends, Jean-Paul and Simone. "My mother's a professor." I take a long inhale: "And my father's a madman."

Didn't sound quite right. I try it again, staring full at my face in the mirror: "My father's a madman."

"Who the hell are you talking to?" Suzanne hollers.

I open the door, stick my head out, and shout quickly back: "I'm practicing a book report."

I flop myself across the bed, start reading "Facts About Love and Sex for Teens" which just arrived in the mail today. I don't want you to think I'm a sex maniac or anything — I just want to know a few things. Like what happens when people do it — I mean besides all the moaning and gasping with pleasure.

"Facts About Love and Sex for Teens" begins with a run-down about the old Curse and how it's "not an unpleasant event in a girl's life" (could have fooled me); I'm skimming along, trying to find the good stuff. Here it is: "Sexual intercourse is a time of great sharing and love between two married people." That's it. I can't believe it. Fifty cents. Fifty cents for that.

"Hey," Charlotte says, "will you do me a favor? I got this

catechism test tomorrow. Ask me the questions out of this book — see if I know the answers.''

She hands me this blue and white book that's got all these drawings of Jesus and angels with haloes floating through the sky.

"Just flip through," she says. "I've got to know *everything*."

" 'Why are we on earth?' '' I begin, a question I've often asked myself.

"We are on earth," Charlotte recites, eyes rolled towards the ceiling, "to learn to know God," she ticks off one finger, "to love and to serve Him," she ticks off her next finger, "and one day to live with Him forever."

"Right." I'm impressed. " 'How did suffering and death come into the world? ''

"Suffering and death came into the world through sin.''

"But how did sin come into the world?"

"Is that in the book?'' Charlotte asks.

"Sorry. 'Why does God allow us to suffer? ''

"God permits us to suffer because through suffering he wants to lead us to salvation."

"Manic-depressive psychosis," my mother says, as she presses her foot down on the brake. "A chemical imbalance in his brain." She slows the station wagon almost to a stop and we ease over the bump in the drive. Oh, no, there is nothing really wrong with him; just a few chemicals off-kilter, just something in his head a little out of whack. Everything is going to be just fine and dandy!

Butler is green lawns and soft footsteps, a red brick building gloomy in front of us. My father bumbles down the steps: he is shaking, ever so slightly, shaking; a wide grin slices across his face.

"Rebecca couldn't come," my mother says. "She had a yearbook meeting."

"A yearbook meeting," my father says, nodding his head up and down.

"Yes," Suzanne says, "a yearbook meeting."

I wait for my father's anger to lash out, but he is groggy, nodding his head.

"Lithium," my father says when we are sitting on the grass. "They say it's a miracle drug."

"Remember when they invented penicillin," my mother says, smiling, smiling, "and suddenly *all* those diseases... "

"That's what they say. A miracle."

"What do you do all day, Daddy?" Jimmy asks.

"Well, we get up in the morning and have breakfast."

"Breakfast in bed?" my mother asks.

"Yes, in bed."

"That must be fun," she says.

"Then we have O.T., occupational therapy. I painted a picture. Of that tree," he says, pointing, "and then. Sometimes. You wonder if there's anything they can do for you. You wonder if... " and my father, sitting on the grass, draws his knees up towards his chest, wrapping his arms around them, and slowly begins to rock back and forth.

Dear Problems of Young Living Editor:

I do not have a real problem that I need your help with; I just have a few questions I would like answered. Also, I know that you "regret you cannot answer letters individually" but I thought maybe you could, just this once. I really do need to know the answers to these questions and if you published this in Young Teen *then anybody who knew me would realize this was from me. I've enclosed a stamped self-addressed envelope.*

What does manic-depressive psychosis mean? Why are we on earth? Why does my mother always start folding laundry when I want to talk to her? What does 'Like the hully-gully but not so slow' mean? (This is part of a song I hear coming from my sister's radio.)

Also, I sent away for your booklet called, "Facts About Love and Sex for Teens" and while I certainly appreciated all the valuable information there are a few more things I would like to know. (I suppose I should tell you here that even though I'm only eleven I'm very mature for my age; I have a very high IQ and skipped third grade and am in junior high school already.) My question is this: when people have "intercourse" what actually happens? How long does it last? Why is it done in bed? Please don't tell me to talk to our clergyman, because we don't go to church, or to my family doctor, because he looks like Frankenstein and is a real creep. I really do need to know the answers to these questions.

My sister Suzanne used to be a regular person, I mean she read books and talked in a normal tone of voice but ever since she turned thirteen she's been really dopey, baby talking, etc. Will this happen to me?

Just Stories

by jill sager

i used to feel like a storyteller, telling someone else's tale. But they were *my* stories, usually told repeatedly, without expression or feeling. The stories have been vague to protect myself from my emotions. I've denied my emotions so I could survive the situations. Maybe I have needed enough distance behind me and a lot of support around me to remember the feelings the stories bring up, everytime a story is told.

I am being wheeled down to the operating room, more commonly known as the O.R. By the time I get to the surgical floor I am pretty doped up from the two shots the nurse gave me on my right thigh. They transfer me onto the O.R. table and the anasthesiologist approaches me holding the black "gas" mask. I have always been afraid of its smell and the black hole I disappear into as the gas takes effect. I am also afraid of the man coming toward me. His one color surgical uniform covers him entirely so only his eyes show and he hasn't said one word to me. The mummy looking at me does not feel friendly especially to this nine year old girl.

As he places the black mask over my mouth I smack it out of his hand and I can hear it land across the room on the tiled floor. He leaves the room for a moment and I feel satisfied that I have won. Maybe he is looking for another way to put me to sleep.

I start to relax just as the O.R. door bursts open and three uniformed men walk in. Two position themselves at either side of the O.R. table, take my arms, and hold me down. I am screaming, letting them know I don't want the mask, letting them know I am afraid of the ether. They say nothing as I cry and try to pull out of their grip. The third uniformed man approaches me holding the gas

mask. I recognize him from before, and he places the mask over my
mouth as I am about to make one more plea.

I am standing in a room with two beds that have metal side rails,
two empty dressers, two bedside tables equipped with plastic washing
bowls and bedpans, and two tables on wheels that can be adjusted
for height. Very interesting furniture but not what I am used to. The
room is sterile, and only the T.V. set looks like it may be friendly
once it is turned on.

I am taking pajamas out of my suitcase, and putting them into
the drawers of one of the empty dressers. I am becoming more
uneasy. I know that I have come to the hospital for surgery. My doctor and my mother told me that I have come to get an "apparatus"
on my leg. That thought had never scared me before. I thought this
would be like the clinic I'd been going to since I was three months
old: I'd wait for the doctors to come and they'd ask me how I'm doing, examine my leg, measure the length of all four limbs and ask
me to bend over so they could take a look at my spine. Only this time
they would strap this "apparatus" to my left leg and I would wear
it for awhile. But now I am feeling uneasy. The hospital smells
strange. The fifth floor that I am on now looks much different than
the first floor where I have clinic visits. The clinic floor is alway so
busy with people rushing around, even though you have to wait for
hours for them to take you to an examining room, where you wait
for another hour to see your doctor. Up here, it is very quiet and
stark and nobody looks familiar.

My mother helps me finish unpacking and I notice a beautiful
new pair of pajamas at the bottom of the suitcase. I am thrilled by
the gift, but feel uncomfortable when I am told my aunt has bought
them for me. They are a special pair of pajamas, too special, all wrapped up and pretty. It's not my birthday, it isn't Hanukah, I have
only come to get an "apparatus" and my aunt bought me a brand
new pair of pajamas. I am feeling uneasy.

We decide to take a walk down to the playroom. It's deserted
except for the tables and chairs which are perfectly comfortable for
me. My mom pulls up an adult size chair and we sit in silence for
a long while. There are many windows facing us, but the New York
City sky has turned gray and night is falling, darkening our

surroundings.

My father returns. I am not sure where he has been but the three of us walk back to the room where I have left all of my pajamas. It has become clear that this unfamiliar room is now mine and that staying at the hospital is not what I thought.

My parents get ready to leave and I watch them as they walk down the hall until they are out of sight, and I am alone. I am afraid to leave this strange room which now feels more familiar than the empty long hallway. I stay in that room all night. I stay there, afraid to go to the bathroom which is down the hall. I lie in the bed, on my stomach, afraid of all the darkness around me. I am afraid of the nurse who comes during the night. I pretend I am asleep and remain perfectly still, as the clanking sound of the side rails on the bed close around me.

And I wait and I listen, and I am uncertain, and I am scared. And I am thinking about my sister who usually sleeps in the bed next to me. I am thinking about my brother and my parents and I wonder how they feel knowing I am not home with them. I wonder if they miss me and I wonder why they have left me alone.

When I awake they tell me I was in surgery for seven hours. I recognize this room and I know where I am, but I don't know why I am here. I am tired and I hurt. I have never felt such a painful burning sensation before. I can't figure out where the pain is coming from. There are people around me, two maybe three nurses are making a fuss about something. And the burning sensation won't stop. I am confused by all this activity. The nurse on my right asks how I am and I can hardly speak. Somebody else says I am in pain and they tell me they will get me a shot so it doesn't hurt. I can hear them fussing and talking very loudly about my mattress. I wish they'd let me sleep. I hurt and the burning pain won't stop. I see a nurse coming towards me with the shot. And I feel grateful as she plunges it into my thigh.

I am awake. I am lying in bed but I am no longer in my room. I am being wheeled into x-ray. I am told I've been asleep for three days. I am very tired. It is hard to concentrate. I recognize x-ray because I have been there many times during my clinic visits. They pull the x-ray machine over my bed and I am wondering why I don't get on the x-ray table. Maybe they're letting me stay in my own bed because they know how tired I am. They are fidgeting with something behind me. I am lying on my back and I know I can't turn over, but I turn my head to the left and tilt my eyes backward and I can see what they are doing. Behind me, attached somehow to my bed are green canvas sacks dangling by some clothesline cord. I don't understand what they are but as I am watching they move one slightly and the pain in my leg becomes unbearable again. I am quick to realize that if they move those bags I hurt an unbearable hurt. I scream. They stop what they are doing and I beg them not to touch the bags anymore.

I am hoping that they will hurry and take the x-rays. I am hot and I feel sick and I am tired and confused but I am definitely aware that it is my left leg that is burning.

I am awake. My bed is bumping into the door frame as I am wheeled out of the x-ray room. I don't know where I am going. I can't remember what I am doing here or why I am in this bed being wheeled around. As I reach the end of the long corridor of the x-ray department I see my mother and father approaching me. They are smiling. I guess they are happy to see me. I am glad to see them. I can't remember the last time I saw them but it feels too long, and there are many things that have happened to me that they know nothing about. I am glad to see them so they can tell me what is going on. But for a split second I am afraid they won't know and that split second gets longer as I see my left leg for the first time. My parents couldn't possibly know this is what was going to happen to me. This can't be the "appartus" I had been expecting. All of a sudden I remember the reason I came to the hospital. I remember I came for surgery. I remember I came to get an "apparatus." I can't believe they have done this to my leg. I can't believe they have done this to me.

I am scared. This "apparatus" is not what I expected. It's huge and there's a lot of metal and there are seven stitches on the left side of my thigh. I can see dried blood and thick metal pins sticking through my leg. I recognize that both ends of the pins have threads, like screws. I know this because my father has explained nuts, bolts, and screws to me many times. I am the only one of his three children who has been curious about the kinds of things he does as a machinist, and he has always taken the time to explain. But he is not here now and I am confused about what has happened. My mother starts to tell me.

Altogether there are eight pins in my left leg. Four of them start just below my hip and go through to my behind. The other four stick out at other locations along my leg. One is at my ankle, one is below the knee, and two are above the knee. Connected to these pins from the top of my thigh to my ankle on the right and left side of my leg are two long metal rods. Attached to these rods are the green canvas bags containing the weights which are suspending my leg above the mattress. Attached to the long rod of the left side about mid-thigh is one metal "nut". My mother is explaining that every evening the doctors will come and turn that "nut" a certain amount which will make the "apparatus" longer and stretch my leg. The seven stitches on the middle of my thigh is where they broke the bone so the leg will stretch.

My mattress has two levels. My upper body is lying on the thickness of three mattresses. My left leg is hanging over the thickness of one mattress. My mother explains that it took them a while to figure this out, but it was the only way to make sure there was no pressure on the four pins sticking out from my behind. This is the "apparatus". This is the leg lengthening operation.

I hurt. I am terrified. I know this was a big mistake. I know there is no going back. I know I will never be the same.

When I was nine years old I didn't understand the risks. I was born with my left leg ¾ of an inch shorter than my right leg. My left leg worked fine, but it kept getting shorter. By the time I was nine the discrepancy was two and a half inches. One month before I entered the hospital my doctor asked me if I would like to wear high heels for my high school graduation. No more lifts and no more heavy leather saddle shoes. It sounded fine, it sounded easy. I wasn't told that my leg would have many permanent scars and stretch marks and that some areas would always feel like needles and pins if touched while other areas would never have feelings again. They didn't tell me.

My parents trusted the doctor. They agreed to surgery to make both my legs the same size. They were afraid to ask too many questions. My parents didn't know that the "apparatus" I was to wear for five months would eventually kill off all the nerves and muscles in my leg leaving my knee, foot, and toes with limited mobility. They didn't know that this first surgery at age nine to lengthen my left leg would be the beginning of many hospitalizations, procedures, and surgeries that would last until the age of sixteen. They didn't realize my sciatic nerve would be damaged or that my left foot would become one and a half sizes smaller than my right foot. They didn't know that the surgery wouldn't work. They didn't realize that entering the hospital with a two and a half inch lift on my shoe would be better than the three inch lift I'd have to wear the rest of my life. They didn't know that I would always walk with a limp and later develop curvature of the spine. My parents didn't know this was called experimental surgery.

It's a birthday party, mine. A celebration for me, ten years since my birth. And I am so excited, because I haven't seen my best friend Nina in so long. I have known her since first grade; before surgery, we would spend weekends at each others' houses, swapping handmade Barbie doll clothes and making fun of her older sister's boyfriends. It's been seven months since I've seen her and it feels good to be back home where she can visit me.

Other classmates I knew from first, second, and third grade have come, even though they are all attending fourth grade without me. I have a home tutor now. I can't go back to public school until this body cast comes off. The cast is so big and heavy I have to sleep in the living room downstairs, because no one can carry me upstairs to my bedroom. So for the entire time I am in this cast the living room has become my room.

Every morning I am transferred from my bed to this stretcher that my father built out of old baby carriage wheels and plywood. Using the walls, I can get from the living room to the dining room facing front and from the dining room to the living room pushing backwards. The cast is so heavy I need help washing, fetching things, and changing positions; stomach or back are my only choices. It's impossible to sit up, because the cast starts at my chest and stops at the toes of my left leg, and stops above the knee of my right leg. They did cut a hole, so I can use a bedpan fairly easily if I have a lot of help.

On my tenth birthday I am in the middle of the living room, stomach side down wondering what games we will play, and I am thinking about the birthday cake and Nina, but I begin to notice I am alone. All my friends have gone upstairs to the bedroom I should still be sharing with my sister.

And I remember waiting in that living room by myself for a long time. Looking back, I don't remember eating the cake, and I don't remember when they all left, but I do know it was the last time I saw Nina, and I do remember that I didn't cry.

Fifth and sixth grades spent in New York City's classes for handicapped children. Two health classes with two teachers in the entire school. One class, for grades one through three, my class for grades four through six. Two segregated classes in a Bronx Public School. Their attempt at mainstreaming meant you did non-challenging math and English in the morning and played chess and other games all afternoon. It meant we ate lunch one hour later than everyone else and watched everyone else in the school playground while we sat on the school steps.

Attending a regular school in a health class meant being the first class to enter the school auditorium for Friday assemblies. For two years every Friday morning I made that long and dreadful walk from the elevator into the school auditorium. It meant walking past all the other fifth and sixth graders as they were getting into lines preparing for their walk into the auditorium after the nine of us were already seated. Every week we walked in single file in front of the rest of the school while they stared and we tried not to feel different.

But we were different and they wouldn't let me forget that 'different' meant I should feel ashamed. I couldn't feel OK about being different because I felt too abnormal. I was too aware of the clanking of my leg brace. I was too aware of the visibility of my back brace.

Every Friday I felt embarrassed for who I was, and that feeling never disappeared until the assembly activities were under way.

I get depressed. Sometimes I drink too much. I know I'm unhappy too often. It's hard to get close to people. I feel angry a lot. I am afraid to be made love to. I don't like my body. I'm ashamed of my body. I treat my deformed leg like an ''it,'' not a real part of me. My curved back is something to be hidden by my long hair. I do feel insecure with people. Sometimes I feel alone even when I'm with others. I don't know how to be vulnerable and it's hard for me to trust people. I'm too needy. I'm too independent. I am weak, I am strong. I don't fit in. I don't like being disappointed. I don't know how to ask for help. I feel like I've experienced rape. I don't like my lover lying on top of me when we make love, it's too confining. I feel like I've experienced death many times. Everytime I start to have an orgasm I have to remind myself that the lack of control I am feeling is not the ''black hole'' I experienced with ether. Sometimes I don't feel different, sometimes it's all I feel. Everybody treats me different but nobody notices what my difference is.

They are just stories, but they are my stories. To remember them with feeling and clarity is part of my survival. I'm trying hard to remember. I never want to forget.

Seizures

by max dashu

Moira balanced on the railing above a concrete staircase leading to the ground story sidewalk. Almost everyone had gone home, including the teachers. There was no one to stop her. Moira knew that if any adult was around she would have certainly been ordered off the railing. But she wanted to slide down. She whooshed down the steep railing with guilty pleasure. At midpoint her hands hit the rail's centerpost. And she flew.

There was no memory, no consciousness. Gradually she became aware that there were people hovering over her. She turned her head around, completely disoriented, and began to sit up. There were blankets over her. Hands pushed her down. She insisted she was all right, barely noticing the quiet kids watching. There was no pain at all, only a heaviness and a feeling of being far away. "Oh! I fell off the rail, yeah." She realized it was a big deal when she suddenly felt the importance the adults were giving to her injury. Moira fell back, subdued. They were talking in hushed voices.

"God, she's so dumb, she should be in the EMH class." The special initials painted over the nubbed window of that segregated set of classrooms stood for *Educable Mentally Handicapped*. Or as the kids said, the RE-tards. They were a separated humanity — their bouncing gait, vulnerable veiled eyes, their bursts of liveliness between sudden cautious silences that refused to be baited. They jerked when they walked, they twitched and rocked and talked loud. Their classes were in the basement of the school, near the vocational rooms, and they got out early. This gave some protection from being tormented by football heroes. There was still no shield against the pain of being outcasts.

Anyone could hear the "normal" girls on their way to the bathroom to rat their hair, arguing amiably. "Stop acting so retarded, I just want to borrow it for tomorrow. I'll give it right back... "

"*Give* it to me, Barbara — you spastic!"

Moira was a spastic; she even had a tic. She was both ashamed and defiant. Sometimes people just looked at her and stared. Her mother nagged her, "What makes you do that?" She couldn't stop it. Being treated weird made her feel weird. Moira refused to acknowledge any obstacles. It was years before she grappled openly with the feeling of looking grotesque.

———

Their desks were pushed together in the stuffy, almost windowless home room belonging to the English teacher. Moira was explaining math problems to Kathleen. One moment it was clear and the next... Kathleen was asking her a question. Moira was astonished because she had lost her understanding. She couldn't remember the problem. Her mind was like a pool of very heavy water whose surface she could not penetrate. Stalling for time she asked Kathleen again, "What did you say?" Frozen. She could not follow the words. Kathleen was looking at her weird. Moira desperately tried to function: "What — " Her head was getting heavy, like something was pressing very hard on her neck. Kathleen gaped at her. Moira scrambled for words, tried to speak, but she had no words, no brain. The matrix of naming had entirely slipped away. Terror resonated within her. The world hummed and pressed against her head.

Across the room the teacher was sharply calling her name. Moira grappled with the tiny corner of awareness she had somehow been reduced to. *What is happening to me?* No explanation could describe it. She realized that drool had poured out of the side of her mouth. The room was completely silent, but Moira didn't know it. The humming vibration pulsed in her body. She could not see the shocked faces turned toward her, or answer the teacher, though she mustered her last effort to speak. The weight was overpowering and wrestled her beyond all knowing.

———

The kid read too much science fiction, maybe. She was really afraid she didn't know what planet she was on. She had never been in this room before. It felt totally alien to her. She struggled to remember how she had gotten there, what chain of events could explain her lying on a cot in this windowless beige cell. The worst part was, she didn't remember who she was. No explanation for her presence here or for her past. She had to come up with a name, her identity. In panic, she scanned for a hook to hang her memory on. The science fiction memory prompted a survey of the worlds. Maybe she was a prisoner. Adrenalin pumped her breath out raggedly.

An older woman walked into the room. Moira struggled to identify the face as the woman spoke, searching for clues. Finally the moments of confusion resolved into comprehension. Moira recognized the school nurse. Her mind bridged across the vast distance from the mysterious cubby to eighth grade study hall. She pondered the unexplainable happening while the nurse drove her home. Her mom was waiting for them, worried to death, but prepared to show no fear. Very matter-of-factly and affectionately, she put Moira to bed and told her to sleep.

Discovering the causes within her body was purely an intellectual exercise for the doctors, who over the years gave pronouncements on her X-rays and EEG tests. They gave a latin name to her condition, *idiopathic temporal lobe epilepsy, grand mal*, which meant they were ignorant of its cause. She could have been born that way. Her brain could have gotten fried during that long delirium of measles when she hallucinated, her body suspended over a grid of iron. But, to Moira, the memory of that first fall on the stairs had mythological meaning, a way of understanding how she was set apart. It was the first in a series of waking from blackness to search her memory.

She obediently took phenobarb for several years without wanting to think about why. Then a friend asked her, "You have epilepsy, don't you?" She hotly denied it, all the while realizing with shock that it was the truth. Moira was ashamed and shaken. She only knew one other epileptic — what a word! Eric was a large boy, usually quiet but notorious for psychomotor outbursts in school, where he jumped up and began pushing desks around, shouting and foaming at the mouth. This only had to happen a few times to guarantee a reputation for Eric.

———————

It was two o'clock on Saturday afternoon. The supermarket was packed with customers and the lines were busy. The pounding of the cash registers was boring into Moira's brain. With 5/8 of a pound of tomatoes at 29ᶜ a pound, what was she supposed to charge? She calculated and let it go at 17ᶜ. Long lines stretched back to the shelves, carts heaped with food. The pace was always hectic on Saturdays. Moira worked faster.

When the aura came over her it was amplified by the fact that It Could Happen in front of 50 other people standing around the counters. Moira could hardly hold off the blackout that would sweep her brain clean. "Just a minute," she disjointedly told the customer, in the middle of checking a full cart of groceries. She turned, hesitated as a wave of dizziness froze her muscles, and dashed to the booth where Betty, her supervisor, presided over the store. "I-think-I'm-going-to-have-a-seizure — need... get someone on my line... ." Compulsive in working class ethics, she didn't want to blow her job. Betty could be stern. She did not look pleased when she sent Moira to break. Later she told her to go home. "You left your *drawer* open. Never leave your station with the drawer open — someone might take the money and you'll be short." Moira felt humiliated. She had made a huge effort to do right by the store but she had failed.

She lost her job.

Four years later, Moira was fired again for having petite-mal seizures at work. She dropped some plates during the noon rush at the Burger Cottage. It seemed like the plates just jumped out of her hands.

———————

Moira went home from work thoroughly fatigued. She was tight, twitchy, her jaw unconsciously clenched. Sitting in the noisy crowded bus, her mind shot in disconnected spurts. Typing always fucked up her brain. After forcing her mind and body through the afternoon's invoices and coding, she had lost the connecting threads between thoughts and motions. She felt people on the bus staring at her. It made her feel more restless: claustrophobia. She looked out the window and thought how unnatural she must look — too jerky, and how she should try to look more normal — blend in somehow. Camouflage was her life strategy in these situations. Moira was disgusted with the watchers but dissatisfied with herself anyway.

The movement and noise of the bus suddenly produced confusion; she was dizzy: "The aura? Oh god!" A wave of fear drenched her and plunged to her belly. Adrenalin shot to her feet and hands. She dropped her head between her knees, because she had to. "Now they're really staring/don't think about that/deep breathe/hang on." Trying not to think about it, Moira remembered the time on the Boston subway near Filene's — a narrow escape. And waking up in a hospital halfway between Seattle and Los Angeles, realizing it had actually happened on a Greyhound bus. They sent for an ambulance and her stuff went on to L.A. without her.

"I can't wait till I find some other work, this is killing me." Finally she decides to sit up, but slowly. As her head comes up, people's heads shift on their necks. Nobody is looking at her now. Three young men behind her suddenly laugh loudly at something. Moira tells herself it doesn't matter what people think — they don't understand what is happening — but she still felt it affecting her. "You can't let them get to you; bring back your self-confidence." Moira was in the process of overcoming the compulsive desire to justify herself to these strangers. Twenty more blocks. "I'll skip the supermarket tonight."

Moira had certainly not gotten enough sleep. She knew five hours was dangerous for her. But she wanted badly to go to the country and the ride was leaving at 6 a.m. As usual she was relentless with herself once she had set her will. Moira knew she needed to get out of the city, but she was not up to hitch-hiking this month. That was a risk she could face only when she felt strong enough to fight for her life, as the price of getting her non-driving body onto the wild land — an act of self-preservation disguised as recklessness, refusing to be a prisoner of the city.

She woke on a dangerous edge, her awareness splintered on the alarm buzzer. Not surprisingly, Moira was shaken with tremors as they loaded her stuff into the car and drove to Ellen's place. She was trying to concentrate on calm breathing. Her brain waves jumped erratically while they climbed to the second-story apartment. Inside, people talked while Moira fought off her shaking and swift momentary blackouts, trying to appear normal. Without the least warning, the final bolt hit her halfway down the staircase.

She came to lying in the street. LaTonya was looking down at her with big eyes, holding her hand and sort of petting her. "She gonna be OK now?" The little girl was full of comfort and concern. They spoke together while Moira shifted her body in the gutter and reached for her glasses. They were missing, uh-oh. The women standing around her handed her a broken pair. At least she had not chewed her tongue. The little girl hugged her in the sweetest way.

Most people are terrified of epilepsy, its dramatic interruption of social convention.

Nervous disorders carry a special stigma because they affect behavior. Very close to insanity. People are threatened by physical movements with no apparent reason. Twitching, jerking, blankness — or full-scale convulsions.

"I mean, what do you say to people standing next to you in an office when all of a sudden your legs buckle and you fall flat on your butt? One minute, you're standing; the next, you're on the floor?" Moira always had this urge to explain what was going on so that people wouldn't think she was weird. In one sense, it was apologizing for being "abnormal". But it was also a refusal to let her epilepsy be unspeakable. Or invisible; because even when its affects can be seen they are not identified or understood by most people.

It finally began to dawn on Moira that her explanations were not having their desired effect. People gave her strange looks or acted threatened by the subject. Some seemed to believe that to talk about your reality is to complain.

Moira began to attend to herself and work on the shame. She knew what kind of looks to expect, but she picked herself up with dignity. She worked on her own confidence. Went back to her feelings about her body, her seizures, the tension locked into her muscles. She had to chisel through the layers of grotesqueness that coated her self-image.

Dance, which had always terrified Moira as a dead giveaway, gave her relief. She was only able to begin to dance alone, feeling watched by phantom, hostile eyes. In that battle, she recovered something she knew about her body that had been drilled out of her. She unclenched her tendons, unrolled the tension, breathed, stretched and discharged that overload of energy which shook her body and racked her nerves.

Moira had found that herbal teas could sometimes calm out petit-mal blitzes. Exercise helped. But she learned to be careful in seeking alternatives cures, because some people are arrogant. Not all of them doctors. Moira had met psychics and herbalists who claimed with total assurance to have her cure. She tried them; they were wrong.

To keep seizures at bay, Moira drank no coffee, no alcohol, no caffeine or stimulants of any kind. She made sure to get enough sleep to keep on an even keel. But it was natural for her mind and body to rev ahead of "normal" pace under noise, pressure, intense stimulation or concentration. Then she talked fast and sometimes loud, signs of the stress of coping with too much input. She had to work hard then to carry on a conversation.

Carol once said to her at a party, "What are you *on*, Moira?" There was no point in explaining anything. Moira stood up and went to refill her plate, blood pounding with rage and shame. She reviewed the way she had been talking, a compulsive behavior check. But what was the point of that? An instant of lapsed consciousness — was that so bad, so shameful that anyone could casually use it against her?

Realization of old wounds was penetrating Moira deeper, gradually. In no theoretical way but in the most profound emotional remembrance, she had begun to grasp how people's judgments and reactions had shaped her own self-rejection. Of her natural way of being. Unacceptable. To be struggled against, hammered into non-threatening form at whatever cost.

The thing that Moira couldn't get over was how unconscious she had been of her own desperate efforts to adjust her behavior. She had been trying to force herself not to appear *abnormal:* epileptic. Old wounds, half-forgotten, still open.

"You spastic!" It was in the glance, not on the tongue. "You mean you don't *drive*?" The response of unthinking judgment. "Oh." Society had not stopped inflicting its stigma.

But Moira herself was changing.

Life Has To Go On...

an interview with elaine robidoux by bobbie-jo goff [1]

"....I don't mind being retarded. I used to mind it, but all of a sudden those three years came up and I started talking more about it[2]. The more we talk about it the less frightened you are about what you feel and what your feelings gonna' be. I think if... the more you talk about it, the less it hurts. The hurt that hurts when you find out that you are retarded. It hurts you for awhile. And when you start talking about it, you're gonna' find out what it really is all about, because it hurts other people when you tell them that you're retarded... "

Those are the words of Elaine Robidoux, a twenty-eight year old woman who has been labelled mentally retarded. Elaine lives and works in Beverly, Massachusetts. Her home is a minimally supervised residential program, referred to as a "co-op apartment" which she shares with one woman. She has been working full-time in a nursing home as a dietary aide since she was graduated from high school in 1978. As is the case with many people considered to be mentally retarded, Elaine's history is one of institutionalization, "special" training and educational programs, as well as absence of family. In fact, Elaine has no memories at all of a family. She was admitted to a sanitorium for victims of tuberculosis at age two. Between the ages of three and five, she lived with foster parents until her first institutionalization at a state school for the mentally retarded. She remained institutionalized at three different state schools[3] until age eighteen. Elaine was among the first group home

---

[1]This interview was conducted in two parts. Most of the quotes regarding Elaine's institutional experiences were taken from an interview we did during the summer of 1982, with most others from an interview occuring during the summer, 1983.

[2]Over the past few years, Elaine has been speaking to different colleges, community and professional groups about her experiences as a "special needs" person.

[3]The names of the state schools have been changed to read: Grover, 1961-1964, Clintonville, 1964-1971, and Island, 1971-1973.

residents in Massachusetts. It was then, in 1973, that she began her formal education which consisted of special needs classes in a public high school. She remained in the group home and high school until 1978 when she was considered "ready" for a more independent living situation, the co-op apartment program where she lives today.

I met Elaine in 1977 as Director of her group home. I see her as a real "survivor"; others see her as a real "success story". We did some public speaking together about her experiences as a "mentally retarded" person, which created a close and special bond between us. Elaine has been my major source of understanding and humanization in my work with people labelled mentally retarded. She keeps me aware of how very much "professionals" do not know about the people they are intended to serve.

We are both very grateful for this opportunity to inform others about what it means to live life as a person with "special needs". We are hopeful that other women who share Elaine's disability will begin to be included in the efforts being made to secure visibility and recognition of the needs of all disabled people. In addition, we seek to encourage other "mentally retarded" women to tell their stories so that they may establish themselves as contributors in the struggle toward creating emotionally and physically safe and accessible communities.

BJ: Elaine, you have had a lot of different labels over the years. You've been called mentally retarded, handicapped, special needs, developmentally disabled and on and on. Is there a term that you prefer?

ER: My preferred is: I'll take retarded, but I'll take special needs better.

BJ: So you prefer being referred to as someone with special needs?

ER: Yeah, just because I think it's a better word. It's a better word to use instead of retarded thrown in your face or something... saying, "You're retarded" right in the street. That's what most people say. To be on the street and saying, "You're retarded." I don't think it's appropriate. So, I say something like: "Do you know what it means?"

BJ: That's what you feel like saying back to them, "Do you know what it means?"

ER: Yeah, but I kinda' think that they'll only beat you back even worse. And, you know, so I just take it. Sometimes you just have to take it. You hear it no matter where you go; especially if they know that you are. They probably know you are. They just look at you and say, "You're retarded".

BJ:*Do you think that you look 'retarded'?*

ER: [laughing] No, I don't think I 'look retarded', but sometimes, you know, they say, "You retarded?" right on the street; especially in Gloucester because I went to school there. Not too much in Beverly, hardly ever in Beverly.

BJ: *Beverly... where you're living now. But in Gloucester while you were going to high school and living in the group home...*

ER: Yeah, because I went to school with a lot of them and they would call you retarded right in the streets. So, I just don't go to Gloucester that much unless I really have to... I mean, you call me retarded — fine. I just ignore them, but in Gloucester it's really bad because I have a family[4] there and I'll just call my father and say, "Dad, come and get me. Come and get me now."

BJ: *You said you preferred being referred to as someone with special needs; what does that mean to you?*

ER: Well, in school it's a little bit different too because you are labelled for that. And I can take it. But to just be called that — I get very upset. Because, I know I am, but I just don't want to show people that. I don't want to show it. Sometimes I show it.

BJ: *How do you show it?*

ER: By being dumb.

BJ: *Being dumb... what do you mean?*

ER: I mean, not really dumb, but like, I'll try to do something and I can't do it. Like Rebecca [co-worker and friend at work] will say, "OK, Elaine, you can do it." [Elaine says] "No, I can't Rebecca."

[4]Elaine's family consists of a staff person who befriended her during her high school years, and her husband and adult children. They include Elaine in many family activities, holidays and she visits them occasionally on weekends. She refers to them as Mom and Dad and her sisters and brothers.

She goes, "You don't take the chance to try it. Try it first and if you can't do it, then I'll help you. You don't give yourself any credit." Maybe because I was always told that I was [dumb]. And she goes, "You've got to give yourself credit sometimes."

BJ: *What are some of the things you feel you can't do?*

ER: OK, the line-up like they have at work. All right... taking the line-up.

BJ: *I don't know what that is.*

ER: OK. You know like where they set the trays up. Remember when you and me went in there with R.B. [resident at the nursing home where Elaine works.] Well, we were trying to set up the lines. I never do that. I never set the trays up. Because there are instructions and I can never do it.

BJ: *You mean you have to read a chart or something?*

ER: You have to read all the charts that go to that floor.

BJ: *So you're afraid that you can't read well...*

ER: You have to read pretty well to do it.

BJ: *You do read though.*

ER: Yeah, I can read, but not enough he said; Mark [work supervisor] said, I can do coffee or beverages and cereal. I can pour cereal out and give coffees... pour the coffee into the cups. I have all the easiest jobs.

BJ: *Are there other things on the job that other people can do that you can't do?*

ER: Anybody could do my job. It's so easy.

BJ: *How do you feel about that?*

ER: Oh — I have the easiest jobs and they all think it's good that I have the easiest job... How do I feel about it? I like it!

BJ: *How long have you been there?*

ER: About five years.

BJ: *How much an hour do you make?*

ER: $4.60.

BJ: *Do you feel that you're treated any differently?*

ER: Sometimes I am.

BJ: *How?*

ER: I'm treated really differently. I'm treated really special. I mean, I should have been out that door by now. Like, I've gotten about five warnings or six warnings and I'm still there.

BJ: *What were the warnings for?*

ER: Something... OK, carts that should never have been in the dining room. Stuff like that. It's like little stupid things.

BJ: *Did you do that because you're 'retarded'?*

ER: [laughing] No, it's... Probably, it was "careless" or something that they used.

BJ: *Do you think they should have fired you?*

ER: If they wanted to, they could have. But I'm still there. I haven't gotten one at all this year. That's a good sign.

BJ: *Right. Well, obviously, you must be doing something right or you would have been fired.*

ER: Right. I don't think they just treated me like the way they did. But, I mean, three warnings, you should have got out.

BJ: *So, you think you got a special privilege?*

ER: [laughing] Yeah.

BJ: *Sounds like you're glad about that.*

ER: [seriously] Yeah, I am. I just worked on what should have been worked on.

BJ: *So that was a good thing that happened. That was a "good" special treatment. Have you had any "bad" special treatment?*

ER:Rebecca, I'm mad at her today. She doesn't talk to me when I'm in a bad mood. She knows. Sometimes I'm treated special. It's different things. Like, she usually treats me special. Most of them do because, you know, they kinda' know my background. And I kinda' think they feel sorry because I told them. They asked me if I went to school and I said no because you can't. They asked me that. They asked me why I can't do the line, so I told them. And different people do different things. They goes, "You don't look that way." And I said, "Well, you stick a book in my face and see what happens." How else can you describe it?

BJ: *Is that what you think is the major thing that makes you different — your reading ability?*

ER: I found out what grade I was. I was really shocked. I thought I might have been 7th or 8th grade in reading, but I'm in 4th. That was when I was in high school, but it could really be down by now.

BJ: *Because you're not reading as much?*

ER: Hardly at all.

BJ: *Are there others things you feel you can't do?*

ER: Ah… my checkbook. I always screw it up. I mean, I came up with $81. I was off $81.00 It was my adding. It is.

BJ: *So, that's something you need help with?*

ER: Yeah. But, you know, I'm not into that right now. I was hoping that I could try going to the North Shore [Community College] one day a week. I'll have to think about it, but I don't know if I'm going to get there.

BJ: *To do what?*

ER: Take a nutrition course. 'Cause, see, it might encourage reading. I'm hoping it wouldn't [necessitate difficult reading]. I've gotta try it. But, I don't know if I can make it through the course.

BJ: *We've been talking about what your label means in your life, especially things you can't do. Are there other ways that being a "special needs" person affects your life?*

ER: OK Work. Jobs... jobs especially.

BJ: *What about it?*

ER: Anywhere you go to apply... Restaurants especially. They don't ever hire you. They just turn you down.

BJ: *Why?*

ER: Probably because... if you have to be a waitress... I could never be a waitress. Too hard and I don't want the aggravation.

BJ: *What part of it would be too hard?*

ER: When you try and write down what they want. I could never do that work.

BJ: *So you feel that having your special needs limits your jobs?*

ER: Yeah... Really definitely. I tried F's [a chain restaurant] and got... I just wanted to be a dishwasher and they went, "You can't just dishwash."

BJ: *Oh — they have the same person doing all different things?*

ER: I guess. I guess it's mostly like for men.

BJ: *Do you think there are jobs that you should get that you don't get because you're a woman?*

ER: I don't think the United States should have it that way. I don't think F's should have... Well, I'm only guessing 'cause I mostly have seen men in restaurants as dishwashers. But women can dishwash too. Mark [work supervisor] has us all doing dishwashing. I mean, I know how to run a dishwasher. I don't break that many dishes! Maybe they think that they're heavy. I've been lifting heavy things for five years.

BJ: *So, instead of being discriminated against because you have special needs, you feel that sometimes you're discriminated against because you're a woman?*

ER: I don't think just being a woman, but basically F's... is good for that. Well, anyway, what I think is... it's not because you're a woman. I think, basically, because they don't want to take us. I really think that. I think I have great power. I have more power than that. Because they know that you're retarded, they don't want to work with you.

BJ: *Do you ever think about leaving where you are and going for a different kind of job?*

ER: I'd like to, but where do I begin? I don't want to work in a nursing home the rest of my life. But it just seems like... I mean, I can't work in restaurants. So, where do I begin?

BJ: *I guess you have to begin by thinking about what you would like. There must be other jobs you'd be interested in and able to do besides nursing homes and restaurants.*

ER: They're the only ones I can think of. I don't want to work at G... [a nationwide organization providing programs for handicapped people]... or something.

BJ: *No, I know that.*

ER: I'll work for B.J. Goff.

BJ: *You want to work for me?*

ER: Yeah, I'll work for you.

BJ: *What would you like to do?*

ER: Help R.B. [a "mentally retarded" woman I work with who lives in the nursing home where Elaine is employed]

BJ: *Elaine, I want to ask you how you think your being a person with special needs has affected your life in certain ways... like your childhood.*

ER: My childhood... Oh, not going to school. That affects it a whole lot. 'Cause when I went to school... It's like I'm older now. OK, I mean... my childhood. I never went to school. I didn't know what school was until I went to the 10th grade [in "special needs" classes]. I didn't know school was even encouraged until Chapter 766

[Massachusetts law insuring equal access to educational opportunities for handicapped children]. Yeah, when that came, I went and met somebody at the high school who was real nice. But, you know, not going to school... It can really affect people. I mean, I have wished I had gone to school. This guy at work didn't even finish. I said to him, "I wouldn't brag about that."

BJ: *Are there other things you think are different from other peoples' childhoods?*

ER: Maybe if I had gone to school, I probably would have known a little bit more. I wish I had gone to school because you see other people and they have more jobs.

BJ: *What about your living situation as a child?*

ER: As a child... most people live with their mother and father. I never lived with my mother and father. You know — nothing. I didn't even know I had a... I mean, I know where I came from, but I didn't go home. I had to eat with all the other people. You'd have a hundred or something people to cook for.

BJ: *So, you didn't go to school. You didn't have a family life and you didn't live in a home...*

ER: That's right. I didn't live at home. Where I lived was in an institution. Most of the time I lived in an institution, so I didn't go to school. I mean, they had school there, but not like... higher. You know, Sophomore, Junior, Senior, the whole bit. It can really affect you. Now, I'm older. I'm very slow. I would be very slow in it now.

BJ: *Elaine, what did you think of yourself when you were living in the institution? How did you feel about yourself?*

ER: I thought of myself... that nobody loved me. You're going to be really interesting of this one. OK, I thought I was... it's like... People who went home... I used to think, "Why me? Do I have a family or do I not have a family?" And then, I used to think that, if I don't, why doesn't people tell me this? And, and just let it stay back to themselves. Because, you know, I should have been the one to know. When I got to Island, I used to think in my room. I used to sit there and cry and think, "Doesn't anybody love me?" Or did they just put me here to leave me off in a jailhouse, because they have put me here and sat thinking, "Is this some punishment for me, or what is the story?" I don't understand.

BJ: *Did you think you had done something wrong, something bad that you were being punished for?*

ER: I don't... Yeah, I did something bad. I don't know. It used to freak me out. I mean, I'd be in a room and then they used to say, "What's the matter?" And I go, "Well, I'm just down again." I used to get down so much. But then, I used to think, "Why me?" It's like, someone should have told me I don't have a family and this is why you're here. Because your family was sick and... But still today, I still don't know what happened to my life. I have still wished I had known way back. It's like now I'm trying to get over it.

BJ: *Elaine, could you talk more about your feelings at that time: happy, unhappy, good, bad...*

ER: I wouldn't say I was happy there. 'Cause I had my days when I didn't want nobody in my life. I used to think, "Well, maybe I should be dead." And I used to think, "It's not worth the living anymore. I might as well just take a knife and kill myself." I used to be the worst down person in the world. I used to walk like some of those people who belong in [the] State Hospital. That's how I was, only worse. I was not that bad, but bad enough to get me down. I used to think, being in this place, I said, "I don't want to be here." I said, "Why am I here? Did I do something wrong?" See, they should tell you that.

BJ: *Were things any better when you moved to Island?*

ER: I would describe myself a little bit better than at Clintonville. I had gotten to the point I started liking myself. I didn't starting hating myself. I didn't have my frustration days. I had 'em, but not as bad as I was at Clintonville. I didn't go around biting myself everyday, I didn't let things block out of my life. 'Cause I did, at that time, block everything out of my life. I didn't want to see anybody. I used to say, "There's no one see anymore."

BJ: *Sounds like you were very lonely and confused while you were living in the institution...*

ER: When I was in an institution, I was never told that I had a family and that I had no family. I think that's what made a lot of people upset. Made me especially upset. I didn't know if I had no family, or what the story is. I mean, you see all these people going out and then you look around, "I'm not going out." That's sad. I mean, the holidays there is like really bad... Then they finally told me, I didn't have a family. I could accept that. But, you know, why didn't they tell me earlier? You know, I could accept it then too. It would have taken awhile. But it's like any other human being could accept it. I could too probably, but it would just have taken a long while... See, in my case, I don't know why I got there and how I got there. And they asked me that day [referring to her most recent speaking engagement]. They asked me how I got there. I can never answer that question. I never could, I never will... A lot of people don't belong there and they're there because their families don't want them. I don't think in my case my family didn't want me. Well, I don't know, 'cause I was too young to know.

BJ: *Elaine, we've talked in the past about some of the things that happened to you while you were in the insititution. Could you say something about those experiences now?... the cruel things that happened to you...*

ER: Any cruel things... ? You mean in my childhood? Anytime?

BJ: *Yeah, any especially mean things that people did to you because...*

ER: OK. What happened... Yeah, my childhood... Yeah, definitely.

BJ: *Could you give a couple of examples, like the time you were thrown down the stairs?*

ER: Because I wouldn't do their little dirty work. And she said, "If you don't do it, I'll throw you down three flights of stairs." So, boom, I went down three flights of stairs. So I took... and then they came in the next day and she goes, "What happened to you?" I said, "Well, an employee threw me down three flights of stairs." And she says, "Well, you're fired [referring to the employee]." None of us should have been pushed around the way we were. I don't think it was right.

Plus, you had to do your own cleaning work. I mean, they didn't have, like... You know how in the nursing home they have housekeepers who work with diet aides? Well, we didn't have that. We did it on our own. We did everything, including the whole thing. At Clintonville... plus their food came from whatever and all you had to do was steam it up.

BJ: *Was there anything else like that that never should have happened?*

ER: That never should have happened? ...OK, I'll take some of the punishments. I don't think that they should have happened. There's one called 'doing the bridge' and 'donkeys'.

BJ: *What's that?*

ER: I'll have to show you.[5]

BJ: *Somebody made you do that?*

ER: Yeah.

BJ: *Like lots of times?*

ER: Yeah. That's cruel. You had to put your legs up. You know how to do sit ups? Well, it's sort of the same thing. You had to go up and down, up and down.

BJ: *As a punishment?*

ER: As a punishment... It's stuff that should never have happened. I mean, mothers and fathers don't even do it to kids.

BJ: *Hopefully.*

ER: Hopefully, they don't. I would never do it to my kids because I know what it feels like. I mean, if you're going to punish your kids — punish them by going to their rooms. I mean, I got slapped across the face. Abuses.

BJ: *Elaine, do you ever think about getting married, having children?*

---

[5]Elaine demonstrated the "bridge" to be like a push-up exercise, only having to hold the upward pose for a long period of time. The "donkey" was like a deep-knee bend, which she was required to do many times in succession, while tugging on her ears.

ER: I'm not thinking about it. I don't want to get married. I don't want to have kids. I want to be a free woman. I like being free. I love being female. But I don't want — you know, this hassle with guys... I couldn't see myself getting married. It wouldn't last.

BJ: *Why not?*

ER: Because I have to do everything I'm used to doing right now. And if I got married, I'd have to change my whole life just for him. No way!

BJ: *What about sex?*

ER: That's out.

BJ: *Out of the question forever?*

ER That's right. Everyone can go find somebody else. Nope. I never want sex.

BJ: *How did you learn about sex when you were growing up?*

ER: I learned about it when I got to Island.

BJ: *How old were you?*

ER: When I was about sixteen.

BJ: *You had a class or something?*

ER: I had it with B.W. [staff person at Island], only one to one.

BJ: *Did it scare you or were you...*

ER: Yeah, it scared me. But she went over and over and over it and said, "You don't have to get married." And once I found out about it, I go, "Not for me". It's not for me. It's just not for me.

BJ: *Do you ever think about sex with women?*

ER: Women are just friends... only as friends.

BJ: *Do you think you'll ever fall in love with anyone?*

ER: If I was going to fall in love, I would have fallen in love a long time ago.

BJ: *Oh — I don't know. I mean, I'm not in love with anybody right now and I'm older than you, but I wouldn't be surprised if I did sometime. I hope I do.*

ER: [laughing] I would think you would have found out by now.

BJ: *Elaine, how do you see your future?*

ER: How do I see my future? I'm not going that far. Why? Do you want me to... ?

BJ: *I'm just wondering if you ever...*

ER: I never thought about it. What would be my goal next? I never thought about it. I'll tell you one thing: I'm not getting married. That will be my one goal. My second: that I would rather live with the Association [sponsoring agency for Elaine's residential program] the rest of my life — forever... I came to the conclusion that I really made up my mind in the past ten years that I just like living with them. I don't know if I ever want to live on my own. I think being out there is too scary. Other people think I should move out, but that's what I think. That's what I think I should do and I never want to move out. I talked with Rebecca about it and she said, "You like living there? You should live there and don't worry about somebody else."

BJ: *What scares you the most about being totally on your own?*

ER: I just don't want to live on my own. Too many crazy people.

BJ: *Do you feel that you get to do everything you want to do... go places you want to go?*

ER: Yeah. I mean, look it, I'm going to Europe for eight days.

BJ: *So, you feel like if you want to take a trip or buy something...*

ER: Yeah, so long as you have the money you can go.

BJ: *Are you able to live off your salary from the nursing home?*

ER: Yes.

BJ: *You don't have to use your savings that much?*

ER: No. I don't live on my savings. I don't even depend on it. I save enough money to do for myself. I do all right. I don't use my savings.

BJ: *What are you saving for?*

ER: Just saving.

BJ: *You have nothing in mind... ?*

ER: I need new clothes. All my clothes are too big.

BJ: *Are you losing more weight?*

ER: Yes.

BJ: *Is that from running?*

ER: Yes. I've been running since March and now it's July.

BJ: *What's the longest you've run?*

ER: Six to seven miles. Today was only three to four.

BJ: *Do you run everyday?*

ER: I just ran before... that's why my hair's wet. I ran at 2:30 pm. You know how hot it is at 2:30. I don't run at night.

BJ: *Why?*

ER: I always pick the hottest.

BJ: *You like to make it hard on yourself, huh?*

ER: Well, also in the bad mood, I had to do something. Sometimes it gets me out of my bad mood, but not always; so I end up running even more.

BJ: *What about today? Did it help?*

ER: It helped some. I was mad at Rebecca.

BJ: *So, do you think you're going to work this stuff out with Rebecca or just stay mad?*

ER: I might work it out. I might work it out with Rebecca because

I like Rebecca.

BJ: *Who would you consider to be the people you really trust?*

ER: I trust Rebecca the best. I trust Rebecca the best of everybody at work.

BJ: *What about outside of work?*

ER: Outside of work? I trust myself [laughing].

BJ: *It's very good to trust yourself. What about friends?*

ER: I trust my mother and father. I'll trust anybody that doesn't hurt me. If someone hurts me, the trust is gone. That's just the way it goes. When I meet new people I gotta check them out... if I'm going to like them or not. It's just... I have learned all my life almost, seeing people go... Coming and going, coming and going... So, I've seen it all my life. Now, I've got to see if I trust one another.

BJ: *Elaine, if you were to describe yourself now and how you feel about yourself, how would you say it?*

ER: How would I say it? You want me to describe myself today? I have my good days and my bad days, when I want to be a child. I think everybody has their days of different things. I mean, I go from today to tomorrow. I have to take one day at a time; but sometimes I just go back. When I get mad, I go, "I'm moving back to Island".

BJ: *Do you see yourself as generally a happy person or... ?*

ER: I'm an in-between person. I'm not very happy or not very sad. I'm in-between because I have my days when things aren't going right. I get very discouraged. I get very upset if something doesn't go right at work. I have to have everything so-so. And if I don't have it just so, I get very mad and I'll go, "Why does it have to be me?"

BJ: *Elaine, are there any final things you want to say about yourself, your life as a person with special needs?*

ER: Being retarded is really hard for us, because you don't know. Being retarded, it doesn't bother me. It's just the label. I mean, labeling, I don't know much about, all right. As far as I know, I know

I'm a slow learner and I know I'm retarded... We all have a handicap of one kind or another. And that is the truth. We are all... I don't care who it is... that you have one handicap or another. You may do things that I can't do and you can't do things that I can do.

" ...Life has to go on. You can't put it back in somewhere in another time. I don't care who they are. We all have special needs of one kind or another and it's the truth. And I still like it today... "

—*Elaine Robidoux*

Speaking Out

by mary ambo

i 'm Mary Ambo. I'm writing this because I want you to listen to me. I have cerebral palsy. Until a few years ago, I couldn't scream or cry out loud. Everybody around me when I was growing up told me it wasn't good to show my emotions. They told me by walking away. They couldn't deal with it. They made me feel guilty for having feelings.

Now I *can* cry, but people around me have to be able to deal with me. If I think they can't, or feel they shouldn't have to, I'll try to wait until they leave. I think if I didn't cry, I couldn't do what I have to do every day. I could not function. It's not that I go around crying all the time, but every once in a while, things get to me.

I had a really hard time when my parents took me away to the hospital, a place near Boston I am afraid to name. They were not talking to me about what they were doing to me. I think they didn't know how they felt, so they couldn't help me deal with it. I'll always wonder whether they had any idea of what was going on inside me. I was only six, but I had a good idea of why they were doing this, and I had a lot of feelings about it. I knew that people like me got put into institutions. Still, I didn't want to go and I was angry. But I could not show any emotion. It would do no good. I knew my parents couldn't take care of me. They were going to do what they wanted to. As I saw it — or was made to see it — they felt they had no choice, there was no option. I knew I was being sent away to live in that place. I was afraid.

Once I got there, my parents talked with the nurses for a while. The nurses' aides took me into a big room and made me take a bath. While I was taking the bath, my parents said goodbye to me. I thought that was a very unfeeling way to say goodbye to a daughter.

I wondered if they loved me. I still wonder, sometimes.

To survive 10 years at that hospital, I had to turn off all my feelings. Once I had to go to the bathroom and just didn't make it. Instead of asking why I had the accident, they yelled and screamed at me, and took me to my room. All the aides on the floor stood around staring at me. The aide assigned to me was teasing and making me feel really bad about myself. I was angry and said, "SHUT UP!" That was the first time I ever told anybody to shut up. It felt good, but it was scary because I didn't know what she would do to me. I was maybe seven at the time. I never defended myself again — it was just too scary. And because I got yelled at for 10 years for needing anything, even now I still say "I'm sorry" when I ask for something.

When I was 16, I was moved from the hospital to the Northampton Nursing Home. I was really scared because I didn't know what it looked like or what it would be like. But even if they had told me I could stay at the hospital, I wouldn't have. They were doing a lot of *hairy* stuff there and had done it for a long time. I never said anything to anybody about it because I was afraid, and I didn't think anyone would believe me.

The day I went into the nursing home, they took me down the hall to a day room full of kids. Most of them were crying. I took one look at them and I started crying because I was scared and didn't know anybody.

But this was the first time in an institution anyone showed concern for my feelings. When I had to go to the bathroom, instead of just taking me, the aide asked me how she should help. It blew me away! I was in shock that somebody asked me a question, because *nobody* ever took the time to ask. Looking at it now, I can't believe that I lived so long without people talking to me like a human being.

I stayed at the nursing home for five years. While I was there, somebody from Stavros Foundation told me she thought I could live independently. At first I did not believe her — simply because I grew up in an institution. And if I *could* live independently, I felt really angry at my parents for leaving me in the institution. It was hard believing I could do something different, but it was exciting to think that I might.

After living with another handicapped woman for a year I filled out an application to live at Clark House, an independent living apartment complex. There was a good possibility I was going to get in, and they wanted me to pick my own apartment. That is where I live now.

Oh, God! Did my life change when I moved to Clark House! I have had more emotional support, from women, in the last several years than I ever had in my whole life before. Because of that, I find I am more able to give emotional support to myself.

Something made me furious today. Two women from the Clark House management came into my apartment to see if I needed anything. I was not told to expect their visit. They asked if they could look around. I was telling my story to Joan, who is typing it. Joan offered to give us privacy. The women said that wouldn't be necessary. Neither they nor Joan asked *me* if *I* wanted Joan to stay.

After a few minutes they came back and told me I have a dirty apartment and that whoever pays my PCA's (Personal Care Attendants) should see that they do a better job. They stood there and asked me how many PCA's I have. I said I couldn't remember. (It wasn't their business anyway!) They found a list on the wall by my telephone and started reading names and counting my PCA's. "I wish I had eleven people working for *me*," one of them said. The same woman told me she couldn't sign the necessary form that says my apartment is "decent, safe, and sanitary." That is *not* true — my apartment is *all* of those things, and I was furious that they talked to me this way in front of another person.

When I asked what was the problem with my apartment, she told me only that the rug needs cleaning (there are spots on it that I also want taken care of) and that there is an accumulation of trash and bottles under my sink. And she went on, "What about that board — that wooden thing — out there on your porch? What is it, Mary? What do you use it for?" I told her it is a ramp I used to get into a van. I was angry that she couldn't already see what it is. "Well, Mary, do you need to keep it out there where everybody can see it? We'll have Maintenance put it in storage. If you want it, you just ask, o.k.?" I didn't answer her. I felt terribly invaded!

I did a lot to get my independence, and it means a lot to me. I get up when I want to. I eat when I want to. I hire my own people to work for me. That is a big step, because I grew up in an institution and never thought I would know how to live independently. Those two women violated my sense of independence. And for what? Spots on a rug, trash and bottles under a sink — things I can and will take care of myself — and for a wooden ramp on my porch, several inches of which "everybody" can see above the brick wall.

People violate my sense of independence outside my home too. I can go downtown on my own. I can take a walk around Amherst — only when I "walk" I drive my power chair. One day I was sitting by myself in Amherst Center. A woman came up and asked me what I was doing out alone. This has happened to me often. Every time it does, it makes me angry. Just because I'm in a wheelchair, people shouldn't assume I can't go for a ride by myself — or do *anything* by myself. I don't usually show my anger, but this time I did. I told the woman I was on my own and to leave me alone! She walked away quickly.

When I go into a doctor's office, instead of talking directly to me, the doctor asks the person I'm with and why I'm there. Once when a doctor did this to me, I confronted him, "Why do you assume that just because I'm in a wheelchair, I cannot talk for myself?" He said, "Because I see a lot of people in wheelchairs." I didn't answer back, but I'll tell you what I was thinking... he gave a truly dumb answer!

Once I did have a good doctor. When I first met her, she surprised me by talking to me directly. That was most important to me because, in order to trust a doctor, you have to have one who will talk to you.

But she will not be talking to me anymore. I just got her letter saying she isn't taking Medicaid patients any longer but would help transfer my records and would recommend another doctor, if I would call. I called. The recommended doctor is not taking new patients. I have now gone through a whole list of doctors. All of them either are not taking Medicaid patients or they are not taking new patients. I want to find the same kind of doctor everybody needs — one who will talk to me and relate to me as a person.

My experiences with doctors, generally, have not been good at all. When I was young they didn't tell me anything about what they were doing to me. That really frustrated me, and scared me, too. I didn't even know what I was scared of, and that made it even scarier. I was angry that there was nobody listening to me.

I went through a lot of operations without knowing what they were for. They may have helped me, but I do not think so. I think the medical profession is oppressive to handicapped people, especially to women.

I want to talk about my experience in Northampton High School. It was hard for me even to get enrolled. Going to school was frightening and felt really weird, even though an aide went with me, so I didn't have to go alone. It was something I never did before, and I felt different and isolated from everybody else. People didn't know how to talk to me. I wanted to talk with them, but I was afraid.

When I started high school, I was 18. It was hard for me because I felt really dumb. I couldn't read and didn't know my letters at all. I had had teachers at the hospital, but they didn't spend much time with me or teach me skills I could use later on. They did not know how to teach me, and they did not have a lot of patience. They seemed to think they didn't have to teach me anything because they thought I would never go any further than the hospital.

In high school I took a bunch of tests that showed I have dyslexia. All my life I didn't know what was going on or why I had felt stupid. I took reading, math, and history in Special Ed classes. Sometimes I was the only person in a wheelchair, the only person with a visible physical disability. The only class I had that wasn't in Special Ed was art. That was a good experience. Art was something I could do, and so I didn't feel so different and isolated.

My first real teacher was teaching me to read, and I was learning, too. Then he got another job. He taught his wife how to teach me, but then she left to have a baby. She taught someone else how to teach me, but that teacher got me confused because *she* seemed so confused herself.

I went to high school for three and a half years. The only reason I stopped was because, when you turn 21, Chapter 766 won't fund you. I think that is not fair. I don't think anybody's age has anything to do with how long she should go to school if she has a disability.

At the moment I am having trouble relating to my parents. They disagree with what I'm doing. The day I moved to Clark House my mother said, "I wish you would go back to the nursing home." She was worried about my safety. I said, "No! If I go back I won't learn anything, and I will become a vegetable!"

After I moved in, my mother would call and tell my PCA she was coming to see me. One day she called to say she was coming, and it was not an appropriate day for me to see her. My PCA told her to call back and talk to me directly (something my mother *never* does). She told the PCA that, if it wasn't a good day, I could call *her* up and tell her. I tried, but she had already gone. I was angry that she always just assumes I will be here. I left her a note and went out. I didn't do this to be nasty or mean. I still feel guilty for doing it, but I wanted her to learn that I am not always going to be here when she wants me to be. Her assumption is another invasion of my independence.

Some time later, my mother called one day to ask if she could come to visit. I felt good about that, because she had asked me. I felt really good about her visit... until she came into my apartment, came into my room, sat on my bed, and said, "I don't like the situation here." I asked her what the "situation" was. She told me she would be ashamed to bring my grandmother here — my apartment wasn't neat enough — and, she said, she didn't like any of my PCA's. I said, "What's the matter with my PCA's?" "Are they homosexuals?" she asked. (I have trouble with that word — no, actually, I don't. It was just the way she said it.) I answered, "Yes, they are homosexuals." "Are *you?*" she asked. "Yes," I said.

My housemate Viv came in to introduce herself. She put out her hand, and my mother would not even look at her while they shook hands. If I did this to a guest in *her* house, my mother would have a fit.

When we were alone again, my mother cried. Then she asked me straight out, "Will you go back to the nursing home?" It was a plea. "No," I said, "I am very happy where I am." She then placed a call to my sister without asking me if she could use my phone — never mind about asking me if she could tell my sister that I am a lesbian!

I think that was the hardest day in my life. It was hard because I knew my mother has enough problems just dealing with my being physically challenged. She isn't ready to accept me as a lesbian, too. I never thought I would tell her. I am proud of who I am, but I was also scared of what she might do to get me back into the nursing home. At that time, also, I was still looking for her approval. Now I don't look for it as much as I used to. When she was leaving, I called her back because she was obviously having a hard time, and I wanted to hug her. "What do you want?" she said, in a nasty tone. "Forget it," I said.

I sent her a tape recording that told her all my feelings about who I am. I told her what I thought about her telling me that if I come home I cannot bring any of my friends. I felt that, under her conditions, I could not bring my real self either. My mother has not responded to that recorded letter, and she has not been here since. Nor have I been home — not even for Christmas. I sometimes talk with my mother on the phone, but it is like I never sent her that tape eight months ago. I wish it were otherwise.

Now that I am living independently, I do many things for myself. I make dates to go to the movies, or even to the mountains, with friends. I go to concerts and music festivals. I paint. I drive myself all around Amherst. I make phone calls (and it makes me damned angry when peole hang up on me rather than listening more carefully to my way of speaking). I operate my TV, plan my meals, plan my day. I am an employer. I have people read to me because I can not hold a book and can not read myself. Right now, I am reading *Daughters of Copper Woman*.

And now, I write. I didn't know I could. This is the first time I have written anything in my life. I am proud of what I have written. It hangs together and it says important things. It took a lot of courage to write this, but it makes me realize how strong I am.

There are many other things I will be doing for a first time. Each will be a physical adventure for me. That is why I prefer to call myself not "disabled" but "physically challenged."

But what I can do does not make me important to myself. I value people for what they are inside, not for what they can do physically. Don't just assume there isn't anything of value inside me because you haven't bothered to look. And how can I learn what is of value in you, if you don't show it to me?

My Learning Disability And How it Affected Me

by louise avendano johnsen

S ometimes I ask myself: When did it all begin? How did I get myself into so many situations that I so regret today? There are times when I hurt so much.

I spent the early years of my life on Precita Street in San Francisco, in a Victorian flat owned by my grandparents, Juana and Francisco Anguaino. They lived 20 steps up to the first level, with my aunts and uncles who were all teenagers. My cousins lived on the 2nd floor and we lived on the 3rd. The years of the 1950's are my happiest memories. The whole family was always together. I had friends all over the neighborhood. They were good years.

Then came the day we moved to Westlake. I was 8 years old and entering the fourth grade. What a change from the old and friendly San Francisco street I had grown up on.

I was painfully shy and very frightened my first day in my new classroom. My problem in learning became quite evident during that year of my life. When called on to answer an arithmetic question, no matter how simple it was, I wouldn't know the answer. Arithmetic became a nightmare for me. I never got past simple division, multiplication and subtraction. But there were other areas of difficulty as well, such as English grammar and social studies. I couldn't even write book reports, because I couldn't comprehend the reading I was assigned. In no time at all my classmates began to notice this. In this new city, I felt torn apart from everything and everyone I had ever known. I missed my old school, where the kids were warmer. At my new school, the kids were more sophisticated and not too friendly. I was lonely. During lunch, I would sit alone in the schoolyard imagining my old schoolmates right before my very eyes. At times I would cry. But I wouldn't let anyone know. Sometimes the tears were so strong that I'd have to bring my hand to the side of my face to hide them. No one ever seemed to know. I thought I had them fooled. Fifteen years later I learned that they had known all along.

Once I wet my pants in reading class. Mrs. Tubbs, our teacher, pulled up a chair, put her arm around me and sat with me until the class was over. All the while I had a terror of embarassment and shame going through me. I prayed the floor would open up and swallow me whole. My socks were wet. There was a puddle of urine under my chair that the kids across the room could see clearly. But since the other kids never really talked to me or played with me they kept quiet about it. It was almost as if they felt something was wrong with me so they sort of felt sorry for me. No one ever said or mentioned a thing about it. The class was dismissed for lunch and my father came to the school with a change of clothing for me. When he saw me he kissed me and hugged me and told me to please forget what happened. But too many things were happening. I just couldn't forget.

Not that I was an angel. I had a temper. I fought with my sister and my brother. I even stole. One Christmas during the fourth grade, we had the Christmas tree decorated and looking very pretty with all its presents. They were gifts that we students had exchanged. There was a small white box that was so prettily wrapped. It had a large red ribbon around it and red and blue glitter wrapping. I loved it. It looked so pretty, so I took it. When I was alone with the box and had opened it I found a very pretty pen. I was kind of dumb. I used it in class and the child whose parents bought it spotted it on my desk. When Mrs. Tubbs found out, she looked at me with a very stern look and asked me if I would like for my parents to know about this and gave me a good lecture. I stood there with my head down feeling sick and very ashamed at what I had done. I told her I wouldn't want them to know. I don't know, but I think my parents were never told because they never mentioned anything about it to me.

When we rece··ed our report cards at the end of the term, Mrs. Tubbs called me to one side to talk to me about my not passing. She sat me down and gently said, "Louise, you'll be staying in my class for one more year." I sat there with a lump in my throat, having expected this all year. She knew I was breaking up inside and then she smiled at me, and told me that in the fall I was going to do much better, that my arithmetic would be improved by going to summer school.

I didn't say anything, but the pain that hit was very strong. When class was dismissed, all the kids were very happily saying good-bye to one another. I just walked very quickly out of the schoolyard.

All the way home, I had a sick feeling inside of me. I kept wondering, how can I give my report card to Mother? What will she say? Suddenly, there I was. At my front door. I paused for a moment, then I quickly turned the door knob. My mother was sitting on the couch with my brother and sister dancing around her, showing her their report cards. I just stood there. She smiled at me and asked to see my report card. So I handed it to her. She waved off my brother and sister and said that it was my report card she was most proud of. "But, I flunked, Mom. I didn't pass to the fifth grade." She smiled and said, "You just didn't pass to the fifth grade. That's all. But you didn't flunk." I felt a little better. But for the rest of the summer, whenever any of the kids on our block asked how I did, I answered that I flunked, and that I wanted to, so that I could be with my teacher one more year. I explained to them how very much I loved her and that I would miss her too much. Boy! They looked astonished and said "That's crazy!" But I stuck to my story.

I had felt the whole year long that I wasn't going to pass because I wasn't understanding the tests and specifically arithmetic. I had too many problems in spelling as well.

So as Mrs. Tubbs explained to me my problem with arithmetic and spelling, and told me not to worry too much about it because I would do much better in the fall, my deepest feeling was that I was dumb, dumb and stupid. I felt I couldn't understand these subjects simply because I was dumb, for no other reason, regardless of the explanations Mrs. Tubbs gave me.

As the years went on, my mind wandered back to that first year of the fourth grade and Mrs. Tubbs. I often thought of her concern and kindness. Maybe it was because of her that the kids never teased me or made me cry.

I suppose I often thought about it because it was a turning point in my life. Now, having gone through extensive counseling, I know that it was in that year that I began to daydream. It kept me going. I was afraid of reality, and daydreaming was an escape from reality.

One more thing about that year: There was a man that I would meet with in the principal's office in the afternoons once or twice a week. He was tall, with dark hair and dark eyes. I was being tested by placing differently shaped pegs into their fitting places on a board.

During my second year in fourth grade, I began to blossom a little. I was making friends. I even made a home run while playing kickball during recess and my team hailed me as their hero. Also, I was excelling in spelling. In arithmetic, I was still bad. But I was learning division and subtraction a little better. Still in all, the idea that I flunked still bothered me. It haunted me through that year and throughout the rest of my school years. However, the second time around, when the term was up, I passed on to the fifth grade. I was quite relieved, but had I known what waited for me in the fifth grade year, God help me, I would not have wanted to pass. In less than one month the kids in this class found out my problem with arithmetic and they also found out I could not tell time. They called me a flunkie for not having passed the fourth grade. I was subjected to malicious ridicule and practical jokes. My daydreaming increased. Whereas in the second year of the fourth grade, I was beginning to catch on to arithmetic, here, I completely withdrew from it and was finally taken out of it completely. I was given remedial reading instead. When I left that year behind me, I knew for certain that I would never be able to conquer arithmetic. My self confidence, whatever little I had tried to gain from the second year of the fourth grade, was completely deteriorated. Gone.

As the years went on, for some reason, I kept remembering the testing I had undergone in the fourth grade. At the time it had been a relief to be away from the classroom where I felt so lonely and so strange. I never questioned why it happened. I was shocked and amazed to learn that my parents were never informed of this testing I was undergoing. I also found out that my sister and brother had been similarly tested.

It was the 1950's and early 60's. Things were a lot different then. People were narrow minded and very discriminating. Life was supposed to be sugar and candy and lily-white. We were the only Latins at the school. Therefore, we were stereotyped.

Again, I could understand why I was being tested. But my sister and brother tested? You've got to be kidding. They were A students. How could they have been given those awful tests? I say awful because the tests were to be for children with learning disabilities, not for children who had no problems in learning, such as my sister and brother. So now it looks different. It angers me. I know now that we were being tested just because we were of Mexican descent.

My mother made me understand something. She asked me how I would have felt if I had known from the beginning *why* the tests were being given to me. How would I have felt then had I known that I wasn't the only child in my family being tested?

Maybe I still would have found it hard to learn. A learning disability is a very hard thing to overcome. I grew up downing myself for not having been smart in my school years. But that's the breaks. During my senior year of high school one day, I was talking to a math teacher. She told me that one day in the years to come the school system would have ways to deal with children who had learning disabilities, that these children would be recognized as children with special problems.

I happened to be a child who was recognized as being mentally retarded. The teachers felt I should have been in a home for the mentally retarded. This nearly ruined my adult years. I had no independence at all, no self-confidence. I got married twice. Both men dominated me. My second husband dominated my life for seven years. He also felt that I was not a very intelligent woman. Of course, his perception of me was partly my fault. I had downed myself so much that I never dreamed there could be a side of me that was strong and determined. But then again, strength must have been in me all along. It was a mightly struggle. I knew I would have to work. But do what? I just didn't know. But I had to try.

My first job was working in a newspaper office. People would write to the clipping bureau asking for articles from the newspaper. There were cutters, the women who would cut out the articles. Then there were pasters. I was a paster. The clippings were given to me on large sheets and I would paste them onto the headings with the company's name. It was a miserable job. I left there after six months and went to work as a file clerk for an insurance company. As the years went on I worked my way up to being a secretary. Today I work as a secretary for the Federal Reserve Bank of San Francisco. For the first time in all my years of working, I have a boss who has taken an interest in me. She has worked hard to help me understand the technicalities of my job and has always told me not to be afraid of making mistakes. Many women my age (34) have made it way up the ladder. I couldn't go that far, but with my boss and all her support, there is hope for me yet.

My Supervisor has also been a wonderful supporter. She has also made me believe that I can make it. Both women helped me a great deal with my job and made me feel confident.

Actually, I really started learning for the first time in my life, learning to live, after my second husband and I divorced. I finally started becoming strong and independent. I wanted to survive. My problem was that I always wanted to be married because I never thought I was good alone, as a single person. I needed someone to take care of me, because I felt someone else could take better care of me than myself. It wasn't an easy road. I wouldn't do it over again to save my life.

After my divorce, I swore that my 30's would not be like the years in my 20's. I had to make them different. I never had belief in myself. This time to compensate for being alone, I went to night school to take the subjects I never learned in my grade school years. Today I find that learning and concentrating is still hard for me. But it's different this time. The class that I am taking deals with learning problems. Trying to learn arithmetic is not the nightmare that it once was for me. I have also taken to writing. With the support of my instructor, and her belief in me, I decided to write about my problem. It also prompted me to fulfill a dream of mine. That dream was to contact my fourth grade teacher, Mrs. Tubbs.

I traced her husband's phone number and left a message with his secretary. Mrs. Tubbs called me one day later. The reunion with her was the most enjoyable event of my whole life. We were together for 2½ hours during my lunch hour. She met me in the lobby of where I work. I couldn't believe it. She was just as beautiful as I remembered her to be.

When she saw me, she laughed as she put her arms around me,

saying that I still had the same face. We hugged and hugged and then we went to lunch. She showed me the message that was left for her husband and she told me that she had immediately remembered it was me. She had never forgotten me either, and had always wondered about me.

She wanted to know how I felt about her for not passing me? Did I grow to dislike her for having done that? I told her that never could I ever dislike her. She explained to me that she was afraid to pass me because she felt that I could have been eaten up alive. She said she never flunked me for being dumb. That was my thinking. She said she tried so hard for me not to think in those terms, but I was so sensitive and vulnerable that no one could really make me believe that I was just fine, and as smart as anyone else. She said that she could see me sitting there at my desk staring at everything around me. She could see the fright in me and worried about what would happen to me when I became an adult. Mrs. Tubbs smiled at me and said that I didn't turn out to be such a little mouse after all. I smiled back and said that it took some work. She told me that growing up always takes some work. The important thing is to do it.

Being with her opened up so much of what I had always been thinking about those years and, of course, my always wishing that I could see her. I had brought my camera along and took her picture, and one of the two of us together. I even brought her back to the office and introduced her to my co-workers. It was a wonderful time for me. When we parted we promised to stay in touch.

These last two years since my husband and I parted have not been the easiest. The realization of having to deal with my self-esteem was one of the hardest things I ever had to face, along with learning to assert myself, to work for a better life, to learn, and to be more careful of men and love, to never have another broken heart again. I guess it takes a while to let go of the past.

As a teenager and adult, what troubled me the most was the idea that I wasn't good enough, that I was too thin and not intelligent. I felt too small. Everyone I came in contact with could see that I had no self-confidence.

This especially became obvious with the first man I fell in love with after I'd been separated from my husband for eight months. He was everything I had ever wanted. This man was so boyish and charming and so calm. He always made me laugh. But I never felt I was enough to measure up to him. He was going to San Francisco State College studying to become a physical therapist. This put me ill at ease, because my schooling was nothing and I felt my job, being just a secretary, was something too simple. I began to cling more and more to him, feeling I had nothing in my life without him. This all became too much for him. At the end of six months when he told me gently that it was all over, I thought that the whole world had caved in. There was no life left in me.

The heartbreak was a very traumatic experience. But it taught me something. That once and for all I had to stop downing myself. It started in the fourth grade and now I had to put an end to it. All I could do after everything was over was to let time pass. As one month after another passed, I began to breathe again. I took a vacation to Mexico. There I found solace and a peace I had never known.

I took taxis and shopped in Mexico all by myself. My Spanish got better. I had gone with some friends of my family and decided to venture off by myself, and found I could do it after all. I even checked into the most beautiful hotel and found out there wasn't any sadness being by myself after all. I had thought that once I would be by myself in the hotel room that memories of my husband and the recent heartbreak would make me feel very sad. As it turned out I enjoyed being alone. It wasn't so bad after all.

A man I met before my trip started to become important to me. I sent him a postcard from Mexico and when I returned he called me. I began to see him. After three months he began to remind me of the man who had hurt me so much. It was the ways that this man had, his flightiness and care-free ways. This time I was not going to go through it again. So I stopped seeing him. When I did that, I refused to look back. I went on and applied as a volunteer for the DeYoung Museum at Golden Gate Park. I felt I should learn about the arts. What a wonder. Now I'll be working with the Vatican Exhibition and I didn't even know it at the time when I applied. When my interview with the DeYoung was over, I then went to Macy's and had my hair (already short) restyled. The hairdresser liked the new style on me so much that she asked me to be a part of the hair fashion show Macy's was putting on. Me, scared stiff, accepted the offer. To my delight, it turned out to be magnificent for me. It helped me deal with my shyness and sensitivity. I became more self-assured and really began liking and enjoying myself for the first time in my life. I felt a control come over me such as I had never known before.

My writing also helped me. There were things I didn't like finding out about, such as the reason for the testing. Discrimination will go on. The important thing I should look at is the fact that it released the crutches that I leaned on throughout my life since. I should always bear in mind that no matter how hard the going gets, pain, mistakes, and wrong decisions that I will sometimes make as I go on, that no matter what, the world is not going to end. This time, I will not be so hard on myself for failing at times. I have learned that the worst thing about failure or mistakes is to not have learned from them.

I have learned to forgive myself and the wrong choices that I have made during my life. I have learned to understand and to let go.

It's all behind me now.

Glimpse Into
A Transformation

by ernestine amani patterson

*e*ven today, a little over four years after I began having my hair braided in cornrows, a few nervy women still come up to me and say: "Your hair is very pretty. But it's too bad you can't see how nice the style is and how colorful the beads are." And while I'm used to having insults veiled in compliments passing my way, I kinda thought I would never hear *that* one in connection with my blindness and the re-discovery of the African hairstyle which continues to be a source of great personal happiness to me. But having answered so many, many questions like it, I always say nowadays: "But each style has its own shape. And though the beads are a different color, many of them also have their own touch." This is quite true, because they are glass, wood, and plastic beads. These are further divided into varying tactile textures. And although I haven't gotten into them yet, you can purchase semi-precious gem beads, and they have their flavor, too.

And if I am wearing bells in my hair when these remarks are made, I shake my head a little so they can hear the jingle; hopefully they'll get the message. In fact, it was because I had encountered a young woman at school whose braids fairly sang with bells that I vowed I would quit pressing my hair for at least one time and try the cornrows. And as a kind of good omen, my classmate, one day when the lecture was over, gave me a small plastic bag containing about fifty sweet, high-noted pieces of bell-shaped metal. *That* did it. There was no way I was going to let such wonderful objects go unused. In my spare time, I would rattle them, listening to the beautiful notes they made, and was reminded of what I was seeking.

My quest was not easy, though. Beauticians and everyday people gave me a boatload of information, some of it deliberately discouraging, the rest offered out of ignorance. They'd say: "I've never seen anybody I liked that style on. It makes you look — I don't know — just doesn't look right." Others would say: "I heard you lose a lot of your hair, and people say it itches, too whenever you get them — so badly that you have to take them down." But the worst was: "Your hair is too short."'

This short hair business always caused me grief. The people unmistakably referred to the short stubborn crop of peculiar hair in the very back, close to my neck. It was said more than once to me that my being mischievous with the scissors as a youngster stunted its growth, and I had always felt guilty about having done it. My classmate said, however, that cornrowing was just what the back of my hair needed. Nobody paid the least bit of attention to this assertion, least of all me.

By the time I had resigned myself to being trapped in failure, I ran across someone I'd met several years previously. She was Mrs. Eunice Younger, a Liberian women, who owned a most exotic African artifacts shop near my neighborhood. She had married a Black American and seemed to be doing quite well for herself. I had thought her shop sold only imports. But as a friend and I talked with her, and I discovered she did this kind of braiding, I immediately made an appointment with her for the end of that week.

"You know," I said, somewhat disappointed about having to remove my head from the dryer, "I really wish I could have braids. But you can press it as we planned until it grows out." I was admiring the warm and friendly fragances of oil, shampoo, and conditioners that beauty parlors seem to love to stock.

I suspect she was just as eager for me to have braids as I was to get them, because she said: "Let's try it." It was a happy shock for me. I certainly didn't think I'd actually leave there wearing braids. It would come to my mind as she worked: *What if we come to the point where we must break off?* The back *was* a problem, because it really was too short to braid. But since she had already braided the rest, and was such a clever styler — an artist, really — she pinned the back portion into curls with small bobby-pins.

"When you take these out," she said, referring to the bobby-pins, "the curls will last for awhile. Then they'll come out, but that will be because your hair is growing. Next time, I think I'll be able to braid the back."

The compliments on my new look were so overwhelming that, when the curls did come out and I got a few uncharitable remarks about what remained of them, I put it down to pettiness. And though I experienced some itching, I told my hair: "You're only adjusting to this new way; you'll get used to it." Sure enough, the itching stopped. And the best part was the next time I visited Mrs. Younger, the back part was braidable. Ever since that time, this previously troublesome portion of hair has entered into a burst of growing and shows no signs of abating.

Funny thing, though. I can't remember what Eunice and I talked about on that first visit. I must have asked her about her family, what her impressions of America were, and how her business was prospering. I, in turn, probably spoke of my radio show, of going to school, and my ever-amusing cat. And doubtless, I had questions about the care of my new style. But nothing of the talk we surely had remains with me, for I was totally entranced with the little bites and tuggings of the comb as it parted and untangled, and the feel of the motions of Mrs. Younger's fingers braiding up and down along my scalp. Whenever her phone rang, I would sneak a rub and think wonderingly to myself: "I'm going to look this good for about a month? Wow! It couldn't be this easy, could it? All I have to do is get up in the morning and step out the door and not do *anything* to my hair? *Wow!*"

Ever since I was a child having to skip swimming classes in the therapeutic pool for disabled and blind children at the small town public school I attended, I had wished in a vague inconsistent way to find a hairstyle or something which would let me sweat, walk in the rain, or hang out in the bathtub or pool or lake till my skin got wrinkly and I wanted to get out. I say vaguely and inconsistently, because back then I knew no way out of this dilemma. It's true that later on in my life, the natural had come. But it never seemed to suit me too well. In any case, once I got my first braids I realized I would no longer have to smell the peculiar, almost acrid odor of metal combs heating and hair frying. And I could forego the fear of being burned by permanents or anything else. That was fine with me. And halleluia, at least as Cobbs and Greer pointed out in the book, *Black Rage*, I could avoid some of the psychological damage that many Black women incur when they try altering their hair to imitate that of white women.

Of course, people are still the same — inevitable and specific in their cruelty — "Your hair is pretty," or "Your dress is pretty." The lines between womanhood and blindness are never supposed to meet. And with Blackness on top of that, what must people be seeing! And although I seldom hear: "*You* are looking nice," I am not the same, even if they are. Since that Saturday in the shop with the wooden floor and squeaky steps, where the heater had to be turned on against the chilly morning, I have always looked forward to the bus ride and short walk there. Mrs. Younger has not only increased her clientele, other girlfriends of hers from Africa help out with the hair. So it's lovely talking to all of them. And since most of these women are used to me now, we relate as Black sisters who, despite the shortness of time allotted to us, have come together. And though this was not a first step in my growth, mine is actually a case wherein the style of my hair altered the shape of my head within. How many women can say that with satisfaction about *any* beauty treatment they try?

This Script Is Very Private

by nanci stern

I'll haunt you when I'm dead you know
Especially when laughter pours from
   crowded ceilings
Into rooms silly with tingling
I'll haunt you like I do when I am living
With blank eyes that stare inside you
With food too decadent for thoughts
With rhymes of times we will love forever
I shall make an excellent ghost,
For I have studied the subject most
   effectively
Everyone should die at home of course
Covered in patchwork comfort
Pushing the same old tails out of
   your mouth of the
Ever present flea bitten beasts
Pre-Purina stuffed by your own hand
All dignified deaths write wills I'm told
Preserving the sanctity of dignity
   I shall leave:
Baskets of endless ripe cherries
   for all those who will eat them
Trips to everywhere for those who will
   travel

Boxes of love for those who will dare to
   open them and
Healthy days until there are none
I shall watch again with both eyes open
Choosing them, losing them, closing them
Only for sleeping or
Winking one maybe to surprise the eyes of
   Somebody watching me
On some special occasion, in some other
   place
I shall climb up the crow's nest,
   Waving a sword in my hand
Shouting over and over again
LAND HO!

5.

This Body I Love
— Finding Ourselves —

Our bodies are our most precious and often our only possessions. They have also been the recipients of such tremendous pain and anguish that many disabled women have dissociated our bodies from our "real" selves. Our bodies have been the targets of medical abuse. We have been hospitalized and have spent years in doctors' offices and still our bodies have not cooperated. Some of us live in chronic pain, some with chronic unpredictability and others with chronic stares. We have felt the deep personal invasion of surgeries and endless diagnostic procedures. Sometimes we feel as though our bodies are trying to kill us. They betray us in our struggle to resist patriarchal desires for "feminine weakness".

We need to see our bodies as worthy parts of our selves in order to invest the time and energy it takes to care for ourselves. Society works directly against this possibility. We are regarded as "defects", as women with something "wrong" with us. Specialists trained to treat one or another of our body parts have contributed to our dismembered body images. Value judgements are assigned to our "good" and "bad" parts. Health is seen as a virtue, disease as evil and ugly. Our integrity as persons has been undermined.

Feminine beauty is manufactured by cosmetic and fashion industries and changes seasonally. Our self worth suffers when we respond to this sexual objectification. Disabled women have been excluded from patriarchal conceptions of beauty and sexuality. Again, we are encouraged to see our bodies and our selves as distinct. Our beauty is reserved for the inside. Inner beauty is used by our culture as a consolation prize for those it finds ugly. Symmetry, clear eyes, straight limbs and fingers, uniform pigmentation and smooth motions are prerequisites for outer beauty, no matter what else may be popular. People jeer at us. We may not be able to find appropriate clothing for the outside and are advised not to call too much attention to our "flaws" with bright or fashionable adornments. Prostheses, canes, hearing aids, wheelchairs and braces are not designed with aesthetics in mind. Our individuality is not encouraged or appreciated.

We claim our bodies and our integrity as disabled women. We insist on our right to make informed decisions about our bodies. We do not have good parts, bad parts or inner beauty. We come in many sizes, shapes and colors. Our bodies deserve our love, tenderness and pleasure. We are whole, beautiful and sexy women!

"Do Something About Your Weight"

by carol schmidt

"**Y**ou have such a pretty face — why don't you do something about your weight?" "Don't you know the medical consequences of obesity? Do something about your weight," or "We can't hire you until you do something about your weight." The usual criticisms fat women hear imply that it is *possible* to "do something about your weight." I tried. Everything known to medical science: intestinal bypass and stomach stapling and total fasting and pills and shots and hypnosis and diet candies and 15 stints at Weight Watchers and almost as many at Overeaters Anonymous.. No one ever told me to "do something" about my green eyes or brown hair or 5'8" frame, only about the 300 pounds, give or take 100 pounds at any one time, on that frame.

Only the fat liberation movement accepts the idea that obese people don't have much of a choice — except at some stage to finally accept that we will never be thin, and urge people to stop lining the wallets of the diet industry anymore. The side affects of attempting to lose weight by almost every method can be worse than the "problem," which is mainly in the eyes of the beholder anyway. If there were no discrimination against fat people, almost all my problems would be solved — except for the remaining consequences of the "choices" I've made in my life-long struggle to be thin. I've always lost — not weight, but other valuables, mainly my health.

Very briefly in the '50s I was thin as a teenager, when I grew a foot in a year and it took awhile for the weight to reestablish itself. During those few years I lived on lettuce and coffee, and once convinced myself I had had a heart attack because of the heart palpitations from so much coffee. I worked three part-time jobs, raised my sister because my mom was usually in mental hospitals, and got through a Catholic women's college while weighing about 230. It was impossible to keep up that regimen on coffee and lettuce, and I was cooking for a factory worker father and my sister and mother (who weighed about 400 pounds when she committed suicide in 1969). My family fit the textbooks of family therapists who note that there is always one "identified patient" in a crazy-making family, and when my mother died, I became "it". She was always pointed out to me as my worst possible role model — and I rejected a lot of good things about her in my frenzy to be as unlike her as possible. What a choice.

In 1975 I was married and living in Los Angeles with a "hippie" style hubby who worked part-time in a tropical fish store that dealt drugs on the side, and I was trapped in a job at a medical journal publishing house where I could hide out in a back office and interview doctors by phone for my articles. At this point I decided to once and for all "do something about my weight." That something was intestinal bypass surgery, and I was not one of the 1-6% who die outright on the operating table in this surgery, though that was a chance I was willing to take. I was that miserable. More than anything it was the economic discrimination — I was stuck in that back office making $1000 a month less than I deserved for the rest of my life unless I did "something." Who knew the consequences? Who was told all the consequences? But as I said, I wouldn't have cared — I but I did have a choice — I had been able to get a job, and had medical insurance. A lot of fat women have absolutely no chances at employment and cannot be covered by medical insurance. I've had to make a lot of decisions about my life based around how I could still hold on to health insurance; I am sure I would be doing better self-employed as a writer, or at least would be happier, but in this age of massive health costs and due to my past health record, I am tied to my insurance plan. This is a common thread in the lives of differently abled women.

After the intestinal bypass surgery, I wanted to die — from the hemorrhoids. Who would have thought that undigested food racing through only 14 inches of small intestine, in big chunks with pure stomach acid, would rip through the bowels and explode in diarrhea that tore open the blood vessels? I spent three weeks almost non-stop on the toilet crying. My husband went out and had an affair.

Then it was wonderful — I became a spokesperson for the joys of intestinal bybass! I lost 165 pounds, and all was well — until the odor started.

Apparently a lot of bypass patients develop infections in the bypassed 22 feet of small intestine, which is just lying there, waiting in case it must someday be reconnected (today almost all bypass patients have been reconnected and almost no one still does the surgery). The diarrhea had always smelled, but now there was something else. A terrible odor, that came out of my mouth and every pore and drove people away. I couldn't go to the bathroom at work — I had to drive home for every bout of diarrhea. No one came into my office — my editors worked with me by phone. I didn't even know that I had the odor until finally my therapist told me, and worked with me on a plan to attack the problem. My doctor didn't believe the problem existed, in his nicely aerated, air conditioned office — and the odor would come and go, to make it worse. I never knew if I smelled or not. I took a friend to the theatre and had to sit on the steps by the door, because the people around me were gagging and leaving the theatre, and my friend couldn't drive home with me with all the car windows wide open.

After hundreds of remedies, I discovered that one medication, flagyl, stopped the odor — but then it was implicated in breast cancer, and no one was supposed to take more than one or two doses a year. I had been on it for months. I transferred to tetracycline, raising to higher and higher doses, until I was taking 3000 milligrams a day. This was a good period in my life, despite working my schedule around the timing for the tetracycline, which I could only take when I had not eaten or had any milk for many hours, nor planned any food intake.

My husband couldn't take the changes, or my newly awakened sexuality, or the fact that now I was clearly superior to him on many arenas. He moved out. I got a divorce and did a complete changearound and obtained my present job, when I was "down" to 185 lbs, the thinnest I had ever been since age 14.

Then a new lover told me I smelled, and I realized the tetracycline no longer worked. Nothing new worked. No doctor in the country knew what to do about this medical complication of intestinal bypass, which was cropping up in patient after patient. I made an appointment to have the bypass reversed and stomach stapling substituted.

Stomach stapling was the new wonder operation, for those of us who finally decided to "do something about our weight." There are several approaches, with slightly different names, but they all involve the principal of either stapling most of the stomach shut so that only a tiny amount of food can be eaten at one time, or wrapping the stomach or both. I had both. Somewhere during the operation my stomach perforated. This is the same as a bullet wound inside the stomach — gallons of unclean food particles mixed with stomach acids shot through my abdomen. This caused peritonitis.

I almost died. The doctor told my lover and sister I had an 80% chance of dying in the second surgery to repair the perforated stomach, and then I might not make it through the infections to follow. I did.

I don't even want to think about the month in the hospital, the weeks in intensive care, unable to talk because of the tube down my throat, my friends and loved ones trying not to show how scared they were. An attorney came in and had me sign some legal papers in case I died; I didn't have a will (I do now, and recommend them to all women, no matter how healthy.)

I came out of this operation with an open wound the size and shape of a layer cake pan, left wide open down to the intestines, that had to be cleaned out with Betadyne every few hours and fresh bandages applied while the body rebuilt the wound from the bottom layer and edges. I could walk at this stage, short distances, hunched over. I was running for Vice President of California NOW, and before I went up to make my nomination speech I oozed blood and Betadyne from the eight-inch-across wound, all over my new pants suit. I couldn't take the infighting and politicking of the meeting, and I walked out of NOW before the speeches, my life in quite a different perspective from when I had first put out my name as a candidate.

All of my life has a quite different perspective today. The health problems did not end once I healed from that operation — I developed a massive hernia that made me look ten months pregnant, a huge disfigurement. No surgeon wanted to operate, because my insides were a mass of adhesions and scar tissues, but I finally found one who would. I have been ordered not to gain a single pound because the hernia repair (which involved putting in an 18-inch-square piece of strong mesh under the skin to keep in the intestines) could rip open. I am again trying to "do something about my weight."

I do not lack discipline — I work hard, I've accomplished a lot in my life, especially considering my background and my fat. I don't even have to justify to anyone why I do not fit the stereotype of fat women — it's the stereotype which is wrong. And too many feminists and our supposed political allies hold the stereotype just as strongly as those we know do not understand. I go out to dinner with a radical feminist who happens to be thin and I see she is watching every bite I eat and mentally counting calories for me — and it is not my paranoia which makes me think this. I have checked it out with some people, and they shamefacedly admit it — if they don't take the opportunity to tell me *I* should be doing it.

There are no real choices for obese people, and other differently abled people, at least not the range of choices that many others have. We do the best we can with what we've got, considering what we can and cannot do, and stretch the boundaries at all times, attempting to distinguish the real limitations from those which we or others impose on us. Sometimes it is an entirely different ballpark from the game being played by those who tell *us* to "do something" about a problem that makes *them* uncomfortable.

Keep Crying and Screaming — You'll Get More Air

by julie taylor

i was born in Massachusetts. I had asthma but nobody knew what it was then. When I was two we had moved to California and I was sick all the time. The doctors then figured out I had asthma. By the time I was three I would have to go to the hospital every time I had an asthma attack, which varied, sometimes once a week, sometimes once a month. When I would get to the hospital, I would have to get an I.V., which I did not like. I remember once I didn't want the doctors to stick the needle in my arm or foot (I had a choice) and I was kicking all around. So finally they strapped me down on a table so I couldn't move at all and put in the I.V. I was very mad.

I remember small unimportant things like rolling my I.V. over to the window to say "hi" to my friends, who were too young to visit. Or things like, every time I went to the hospital my mom and I would sing the song "Oklahoma."

But there's one thing which I don't remember and that is when I was four, I almost died. My mom just told me a year ago when I was eleven. Before that I didn't know. This is what she told me:

I got really sick, she brought me to the hospital. They gave me an I.V. and paged my doctor. But he wasn't in the hospital so they tried to get him where he was. By this time my dad had come. It took a while to get my doctor and when he finally came everybody was worried because I was getting worse.

The minute he came back he started telling people what to do. He sat by my head and talked to me. I was screaming and crying and he was saying, "Keep crying and screaming you get more air if you do."

Well, I don't know how long this was going on, but it got to the point where he asked somebody to get the (I can't remember the word), which is a thing that they stick down your throat, and it breathes for you. The only problem is that it is very dangerous for kids because it can easily pop an air sack and that would cause more trouble.

Several times they were going to put it on me but didn't. I ended up not having to use it. I stayed in the hospital for a while and got out when I was well enough to leave.

When I was in fifth grade, I couldn't have P.E. classes with everybody else. I would play with this other girl who also couldn't have P.E. because of something with her eyes.

I feel that I would be very different if I didn't have asthma. I think I would be much more active and I wouldn't be as shy and quiet. I would be more limber or stretched out and stronger. And I know I'd have a pet of some kind.

Over the years, I have gradually gotten better and I can now have P.E. classes.* I have gotten so I get sick maybe twice a year, and when I do, I can handle it myself and I don't have to go to the hospital. I also got my first pet (a hamster) six months ago and I haven't gotten sick because of her yet.

I still do have asthma but I'm going to an acupuncturist who is helping me get rid of my asthma forever. I am learning to understand my asthma so I can help myself get better. And maybe the next time I do something like this I won't have a handicap.

There is a game that I have, and you have to pick a card. One of the cards says: "If you were a doctor what would your practice be? Why?" I would always say that I would help people with asthma because I know what it's like and I can understand their feelings. I would know what to do to make them more comfortable until they get well. If I ever do become a doctor, I will help people with asthma.

*I'm twelve now but I will turn thirteen on November 10.

Remembering

by jill lessing

*a*lone with myself, I'm aware of remembering, and the need to write something down of an old experience. To get it out. To get it out of my body. Lift it out. Transform the pain. Lift the pain from all our lives.

Lost. Left alone in a corridor.

I remember my first strange and terrifying night in the hospital. I am a big girl now, almost five, and suddenly I'm trapped behind these bars. This bed's so big, so high off the ground. I'm alone and it's dark. I've been crying and screaming for a long time, but it does no good. I'm a trapped prisoner here, my freedom and my dignity stripped away. Why, oh why did they leave me here like this? Mommy! Daddy!

Where are they taking me? Wheeling me in this dreaded bed in the middle of the night. A nurse comes, without much reassurance.

I'm still crying, an exhausted kind of whimpering now. This bed is such a disgrace. I feel degraded and ashamed to be in it. How could they do this to me? I'm indignant.

Later, I somehow manage to sleep — worn out from pleading for help with no answer.

The next day is warm, the sun is out. But I am stuck here in these stupid clothes. Everything is new and frightening. I don't understand all the things they're doing to me. None of it feels good. Most of it hurts, invades, pricks. I'm completely dazed by now — can't keep awake.

Suddenly everything is moving so fast. White, starched shuffling. Flat on my back, whisked and wheeled down halls. The motion of the gurney exhilarating. My legs are shaking and so are my arms and my sides and my belly. My legs are shaking so hard I'm afraid everyone who looks at me will see the white sheet shaking. The sheet is shaking so hard I'm sure they think I'm crazy. I'm so scared I can't stop shaking. My body has her own mind.

Nurses keep coming over to check on me. I'm stranded here in the hall waiting and shaking.

[Years later, a shrink tells me I had been "hysterical".]

Finally, I'm being wheeled in. They lift me onto a table. Cold. Lights. Mirrors. Lights all over me, lights in my eyes. People moving in over me, talking. My doctor is so sterile and strange looking as he bounds into the room. he shouts happily, "So here's my little Jill!"

Before I know it I'm strapped down. I can't move my arms. A large, dark mask slowly begins to descend over my face. I'm terrified — over my mouth, over my nose. I can't breathe. I hold my breathe. Don't breathe! This stuff stinks. Hold it. Hold your breath... hold... it... a spinning, swirling vortex is drawing me in. Pulling me down, down under. Wave upon wave of a sickening churning at the pit of my stomach. I'm being swallowed. Devoured into a great void of nothingness.

A thick, cloying blackness surrounds me. I'm caught in it's web, the weave only seems to expand with my breath. At each exhale the strands wrap tighter and tighter, pressing me down with a vice grip on my chest.

The medical squadron checks my bodily functions. My vitality shouts back at their calm, poised, ready-for-action theater. Draped and covered, cordoned off, my body now in sections, there for the taking.

The blackness seems to be receding and I'm aware of swirling colors creating an opening at the bottom of the vortex through which I am being pulled. Suddenly, I am floating weightlessly, hovering above the operating table. I feel scared as I don't think I want to be seeing all this. I hear them talking but I don't really understand. I look over and see through the set of open double doors. There is an operation going on in the next room. My fear mounts as I realize there is also an operation going on in here.

The cold, steel blade slowly descends, skillfully wielded in the hands of a hundred years of medical heritage. My doctor artfully etches a foot-long French curve into my skin, extending from around the top of my hip socket down to my thigh. As the layers of flesh are peeled back, rivulets of thick, red blood spurt and pour, spilling my life's mystery with a flowing force. The medical team races to hold back the rushing tide. Stopping, clamping, sponging.

Mommy! Mommy! How could you leave me here like this?

For a moment I imagine myself back at home, playing and having fun. I remember how it feels when I fall down, my hip dislocating, and I have to lie on the ground for a while, wiggling and twisting, until my hips goes back into place. Maybe now, the doctor can fix my hip so I can walk without falling — like other kids.

I begin to feel calmer as I notice that I actually feel okay up here on the ceiling. I can just hide and watch.

I look down, against my better judgement. Large metal contraptions are now poking out of my hip joint and I see the bones being pulled apart. Hammering. Scraping. The chiseling of bone chips. My doctor looks like a sculptor wielding his large mallet. I can't believe the child on the table reeling against each blow is actually me. Pounding. Pounding. The bones are being molded into a new setting. Pounding. Pounding. I feel the shocking blows, the earth tremors in my bones.

Slowly I'm aware of waking up, though I can't open my eyes. I hear voices and I feel something hard all around me. They're talking but they don't know I'm listening. I try to speak but nothing comes out. I need them to know I'm awake! Maybe they're still operating! My hands are strapped down to the sides, which I discover because I can only wiggle my fingers. My legs are paralyzed inside hard casings. I can't move at all; I can't speak at all. I listen. Maybe that way I'll discover what's going on. I listen. I listen hard. I realize they are still covering me with this plaster casting.

Finally — the words I've been repeating over and over inside my head burst out — I'm awake! Hey! I'm awake here!

The doctor reassures me that it's okay. They are just finishing up. My panic subsides for the moment.

I fall in and out of sleep then. The merciful, healing sleep of the traumatized.

After sleeping in the recovery room, the nurses wheel me to "my" room. The nurses here are nuns and wear special white habits. This is a Catholic hospital. At home we don't think much about religion, but when we do we're Jews. The huge pictures of Jesus in the halls are dark and strange.

Mom and Dad are waiting for me in the hall. When they see me, my mother just about goes nuts. No one told any of us what to expect *after* surgery.

I'm spread eagle on the gurney. A plaster cast covers my body from my waist to my toes on both legs. The front and back are cut away so I can use a bed pan. My mother is crying a lot now — for her baby. Me. My only concern at the moment is the mounting nausea growing in my stomach. Just as I get to the refuge of my new home, the hospital room, I can no longer hold back the force of the sickening feeling inside.

I heaved and retched for hours. Throwing up even when there was nothing to come out but the burning memories of the vile ether dreams, the stench of my body's rebellion, searching for survival.

As the waves subsided I could taste my own exhaustion which was driving me to seek the sweet oblivion of unconsciousness, of sleep. It helped that my mother made them take down the large dark cross with Jesus on it that had hung right over my bed. It made me scared and sad. But my dreams were still uneasy, filled with the strange sounds and shapes of fear, of pain. And, in fact, when the ether finally wore off the searing reality hit full force. I couldn't move from the waist down for one thing and the burning pain was excruciating, almost to the point of madness. I soon learned to cry and scream at great length to be able to receive the sanity-inducing injections that brought me release. And soon enough I developed the need for sleep to wipe away the pain, even if only temporarily. If I could only sleep — it wouldn't hurt. Dreams wove in and out — of my mother holding me, stroking my back, whispering that I would be all right. Making me safe with her presence, her love.

Oh Mother, please don't leave me! I'll be good. Don't leave me here all alone. I won't cry and make you feel bad. Just keep me company.

In my dreams my body and mind remember. I bargain with the fates to let my mother and father stay with me in exchange for which I'll be strong. I'm so mixed up, Mom. I only know that I feel pain when I see the pain on your face and it's too much for me. I need to hide, to stop it, to make it go away from both of us. I will be strong for you, Mom. I won't let it show. We'll both be safe and I know you'll stay. Please stay.

I cried so loudly an actor from a nearby room sent me flowers. Years later now, I look back at the strength of that little girl me, and marvel at her endurance. Olympic champions, all of us, without medals.

And, sometimes, even yet, with as much ferocity as then, my body's enduring anger clamps shut tight against the onslaught remembered.

When I was seven, I asked God why I had been chosen. The answer came: to understand the pain, to help others. And now I know it has also been to love. To love life with the same intensity I once used to survive.

Age and Image

by rene ungerecht

*M*orning. I'm awake too early, like always, awaiting the sound of the key entering the lock; the scratch-clack of metal against metal interrupting me. He comes on time, like everyday, starting the tireless routine.

I come back away from the night-world or whatever it is since I go there when I can, not just at night. He greets me. I respond automatically, unconsciously. I'm still not ready to leave the night-world and start the pain. But he's ready; it's his job.

He bitches about his fatty gut. I look at his body, thinking about my first life. If I had his body, I would run like in my first life: I can feel the ice-cold pain in my lungs, the grabbing twisting of my shin muscles, and the only sounds I hear are my even breaths, the drum-ming of blood gushing in my head, and pound-pound-flop-flop of my shoes on the feet-beaten grasses.

But I died eleven years ago. The runner legs are still connected to my body but dead, immobile. He turns the runner-legs over, straightening the left one that spasms almost away from him. Chit-chat as he bathes my fattening, spreading body. The rough wash cloth scratching across an unfeeling body, my body. He's going wallpaper shopping today.

I try to remember what I'm doing today; sometimes it gets hard to separate my first life from my second life: quad life. I keep thinking how I'd like to stand up and walk away to a shower, wash away my night-sweat, drown the intrusive memories. But I'm a quad now. An eleven-year-old quad. We don't let the first life hurt us at this age. I have a position and identity to reflect.

The shine of the wheelchair in the corner catches me. I forget the conversation; he remembers that I forget and lets me go. Hateful shine.

A paradox: the electric monster with wheels and cushions, my machine to freedom or the technology of slow psychic death?

Tubes to let me piss, gloved fingers to let my shit, pass me by as I focus on the wheelchair. He laughs and teases me about the cloudy urine, the tenacious feces; he doesn't want to remember how real it is; he doesn't want me to cry. He knows that old quads don't do that. We no longer feel dehumanized that we can't even shit by ourselves. Old quads are too mature for that.

He finishes dressing me and sets me in the electric monster with wheels and cushions. He scrubs the night sweat from hair, brushes it, and dries it. Glancing critically, then questioning, he adjusts a sweater, puts in an earring, or brushes the hair again. Finally he's proud of his quad and steps away. I look in a mirror seeing the ghost of the fifteen-year-old me. What would she be doing today if she were alive?

If there is snow in the mountains, she'd be traveling it, stabbing a mogul with her ski poles as if an enemy, fighting to get to the bottom of the hill, and then wait a colored line of other puffy-parkas to return to the top again. If there were no snow, she'd be running to the mountains where she could play with Candy's goats and listen to her strange mandolin. Green and good, cold and now forbidden... the rubber tires know no love for the snow and terrain of goats, only fear.

I always wondered if my mountains were taken from me, and her, because we stopped running that one time. It was so strange on that desert plateau with the pink-rocked running ring. We looked at it half awed, halfway disgusted. Our team had never seen such a track, but none of us had ever gone to a Girls' State Track Meet. We had three pairs of spiked addidas to share among the eight of us; we were so out of sorts that we didn't even have matching uniforms! Just these red shirts that we had bought for $3.00 at the same store. "Short spikes only," they kept announcing. We had lost some of the short spikes so some of the egg-shell light adidas had a couple missing. My heat of the 880 came, the strange, high-heeled-no-heeled shoes were given to me so I could run on the pink rocks. It was all so beautiful but all so wrong; the running seemed wrong. The race was almost over, my kick was coming, I stopped and walked off the track. Later I cried and told my teammates that I had become too winded because I knew they'd never understand what really happened. How do you explain how incredible it is to run around a corner and have a mountain like Rainier loom up into your vision? turn another corner and you face the whiteness of a docile St. Helens? and realize you don't give a fuck about some stupid race run on stupid pink rocks?

I thought that because I didn't follow the rules, again, that the car accident was my fault. I never thought that the death of our coach who drove the car was my fault, well, not for very long anyway, but I knew I was responsible for the loss of a fifteen-year-old runner. I can't remember my neck snapping, the bone breaking away from the spinal column, my cervicals crushing against one another, though others say I was conscious. So much is forgotten when the runner left me and too much remembered when the quad awakened.

My mother had left me to fill out insurance forms. We had just been transported from the warm, old hospital in Yakima to this cold structure of learninglessness: University of Washington Hospital, Rehabilitation Ward, Four North... I was still on the stretcher they had used in the helicopter, alone in the hallway, staring at the lights of the ceiling, my peripheral vision catching sight of a white cloth now and then floating past me. Nobody came to move me or ask who I was. I kept waiting for my mother to return. I don't know how much time had past, only that too much had. I cried. Quietly so as not to attract the white clothes passing me because they scared me. The fluorescent lights scared me. The loneliness scared me. Where was my mother?

Purple-Eyes, head nurse, rushed to my rescue: "Stop that crying, now. You are paralyzed and will be for the rest of your life and crying will do no good. So stop." Her indoctrination to Quadom was brisk, cold, but not without merit. Eleven years later I don't cry because quads that old don't and I am not one to break rules.

Journal Piece

by stephanie sugars

Feb. 7, 1975 I am floating away. Experiences I have tire me of my body. Set me off into my mind. It is fun here in my mind. It is fine and clear like light.

July 7, 1978 Scars are lessons to remember. Scars for feeding, for no more babies. To cut out a part of me, to remember adolescence, to remember childhood, to remember what is right in front of my eyes.

Scars seem OK so long as there is no gathering of pain or tension. Scars hurt when it rains, when tears come.

I never want to have surgery again. Knocked out and torn apart and put back together in a different way.

July 24, 1979 Forcing myself into humility — negating myself — not worshipping myself. I can't do this. I won't. I am in need of validation. I choose myself. I will/I must be here for myself. I want to live. Oh goddess, I want to live. The cancer in my belly is a monster reflection of self hatred, self degradation. I want to live. This is so important. I need my body.

July 28, 1979 I've been having motion sickness for the last couple of weeks. My life is neatly tucked away in boxes. Having checked to see that I am neat and orderly, I lid my boxes. The lid becomes a door, a door in the wall, becomes a wall. I am contained in finite structures.

August 5, 1979 You speak to me of violence. Of things "they, those boys" do to us.

And I am forcing myself, my body and my beliefs. The enemy

is inside me. Facing me, facing me, facing me. I am wracked with sobs. There is little water left in my body, yet it arises within me. If wanting could make it be. I'd be bionic woman. Who, as I understand it, knows and creates and recreates her body and being. Suitable relative forms.

I feel so helpless though. I don't want to listen outside anymore.

I am in pain. I am suffering. And I don't want to suffer, every cell is rebelling and I keep on suffering. Twenty three years. I force myself to go on living. I force myself not to pull the plug. I force myself. I am shoving myself.

Jan. 1, 1980   I feel like another shell is falling away. My snake is dropping another skin. Through passivity, through illness, through deadness, dullness, depression. Another layer of gray evaporates before my eyes.

Jan. 26, 1981   Hospital traumatic. I survive as best I can. X-rays again today. Tests. I'm OK. Survival.

April 22, 1981   Feeling insecure when I'm feeling sick. Feel self-hateful too. I don't understand how anyone could like me, much less love me.

Feel terrible for a couple of weeks now. Fever, runs, depression, cramps, aches, shakes and tender skin. Suicidal when I think of it never ending; of it always being this way.

May 24, 1981   I'm afraid to express my emotions when I'm ill because everything feels out of proportion. Yet if I don't I'm stuck with everything inside.

The disabled lesbian group has let me hang out with my disability, to touch it in different ways, to understand myself through touch. To understand through sharing our differences and our similarities. The humanness of disability touches me deeply. I have felt for a long time that survivors have deeper understandings of all reality. One of the first steps of being a survivor is identifying that something happened that was survived. I begin to understand how my denial has helped me to survive. I have attempted to assimilate myself by insisting that my life is no different than anyone else's. I needed to blur over the differences, to be non-threatening.

I feel now that it is important to express the differences. Only through understanding other women's lives can I begin to understand how truly connected we all are.

Freaks. I never wanted to be a freak yet I always was. Body, mind, emotions seemed to keep taking a different path. At times I pass straight, able-bodied, middle-class. Then the passing invariably breaks. Survival is a precarious balance.

July 12, 1981   I would that I could start my life over. I would be born without a sickness within me. It had always appeared easier to me to have a sickness of the limbs, eyes, ears. A sickness that could have been caused by something outside me. A sickness visible to the naked eye. My insides are the traitor to my body. It seems so grotesque. My body came with this disease.

Sept. 23, 1981   Reading about Nagasaki. Too big to ponder. Bye bye San Jose. Eyeballs bleeding down cheekbones. Loss of power. It makes me not want to live. Sometimes I seem so frail to myself. I can see between the atoms that currently make up my body. I can see only shadow where there should be light. Feel only numbness where before there was pain. Depression, anger, despair. Sits inside me. Sits and feeds. Parasitic monster. My despair turns my body into food for the living death.

A disease of the digestive tract. Unable to digest, assimilate. I write so I can understand. I am driven to understand. Being a lesbian is very hard for me right now. It seems to mean a life of questioning, a commitment to going deeper and deeper while being as comprehensive as possible.

Now my body seems solid and firm, smooth light skin. My muscles are returning. I am filled with hope for change inside of me and in the world.

May 9, 1982   So much love. So much rage.

Memories of burnt and blistered skin peeling away. My eyes melted. Future memories. I live far enough away from what I suppose will be the epi-centers that I won't be the first to go. There is no safety. Tomorrow we go to Livermore Labs. And they are trying to kill me. I am trying to love my body. I spend these years reclaiming my body from abuse, medicine, illness. They are trying to kill me.

I have worked so diligently. I've learned to turn myself over. I open to myself, stretching, and growing, loving.

The image returns. Slow death, burns, blisters, hemorrhage. I am enraged that deep within me this image lives. That the threat of annihilation turns self-love to terror. So I die. But will I incarnate next on a radiated planet?

August 20, 1982   Healing has been my primary objective for so long. Sometimes I measure my life in terms of where I've gotten. I have tumors still. I am changing how I perceive and relate to my health. Watching how I live in the world in my body, I see how incredibly far I've come. I am coming to trust my body's integrity.

October 5, 1982   I have a place deep inside me. I feel it when I feel pain/suffering. I run away from that place sometimes trying to be well/healthy. But I'm pulled towards it when all I know is the pain.

Deborah says we are gifted with the pain. I don't know. I fluctuate between wanting to be normal and treasuring myself as I am.

October 20, 1982   Awake in the night. Lying here thinking my life is traveling so fast. My belly aches. So I wake up wondering, worrying about getting sick, about overdoing it and losing it again. My body is such a sensitive indicator of my being. If I refuse to respond to my intuition, my body steps in with pain/discomfort/illness. I have a gate to my unconscious mind through my body.

Nov. 21, 1982   My body has been demanding lately. Six days of flu-like symptoms followed by acupuncture and then emotional upset. Feeling quite queasy and upset intestinally. Anyway, I cancelled all appointments last week except work, acupuncture and J.'s birthday. Taking it easy is hard for me because friends are the first axed and they help keep me healthy. Sense of loss. I feel like I'm just beginning to deal with my life in terms of coming loss. Because I'm so sensitive, I don't see myself as strong or resilient. I see myself absorbing and containing all possibilities until I implode. Destroy myself.

The pain is so great and I am living in no great adversity currently. Except disease, pain and fatigue.

April 11, 1983   I don't feel very well. Toxed out would be the description. I'm feeling a lot of physical and emotional stress. Read Audre Lorde's *Cancer Journals* last night. She hasn't said anything that I haven't deduced on my own except — and this is a very major exception — she takes herself and her experience very seriously.

May 31, 1983   I feel so cynical about disability and illness. My beliefs run both counter and parallel to the Sonoma County hip holistic healing scene. Anyway, I'm feeling very cautious of involving myself with them.

Have I written an environmental illness poem?

Being so ill today. All the classic symptoms of toxic reaction, yet I plunged ahead moved by my mind.

July 28, 1983   The lumpy woman is me. I can feel them growing. Parts of flesh, muscle, lymph breaking off. They gather in soft flesh. Clump together tightly, holding onto sister cells. Knots. I am reminded of the knotted thong penitents used in payment for sins. My body has lumps close to the surface and far below. I am scared today by a lump on my cervix, a dimple and a lump hard near my os. Cathy's voice keeps coming back to me "feel the feelings". I am racing to deny. I am hoping for scientific refutation. My true feeling is that my body is trying to kill itself; that I'll keep producing lumps and diseases until there is no body to take it. I fear that I will be worn down.

Tale of a Pretty Woman

by cheryl wade

S he awoke one morning with her right foot gone. Not actually gone from sight, just not there when she stood on it. "Oh, what am I to do without a foot?" she wailed. "I have never been able to endure looking at poor creatures who hobble — they depress me so. Besides I am far too pretty to be hobbled." She was truly miserable and wept and wept at the injustice of life — that such beauty should be tainted.

Of course she could have saved her tears for God did not mean for her to be so miserable. He agreed she was, indeed, far too pretty to suffer such a fate, so He performed one of the many delightful miracles that has kept Him so popular with so many for so long.

The very next morning she awoke to find her left foot gone to match the right. Attempting to arise from her bed she fell flat on her face on the floor, splattering her delicate nose from ear to ear and although she was now more hobbled than ever it mattered not half as much. And such be the glory of the Lord. Amen.

Five Reasons I Play Wheelchair Basketball

by jill sager

1.

Because I enjoy the competition.

I never played sports growing up. I didn't have the opportunity to. I was excused from physical education all through Junior High and High School. The assumption was that I couldn't compete, couldn't do the activities. And it was true, I couldn't, especially in the environment and structure that was always offered to me. If I tried any sport at all I ended up feelng inadequate because I couldn't run or kick or keep up. The first time I got in a wheelchair to play basketball with other disabled women who were also in wheelchairs, was the first time in my life I felt I could play a sport and play well. I can keep up and I have an equal chance to compete.

2.

Because I enjoy the speed.

When I'm sitting in that wheelchair I can run. I move fast. I have power.

3

Because I like how my body feels.

After every practice I'm sore and my muscles ache, but it's not because of my disability, it's because I'm working out and working hard. And it feels great to give it everything I have and sweat and feel tired, and ache and feel the exhilaration of another good practice session.

4.

Because I like calling myself a jock.

I always thought that word was for people with well developed leg and arm muscles, who stood up straight and tall showing off their strong backs. Well I'm thrilled to be able to think of myself as that person.

5.

Because it makes me feel good about myself.

When I'm playing wheelchair basketball I'm not thinking about the deformities in my leg or my curved back. I'm thinking about how good I feel. And I'm thinking that I do look beautiful. That who I am is OK. I'm not ashamed or embarassed to be me or to be in a wheelchair. It's because of that wheelchair that I have learned about a part of myself that I have always felt disconnected from: my body. And I have learned about a part of myself I didn't even know existed: the love of participating in a sport.

This Body I Love

by deborah s. abbott

i am standing in the shower, in the large common shower after seventy-two laps in the public pool. The water scalds my skin after the cool night air. I peel my suit down; stubborn over breasts and bottom, it suddenly slaps the tile at my feet. I step out and begin soaping, rubbing the almond-scented liquid over my shoulders, my arms. I am proud of these arms, growing broad after three weeks of swimming. They have propelled me through a mile of water tonight, arcing and scooping and pulling at the tremendous weight, and still they are not tired.

I raise my arms by turn and make a great lather in the hollows, in the thick, black ovals of hair. This hair which gathers the scent of me, blots it outward like a wick, and announces me to my friends in the heat of the day. I think it's been ten years since I've stopped shaving it, since the pits of my arms prickled with insistent hairs, since blood beaded at the surface and clotted against my shirt. Ten years now of this hair, tangled as the twigs of a nest. Hold up my arms and small birds fly.

Oh, and then lovely, left arm still raised, suds careen down the slope of breast, heap on my nipple like cream on warm pie, then edge over, splatting the tile. Such fondness I have for these breasts, such pleasure they have known. Babies have choked on the milk of them, lovers have been finely sprayed, and I, too, have tasted and touched. My breasts are those of a woman who has lived long and well. I call them lazy breasts now. They have done their work and lie on my chest like fruit upon the ground.

Now lower, soapy hands on my belly. Belly remembers these babies which rose from beneath until the skin was firm and resonant as a drum. Belly rounds, nostalgic. Fleshy, it makes a cushion for the cheek of a child.

Oh, then down, down, into the other nest, over Venus' gentle mound. In this great tiled room there are four high spigots and a low one as well. I smile, remembering my young son discovering the one low-set in the corner. "Oh, they made one for kids!" he exclaimed, his naked body delighting in its spray. "And one for women in wheelchairs." I added, aloud. To myself I remember thinking 'For women's genitals as well.' I wanted to slide the soap between my folds then, to part my lips and let the water hum over them until they broke into song, but I reminded myself this was a shared space and mine a private tune. This time I rinse for half a minute, the fantasy as sweet as before. My fingers release and my labia settle together like petals of moonvine into the dark.

I lean over. My legs are long; one longer than the other. There is no symmetry in my legs and, even after thirty years, this sometimes disturbs. After all, dutiful daughter that I was, I learned to part my hair precisely down the middle, with neither more nor less falling to either side. I cannot talk of my legs as one talks of eyes or ears or arms, usual pairs of these. I have always needed to buy two pairs of shoes, in different sizes, in order to have a single set which fit. My legs do not match. They will not match. They have not matched since a virus crept along my spine, consuming synapses as an insect chews it course along the nerve of a leaf.

My left hand grips the steel bar, steadies me, while my other squirts soap onto my great left thigh. 'Thunder thigh' a lover called it once, as I wrapped it, vine-like, around a belly in the heat of love. This leg is thick with muscle. The Balancer. The Protector. The one which anticipates, compensates, takes the stairs, takes off in the pool, churning water behind like the wake of a whale. I hold onto the bar with both hands and lean back. The soap flows down, making rivulets through the forest of hair on my thigh, bubbling down my calf, over my toes, and onto the tile. It swirls round the drain and is loudly sucked down.

Now to my other. I stroke this slender limb, along the pale sutures whose indelible ribbons mark times the skin has been incised and peeled open, the bones broken and re-arranged, the flesh stitched shut and left to mend beneath a wrapping of plaster. I am tender with this leg, forgiving, soaping it as I did a friend, fragile in her dying hours. I lift it a little, reaching the undercurve of foot.

I have never known how to name it. To make reference without causing further harm. The Small One? The Weak One? The one which bows like a sapling in a climate of winds? I am a writer found inarticulate in the naming of a body which will not conform. Which will not conform to the body of words a language holds. Perhaps the hands could make a sign which tells.

I turn and fill my mouth with water, spitting some, swallowing the rest. I wet my face, my hair. I am wet all over, warm and clean. I reach for shampoo. I make a lather in my hands, then pass it to my head, fingers massaging my scalp.

Two young women have entered the shower. They stand along the opposite wall, talking while they wash, all the while with their eyes closed. The force of their showers sends a cool wave of water over me. I shiver; my flesh puckers against the cold. For a moment I falter, then I catch the bar and hold fast.

I am not ashamed of looking. These women's bodies compel me. I watch them as though I were in a museum studying sculpture, as though I were eyeing shiny photos in a magazine. Perhaps these bodies are well-polished stone and mine the only blood-warmed flesh. Perhaps mine is the image fixed in the frame of a camera and theirs the flesh that is real.

I am not certain whether the water warms or my body accepts the water's chill, but finally my nipples lose their tension, the goosebumps leave my arms. This shower is like an enormous collander in which we all are contained and rinsed clean. And I am the ripened piece, irregular in form, yellow and softened and sweet. It is common knowledge that they too, will ready with time.

6.

Becoming Mothers
— Raising Our Children —

Fear of disability and the belief that disability is inherited have led to judgments that disabled women should not be allowed to have children. We are actively discouraged from even considering the possibility. This is accomplished through the lack of appropriate sex education, forced sterilization, and the promotion of stereotypes that we are either asexual or sexually promiscuous. The negative aspects of parenting are exaggerated while the benefits and joys are minimized.

It takes great courage and support to consider the possibility of choosing to have a child or to decide to continue an unplanned pregnancy. We venture into unknown territory with no role models. We must deal, not only with our own doubts and fears but those of others. Emotionally and physically disabled women are in jeopardy of losing our children when society backs up indiscriminate accusations that we are unfit mothers. Disabled women are mothers. We may be single, partnered, lesbian, heterosexual. We need access to each other so that we can have realistic images of what is involved in raising our children. Together we can learn about resources, fight for what we need, and share the joys of mothering. Perhaps it is the children raised by disabled mothers, in environments where limitations and interdependence are acknowledged as normal, who will become adults able to face and deal with the realities of disability in all of our lives.

The Lois Anderson Story

by lois anderson

My name is Lois Marie Anderson, born Feburary 25, 1942. I attended the Christopher Rose Elementary and High School. I was married on my eighteenth birthday to Thomas Pine. We were married for six years. During the marriage we had four children, two sons and two daughters: Derrick, Glenn, Steve Curtis, Marie Louise and Pamela Denise. The marriage ended in divorce on May 15, 1966. At the young age of 25 I became a single parent. During those very difficult years from 1966 to 1972 the children and I managed to get through some hard times with very little income.

On July 27, 1972 my life took a complete turn. I was shot. The bullet entered my left side at close range, traveled through my left lung and lodged in my third vertebra. The bullet was pressing on my spine and I was bleeding in the chest cavity. My life was saved by nine operations. After five months in the hospital I was able to sit up in a wheelchair for about ten minutes. Those ten minutes were hell. I hadn't realized how small my body was. I was very weak and in pain, with headaches, stomach pains and intense heat throughout my body. I wondered, "Oh God, will my body ever respond enough to sit in a wheelchair without any balance?" I was hoping I could be able one day to return home to my children of 7, 8, 9 and 10 years old. I didn't allow myself to fall apart, thinking: "I've got to keep myself together, because if I give up now, what will happen to me? If I get put in a nursing home, I will never be able to see my children. I've got to take care of myself."

Looking at myself in that big water and sand bed I saw a body so horrible looking. I started thinking about the three wonderful years I spent with my boyfriend before this accident. What was going to happen to me now? I loved him and wanted very much to keep him, but I gave up my relationship. My hopes went down the drain. I had to give him up. I knew I was the same person in my mind, but my body kept telling me it would not work out. I felt I could not give him what he needed. I felt that my sex life was over. I thought I would never be able to sit up or walk on my own again.

During this period I became very upset, scared and worried. I did a lot of crying during those long nights in the hospital. Dr. Wells and Dr. Kene knew I wanted to see my children. Dr. Wells made arrangements for me to see them for about ten minutes. I saw four small children that needed their mother. I started to ask lots of questions.

That's when I met the social worker at the Thorpe Hospital. Bobbie and I started talking many hours about various institutions. She referred me to the Rehabilitation Center, I believe because my feelings were sincere and I wanted to work hard to better myself and learn how to deal with my handicap.

In December 1972 I was transferred to the Rehabilitation Center. When I arrived there I became irritable, hostile, argumentative and just downright mean. I remember hating the institution, but they did not hate me.

At that time, the Rehabilitation Center was a very small building of five or six floors. Mrs. Sommers was the head nurse. Dr. R. Benson was my doctor. Bonnie Bate was my physical therapist and Vear was my occupational therapist. These wonderful professional people started working with me. Bonnie and I went through hours and hours of therapy. I had hours of pain everyday. Days turned into weeks and weeks into months of physical therapy, but Bonnie was with me all the way. There were many times I wanted to give up, but not Bonnie. We worked hard. She made me proud of myself and would wipe those tears away. Bonnie knew I would make it. I would scream a lot so she would tell me: "Lois, when the pain starts, call your children's names as loud as you want to." So I did! My muscles started to rouse. I started to look human again. Some of the positions Bonnie and I would get into were so funny the other therapists would laugh. She and I would just lay down on the floor and have a big laugh ourselves. Even when I was in other classes, she would stop by in the morning and say "hi" and give me that big smile. I knew I would lose Bonnie and I cried happy tears. I never did lose Bonnie and she will always be in my heart.

Mrs. Sommers was my nurse and it took a strong nurse like her to deal with me. You see, I did very little talking. Mrs. Sommers would tell me: "You will start talking when you want to." I had a very bad skin breakdown while I was in the hospital. Mrs. Sommers was aware of this and knew it might require more surgery. This operation consists of grafting skin, 12" long and 8" wide, from the back of my thigh, cutting out a hunk of muscle, moving some muscle tissue over the buttocks, packing it with my own muscle and covering it with my own skin. Being a concerned nurse, Mrs. Sommers took good care of me and would check me four to six times a day because the skin was raw. When I went to see my doctor, Mrs. Sommers never forgot to take time out to check me and talk with him about the breakdown. I've known Mrs. Sommers for the last eleven years.

Vear, my occupational therapist, was Johnny-on-the-spot. Working with me, she taught me many things in classes like rug hooking, making picture frames, all kinds of necessary work and interaction with other patients. I met some delightful people and I loved going to occupational therapy every day I could. I started to blend it with the other patients. This was a wonderful feeling along with the reactions I received from the other people. Being a friendly person most of my life, meeting new friends was one of the happiest times I spent at the Rehabilitation Center. I found that I was not alone and all of us shared and helped each other with different projects in occupational therapy. This became one of my most important activities. I had lots of new friends. They were just super great.

This is when I began to accept my life as a handicapped person. I was no longer mad at the world or blaming everyone for my accident. Instead, I was thanking God that these people cared about me.

The Rehabilitation Center helped my children to understand what mommy was doing and they kind of grew along with me. They could come during dinner time and they loved it. They knew Dr. Benson, Bonnie Bate, Mrs. Sommers and Vear. The children became more popular than I was. Thanks to that remarkable institution, each day put me closer and closer to going home. This is what the children and I looked forward to. Promising to follow all the rules, I was released in May 1973.

A visiting nurse came in twice a month to see me. Mrs. Ellis would examine me and change my dressing. She would tell me, "Lois, you can get infections living under the conditions in this apartment." It was unliveable. I was gone ten and a half months, so how could I possibly find things as I had left them? Things didn't come easy. Rats, mice, bugs were everywhere. I had to sleep during the daytime so I could be awake to watch the children at night. I didn't want the rats to bite them. It was me and my broom and those rats at night. We were all sleeping in one room. The children had bunk beds and I had a hospital bed.

At their young ages of 8 to 11 years old, the children saw the raw areas on my body. When the visiting nurse came they would ask her many questions: "How can I help my mommy? Why can't she get out of bed? Mrs. Ellis, would you sit down and talk to us please?" Mrs. Ellis would tell them why I couldn't get out of bed and many other answers to questions she felt they could understand.

We lived in that apartment until July 1973. We moved with very little furniture and clothing, but the children were happy. I've never had a housekeeper or a personal care assistant. The children would tell me "Mommy, we dirtied the house up, can we clean it up?" I was shocked! God gave me the strength I thought I would never have. In 1977 I weaned myself of the indwelling catheter tube that was in my bladder. The Rehabilitation Center admitted me to remove the tube when I felt I no longer needed it. We have been in this apartment for ten years now. There are lots of memories here.

School wasn't any problem. The children did not give me much trouble. Yes, I went through things during the children's growing years. My daughter came close to being a teenage alcoholic. It took time for me to understand the problem. It became so bad I had to call the police because she became very violent. I made up my mind that I needed help with my daughter. Jeanne Marvin is my social worker now at the Rehabilitation Center. We worked hard trying to get my daughter to overcome her drinking problem. My daughter started to come around. Without Jeanne I couldn't have handled this problem. Now my daughter doesn't have any more problems with alcohol.

My son was going through some changes. I practically had to pull him out of bed some mornings when he was in high school. Stealing became a problem with him. When he was caught for the fourth time, it would have cost me $100 to get him out of jail. I was not going to let him get me down or keep me worrying anymore, so I stopped getting him out of jail. It hurt me but he had to learn you can't constantly take other people's property. It's wrong. With the help of God and me talking many hours to my son, he stopped stealing. It doesn't matter whether you are crawling, walking or in a wheelchair — raising children is not an easy job, especially when you don't have any support from your family. Being alone is *hell* but you can't give up.

Today, all four of my children are working. I am proud to say that they are very independent adult people. Derrick is 23 years old. Steve is 22. Both of my daughters are married. Marie is 21. Pamela, now 20, is a proud mother of a baby boy.

Now it's time for me to get on with my life. I am living on my own in an accessible apartment. This is my second year attending classes, facilitating groups and volunteering at Access Living, an independent living resource center. We created a new group at Access Living, Handicapped Independent People. Our concern is accessible housing for all disabled people. My dream is to return to school and become a social worker. With God's help, I know I can make it.

To Choose A Child

by donna hyler

i found out I was pregnant on June 6, 1979. I had gone to the doctor complaining of swollen feet and a state of constant sleepiness that bordered on narcolepsy. "Are you pregnant?" he asked. I laughed, nervously. I felt embarrassed, as though I'd been given credit for something by mistake. I wondered if he was joking. But then it dawned on me that his question was perfectly reasonable. I had even made a joke about the possibility to David, my partner/helper, the day before. I left a urine sample for the test and went home to await the results.

It was very quiet on the way home. Suddenly I was face to face with a question I'd never asked but wondered about, ever since I could remember. Could, should I have children? Of all the doctors I'd seen, none had ever discussed this issue. I'd just assumed the answer was No. The fact that I had an adult relationship had exceeded my parents' expectations for me, and everyone in the family was always telling me how lucky I was. I had decided this was true, and had always taken precautions to assure that there would be no baby. This was fine with David, too. Now, the chance that I might actually be pregnant brought in conflicting emotions, scared and depressed me, and threatened my not-so-confident sense of self. I considered the "inevitability" of an abortion. Finally, despite all the "rational" arguments against my having a baby, the possibility that I might be pregnant awakened in me a growing sense of joy that I had never before felt. A previously dormant part of me — spiritual, physical and psychological — was heralding its existence and making friends with the rest of me. I felt suddenly more integrated within myself. Somehow more complete. Had I not been pregnant, I would still have gained from the waiting experience a delightful introspection. But this moment would only be the beginning of a life-long period of new discovery and change. When I checked with the doctor two hours later, I found out that the test read positive. Based on the dates I had given him, he determined that I was five weeks pregnant. The doctor said, "What do you want to do?" I told him that I really didn't know, and I started asking all the questions I'd never asked. "Will this make my arthritis worse?" I learned some women have increased symptoms post-delivery, due to naturally occurring chemical changes. But, medication, adequate rest and other common sense solutions would reduce or eliminate any flare-up. "How would the baby be affected? Would he or she be pre-destined to have arthritis?" The doctor answered that this was never proven. There was no reason to assume that my baby would ever have arthritis, any more than any other woman's baby.

I sat with these facts. Every woman has the right to choose an abortion. I knew I had the right to choose against one. I also had to think about David. He would have to help me with all the things I could not do for the baby by myself. He had never planned on having children; at least, not for a long time. He was shocked by the news, especially when he heard that I was considering going through with the pregnancy.

He didn't know what he wanted to do, how it would affect our relationship, how it would affect our even being together at all. It was a very sad time for me. Somehow I knew that I wanted to keep the baby. I always knew, from the moment I found out I might be pregnant.

When we went to the gynecologist he had a long talk with us. When I look back on it now, I can't help but feel a little bit upset about what he had to say. Basically, he gave us as much negative information as he possibly could. On the other hand, he assured me that if I wanted to go through with the pregnancy, he knew that it *could* happen. I think he was trying to hit me with some stark realities that I felt I was already in touch with. David, however, who was already doubtful about the whole thing, was very frightened. I had quite a time getting him to realize that there was another more positive perspective. Finally, after about two weeks, David agreed that he would participate and do his utmost to feel positive about the coming baby. From the moment that he decided to be supportive, he *was* supportive. I was deeply relieved, and I really fell in love with him again at that point in our life together.

The next step was talking to our families. We expected them to be concerned. After all, we were concerned ourselves. There are no guarantees when one is pregnant. No one knows — even a healthy woman — whether her baby will be healthy, and whether or not she or her spouse can cope.

We telephoned David's parents first. They were surprised and quiet. David's parents have a policy of non-interference, trust and respect toward their children. On the other hand, when asked, they will come out with a very straight-forward appraisal of a situation according to their perspective. This is what I asked for when we spoke with them. They were concerned about common sense things, the kinds of things I had discussed with the doctor. They were also concerned about David caring for the baby. When I assured them that we had discussed it all, they were very accepting and reassuring.

The next people we told were my parents. Now, my parents have a history of not being able to deal very well with me in relation to my disability. Although I know that they love me dearly, I don't feel that they have always been able to respond realistically to my needs and my actions. When I told them, the reaction was less than positive. In fact, they were quite shocked. Later that week, they wrote us a long letter. I know that it was meant to be helpful, but what it turned out to be was a long list of reasons why we should not have children, why *I* should not have children. One of the reasons was that the child would suffer psychological damage as a result of having a disabled parent. I read that, knowing that they were still uncomfortable with my disability. I put the letter away and cried. There wasn't anything else I could do. As it turned out, seven months of my pregnancy went by before my mother even spoke to me again.

I had also contacted other relatives on my side of the family. I found out that they were able to give me the kind of encouragement, enthusiasm and positive feelings that I so deeply missed from my own parents. Not only were they supportive of me in a way that I had never anticipated, but they also helped me feel as though I had a right to go for as much joy in my life as anyone else. I felt they would be behind me, no matter what happened. In the process, I discovered I had real family ties. I was more than a paper relative. I will never forget their encouragement and love.

Amy Robin was born on January 24, 1980. Together the three of us have grown as a family. David and I have learned as much from Amy as she has from us. David is a loving, caring parent and teacher. I am more capable than I had ever thought possible. Amy, now five, is a bright enthusiastic child who, in addition to the regular activities of childhood, enjoys sharing household responsibilities and the good feeling she gets when she's helpful to me or her dad. She is particularly sensitive toward people with special needs. I am moved by her understanding and awareness of others. I have great hope for us as a family, and for Amy in particular. I look forward to seeing her assume her role as sibling in the coming year as we plan the birth of our second child.

Parenting

by joann leMaistre

1983

was simply a disaster. Most of my my daughter's six years contained some element of disaster, but this year it was nearly as pure as one could imagine. Ironically, 1983 was also the year I was named mother of the year by my county multiple sclerosis society. Society officials had energetically searched their records for someone who was a single parent, who was the family economic provider, who had full-time responsibility for her offspring, and who had some of the conditions which *guarantee* entree into the society. They also told me they had looked for someone whose child had the sparkle and resilience characteristic of children who have benefited from adequate parenting. When I won the award, I was thrilled — I was receiving acclaim for parental qualities I wanted to have, even if I was not all that sure I possessed them.

In truth, during this year I was far less able to be the good mother that I had been in preceding years. I was very ill for eleven of the twelve months. My baseline disability is major visual loss. When the multiple sclerosis kicks up, the rest of the disabilities — trouble with walking and balance, problems with speech, loss of all fine motor control — quickly come into play. Nineteen eighty-three was not the year to be a mother at all. I needed to rest and mend, not to work and shoulder major responsibilities for child rearing.

Long ago I decided that something I can give my daughter is an example of how one can manage when objective reality is the pits. This year, I showed her what happens when someone is really pushed beyond what can be handled. With a lot of help from friends and my own mother, we got through. The price to my self-esteem and my sense of competence would have been astronomical without the almost absurd juxtaposition of my mother-of-the-year status. After all, I wanted to live up to that honor.

Motherhood, of course, was never what I imagined it would be. I had planned well, I thought. I was sensible and ambitious and knew I needed to satisfy my own career aspirations before tackling motherhood. After nine years of graduate and postgraduate training, an equally long marriage, and two years of getting myself in the best physical shape possible (at what I considered to be my rapidly advancing age), it seemed the time was right. I can laugh now at the naivete of this approach. I had so much to learn yet about my priorities, my capabilities, and the limits of my competencies.

Parents who take on the demands of child rearing while already struggling with the complexities of physical disabilities learn to keep priorities and self-definitions very clear. The physically limited parent need not be a disabled one. She is just a parent who must approach the delights and difficulties of parenting with fewer physical resources than parents enjoying unimpaired physical health and function.

In truth, our society is not adequately supportive of any parent. There is no real training for parenthood, so the reality comes as a surprise to most of us. Parenthood is the hardest job anyone will ever have. Yet the physically limited parent may be the only parent in the neighborhood toward whom the community directs its anxiety about the difficulty of the job.

In its worst form, this anxiety creates overt prejudice against such a parent; the opposite attitude of helpfulness may also exist. In either case, it is very important for the individual parent to figure out what her own particular strengths and weaknesses are. Parenthood never works out exactly as we expect. It is both more gratifying and more depleting than we anticipate. Surprises are par for the course. We need not be thrown by the surprises and can still be adequate parents if we are sufficiently flexible in our approach to child rearing. We are inadequate only when we are so stressed that we cannot see the child as separate from ourselves, cannot control hostile impulses, or simply have no physical energy for, and no alternative to, the rigors of parenting.

My first surprise as a mother was that my daughter was so pretty the moment after she was born. She was given to me right away, and I saw only that she was adorable, even before she had been cleaned up. Within hours it occurred to me at a rational level that she could not have been all that cute; she hadn't even been bathed yet, but I had absolutely no realistic memory of her at all. Nature is truly marvelous, I concluded.

I was to conclude that over and over again. The baby was born several weeks early after a wonderful pregnancy. I had had only one day of morning sickness; I fainted once, and my right leg had occasionally been numb at unpredictable times, but overall, I felt healthy and high-spirited and was very active physically. Part of the reason I felt so well, I was to discover later, was that the normal hormonal changes of pregnancy were protecting me against major trouble from a disease I did not even know I had. But by the time my daughter was a month old, I was in the midst of a raging attack of multiple sclerosis. Translated into practical terms, this meant I was too weak to hold a five-pound infant and I could not make eye contact with her because I had lost most of my vision. I could not nurse her because my body would not produce adequate milk, and even if it had, the medication I was taking would have been detrimental to the baby.

Knowing how important early contact is for an infant, I talked to her, sang to her, cried right along with her, and kept as physically close to her as I could. There was no disruption in the early bonding, and I found myself very annoyed with doctors and friends who wanted to blame my physical predicament on the baby. It is true I would have rested better, worried less, and felt less incompetent had I not just become a mother, but that is true for all parents. I would also have been more frightened and depressed. The baby, endlessly changing, provided stimulation. I had a wonderful baby-sitter who kept me involved with every aspect of my daughter's life and turned parenting tasks over to me as my strength permitted. The pediatrician was sensitive and made well-baby visits at home so I would not have to be left out of that pleasant experience. Friends were glad to be able to do something useful, and when the baby needed to be fed round the clock every two hours, there was no shortage of helpers. Everyone realized that infant care is very demanding, and so much help was readily available I did not begin to feel intensely guilty about all the things I could not do for my daughter until she was about a year old. It took me a long time to discover I was much more direct and comfortable asking for help with the baby than I was asking for help for myself. But as my daughter grew, it became much more painful not to be able to play with her for more than five minutes at a time without exhaustion. I was always convinced she would seriously injure herself on something I was unable to see and move out of her grasp. Fortunately, it turned out that a house safe for my physical limitations was also safe for a toddler.

There are ways my daughter's early childhood has been limited by my own restrictions. Unlike most of her school chums, my child does not come from a two-parent home. I am not like other mothers who can dash around taking children from place to place. I have to rely on household help to tell me if my daughter is dressed nicely for school. I am often at a loss about how to be helpful to her with her school work. At times, it is not clear whose tantrums are more childish — hers or mine. I think they probably do us both some good. I find myself vastly reassured by the observations of other adults — my daughter is healthy, happy, bright, and socially engaging. And then I think to myself, "you wouldn't even be listening to other people if you weren't so unsure of yourself." I suspect I will have a long struggle with that one.

The children of physically limited parents are likely to have more responsibility than their peers. This is only a problem if the child does not have adequate time to play. This very necessary play experience can be expanded into a network of neighborhood play with other children — and there is no reason the parent cannot be playful herself when she is feeling well. My home will often become a meeting place for children who are more mobile than my child. We import children from all over town who have parents willing to chauffeur them. The tea party has not lost its magic any more than storytelling or puppets have, despite all the plastic nonsense and video games available for children in arcades. Encouraging imagination may lead to a messy house, but the children are remarkably good at putting things back because they know I might fall on something I don't see.

Children can never have too much in the way of age-appropriate learning and play opportunities. Baking cookies, traveling, or learning to walk along the street holding onto a parent's walker may be an adventure or an unpleasantness, depending on how the task is addressed. After I discovered that the introduction of any new equipment I needed for my well-being was easily accepted once my daughter and I decorated it, life seemed less complicated. Having the house festooned with bow-bedecked white canes, crepe-paper-covered walkers, and wheelchairs elegantly covered with cloth scraps created so much excitement that decorating was best done on a weekend. Then the aids could be reinstated to their normal appearance for weekdays. Whatever equipment became unnecessary remained decorated, lending the household the look of a perpetual birthday party.

One's own children can and do encourage discussion of your physical problems. This is good. Their friends will follow suit. Even children who are strangers are apt to be more curious and more honest in their reactions than are most adults. I had taken a friend out for ice cream, I remember, and we met a little girl who gazed with great wonder at my companion's prosthetic leg. The child came up to her and simply asked what this strange leg was. My friend explained. The little girl, curious but content with the answer, showed no fright; but her mother was embarassed and shocked. She hurried the little girl away. She could not allow her child to discover and master an aspect of reality. Nor am I likely to forget the three-year-old boy standing with his mother in front of me at the bank. He was fascinated by my cane, and we developed a hide-and-seek game whereby he was discovered by the cane. This produced gales of laughter. The mother was uncertain at first, but she eventually began giggling too. This mother was teaching her son that although new things might seem different they need not be frightening.

Parents and children are a team. If they approach life's upheavals and problems in sympathetic step with one another, their course will be easier than if the name of the game is power — where one or the other must "win." In such power plays there really are only losers. If parent and child are fortunate, each has a temperament appreciated by the other. It does not always happen. There are difficult children and difficult parents; there are difficult times. If there is a basis for harmony, however, it shows up early and sometimes strikingly. One of my most interesting parenting experiences occurred when my daughter was five months old. She was very attached to her pacifier and would cry if she dropped it unintentionally. By then, I was well enough to sit near her on the floor as she lay in her basket. I was very slow at finding the pacifier and returning it to her, but she would lay absolutely still, mouth open wide, until I managed to get the pacifier in her mouth rather than her ear. If anyone else was returning the pacifier to her, she was likely to thrash about impatiently. The implied level of cooperation was stunning, because it was not a rational act on her part as much as a type of synchrony more basic than words or cognition.

Parents need to remember that it is likely children will be easier at some ages than at others. With each new stage of a child's life, any parent has to learn the new limits of both the child's and the parent's competence. Not every parent can be a math tutor or swimming coach. When the child needs more than a parent can give, then some thinking needs to be done about locating a tutor, baby-sitter, or recreation director.

The basic goal of parenting is to foster independence from the parent. Sometimes to do this, parents must first become independent beings themselves. The means to self-confidence and self-reliance is love. That covers a lot of ground, including how to set limits that are age-appropriate for the child. For example, the two-year-old is at an age where she is striving for more autonomy and is often overcome by frustration at not being able to do something (the terrible twos are really the trying-new-things twos). If the parent has decided on eggs for breakfast and knows that her child will say no to anything that does not seem like her own idea, then one approach is to ask would the child like eggs scrambled or fried today. There are lots of ways to say "no" to undesired behavior while still saying "yes" to independence. A child, age ten, wants to try driving the car. "Certainly," says the parent, "when you are sixteen and the law allows you to take drivers' training." The parent who has to say no because of her physical impairment can provide the logic for the response. "Mama, why don't you ever drive me anywhere?" can be answered by saying, "I cannot see the road, and I would never do anything that is dangerous to you."

The physically limited parent may have fewer moments to relax and enjoy her children's development, but she can have a satisfying time helping them along their way. There is certainly no smooth road — anything but that. Guilt, dread, sadness, fatigue, constant awareness of one's limits are very much part of the picture. The struggle will be arduous. A physically limited parent benefits tremendously from predictable routine; a break in routine, such as that caused by a child's minor illness, is sufficient to bedevil the parent with feelings of inadequacy and anxious self-reproach. Or she may feel unjustly overburdened in an already difficult life. There is no justice. There may not even be any attainable goals, if these are set too high. I am convinced, though, that a child learns much from the way the parent approaches the struggle. The mother or father who honestly admits to difficulties, avoids playing the martyr, and avoids attempting to be superparent, teaches the child how to meet all manner of realities with steadfastness. If the parent is able to ask for the help she needs, parenting tasks are less overwhelming. Those who can give a mother a few hours babysitting respite will allow the parent to reengage with the child feeling more energetic and emotionally nurtured — able to give quality attention and time to the child. Time away from parenting is very important so that the parent can maintain her own flexible, creative reactions to physical stresses.

Under the best of circumstances, parenthood can be burdensome. Like any creative endeavor, being a parent touches a core part of ourselves. And if we are honest, we can see that the core contains negative feelings as well as positive ones. It helps to know these negative feelings are there, for once known, they lose some of their power. Contending with physical disability will diminish our reserves of optimism at times, but during the good times, when we are feeling emotionally settled, we can take pleasure in the increasing complexity of our children and their needs, while feeling whole and capable. I think the goal of any parent is to find ways of increasing these moments of true well-being.

When I was a healthy teenager, my father told me about a woman friend confined to a wheelchair. She had watched with horror as a poisonous spider made its way toward her baby's crib. She was not sure, confined as she was, that she would be able to defend her child from this threat. She was able to rescue her child, but was badly shaken by the experience — as any parent would be. In the innocence of health and the naivete of youth, I vowed I would never have children if I were physically impaired. I did not think I could withstand such a fright. In those days, of course, I could not really envision myself slowed down by anything until I was old. Clearly, life has taught me to overcome that exaggerated fear of physical limitation and has forced me to change my attitudes about parenting. Indeed, I've come to realize that we may give our children something which is uniquely the result of our physical disabilities. If we are self-accepting, our children will learn not to be afraid of disabled people, will admire and wish to emulate the strength in our daily struggle, and will accept for an entire lifetime the simple but too often hidden fact that there are no perfect people, no perfect lives, and that physical distress is very much a part of living.

To our children we can give a zest for human contact and the examples of myriad ways in which it is possible to get going productively when the going gets very tough indeed. To have a hand in producing emotional resilience, compassion, and the willingness to set reasonable goals for oneself is a very fine expression of parental love.

Claiming All
Of Our Bodies
Reproductive Rights
And Disability

*by anne finger**

*j*ust as I can't remember a time of my life when I wasn't a feminist, I can't remember not believing in disability rights. From the time I was a very young child, I understood that I was "more handicapped" by people's perceptions and attitudes towards me than I was by my disability (I had polio shortly before my third birthday). Although as a child I didn't have the word "disability," never mind "oppression" or "attitudinal barriers" to describe my experience, what I *did* have was the example of the black civil rights movement, then beginning in the South. From about the age of five or six, I used to think, "People are prejudiced against me the same way that they are against Negroes."

While increased understanding has led me to see the differences as well as the similarities between Black experiences and my own, my belief that disability in and of itself was much less of a problem than social structures and attitudes towards disability has never changed. In part because I was exempted from traditional feminine roles — *no one* ever so much as mentioned the possibility of my having babies when I grew up — I was also a feminist, at least in

*I would like to thank Adele Clarke, Judy Heumann, Susan Hansell, Jean Miller, Kim Marshall, Carla Schick, Lisa Manning, Susan Dambroff, and Sex Education for Disabled People in Oakland, California, for their assistance in preparing this article.

some incipient form, as far back as I can remember.

But it has not always been easy building a politics that connects these two parts of my experience. The feminist movement — the movement which has been my home for most of my adult life — has by and large acted as if disabled women did not exist. For instance, the 1976 edition of *Our Bodies, Our Selves* mentioned disability only twice — both time speaking of fetuses with potentially disabling conditions, not disabled women. (Boston Women's Health Book Collective, 1976). In the early years of the feminist movement I heard constantly about how women were sex objects — I could see that that was true for a lot of my abled sisters, but there were no voices saying that being stereotyped as asexual was also oppressive — and also was part of our female experience. More recently, the disability rights movement and the women's movement have seemed to be at loggerheads with each other over issues of reproductive technologies, genetics, and fetal and neonatal disabilities. I hope this article will be a step towards helping us to claim *all* of our selves.

Most discussions of disability begin with a laundry list of disabling conditions. Disability, we are told, does not just mean being in a wheelchair. It also includes a variety of conditions, both invisible and visible. These include being deaf or blind, having a heart condition, being developmentally disabled or being "mentally ill." While this is necessary to an understanding of disability, thinking about disability only in medical or quasi-medical terms limits our understanding: disability is largely a social construct.

Women, like disabled people, can be defined in terms of physical characteristics that make us different from males (only women menstruate; only women get pregnant; women tend to be shorter than men). We can also be defined socially. A social description would include all of the above physical characteristics, but would emphasize that, in our society, we are paid far less than men; we are less likely to vote Republican; and more likely to be emotional and empathetic.

In the same manner, when we start looking at disability socially, we see not only the medically defined conditions that I have described, but the social and economic circumstances that limit the lives of disabled people. We look, for instance at the fact that white disabled women earn 24 cents for every dollar that *comparably qualified* nondisabled men earn; for Black disabled women, the figure is 12 cents. (Figures for other racial groups were not reported.) Media images almost always portray us as being either lonely and pitiful or one-dimensional heroes (or, occasionally, heroines) who struggle valiantly to "overcome our handicaps." Many of us are still being denied the free public education that all American children supposedly receive; and we have a (largely unknown) history of fighting for our rights that stretches back at least to the mid-nineteenth century (and probably further). To understand that disability is socially constructed means understanding that the economic, political, and social forces which now restrict our lives can (and will) change.

The Eugenics Movement And Sterilization Abuse

The reproductive rights movement has, by and large, failed to address the ways that sterilization abuse has affected disabled people. Compulsory and coerced sterilization of the disabled began in the late 19th century. The eugenics movement provided the ideological basis for these actions (as well as providing a similar rationale for racist actions). The term "eugenics" was coined by Sir. Francis Galton; the Oxford English Dictionary defines the word as "pertaining or adapted to the production of fine offspring, esp. in the human race." The aim of this movement was to apply the same principles of improving "stock" that were used for horses and vegetables to human beings. This movement has strong roots in Social Darwinism — the idea that life is a struggle between the fit and the unfit. The unfit — which includes the "feeble minded, insane, epileptic, diseased, blind, deaf, [and] deformed" were to be bred out of existence. (Bajema, 1976).

Based on the mistaken notion that all disabilities were inherited, there were several factors that contributed to the growth of the eugenics movement at this period. One factor was the prevalent assumption of 19th century science that human perfection could be achieved through a combination of technological and social manipulation, an increased understanding of heredity, and the fact that surgical techniques for sterilization had become available. But any discussion of the eugenics movement which leaves out the changing social role of disabled people at this period fails to grasp the true nature of this movement.

As America industrialized, there was less room for those who had physical or mental limitations to adapt their work environment to their needs. Our history as disabled people has yet to be written. But from what I have been able to glean, I believe that in rural societies disabled people had far more of a social role than they have had in the more urban and industrialized world. The fact that folk tales and rhymes refer to "the simple;" that "the village idiot" was a stock figure; that blind and other disabled people appear in the myths and legends of many places, all indicate that in the past, disabled people had more of a daily presence in the world.

As work became more structured and formalized, people who "fit" into the standardized factories were needed. Industrializing America not only forbade the immigration of disabled people from abroad, it shut the ones already here away in institutions. The growth of social welfare organizations and charities which "helped" those with disabilities did provide jobs for a certain segment of the middle class; and volunteer charity fit in with the Victorian notion of women's duties and sphere.

This change in attitudes towards disabled people can be traced in language. The word *defective,* for instance, was originally an adjective meaning faulty or imperfect: it described one aspect of a person, rather than defining that person totally. By the 1880's, it had become a noun: people were considered not merely to have a defective sense of vision or a defective gait — they had become totally defined by their limitations, and had become *defectives.* A similar tranformation took place a few decades later with the word *unfit,* which also moved from being an adjective to being a noun. The word *normal,* which comes from the Latin word *norma,* square, until the 1830's meant standing at a right angle to the ground. During the 1840's it came to designate conformity to a common type. By the 1880's, in America, it had come to apply to people as well as things. (Illich, 1976).

Close on the heels of the rise of institutions for disabled people was an increase in forced and coerced sterilization. Adele Clarke has pointed out that "the intentional breeding of plants and animals is almost exclusively undertaken to improve the products... [to increase] profitability from the products, whether they be Arabian horses or more easily transportable tomatoes or peaches. Eugenics applies, I believe, the same profit motive to the breeding of people." (Clarke, unpublished paper). Since disabled people were of little or not use to the profit-makers, and since they were thought likely to become burdens on the state coffers, they were to be stopped from producing others like themselves.

Compulsory sterilization laws were passed in the early 1900's. By the 1930's, in addition to sterilization laws, 41 states had laws which prohibited the marriage of the "insane and feeble-minded," 17 prohibited the marriage of people with epilepsy; four outlawed marriage for "confirmed drunkards." More than 20 states still have eugenics laws on their books. (Clarke, unpublished paper).

Coerced sterilization is still very much a reality, especially among the developmentally disabled. "Voluntary" sterilizations are sometimes a condition for being released from an institution; there has been at least one recent case of a "voluntary" sterilization being performed on a six-year-old boy. (Friedman, 1976).

It is important to understand the connections between sterilization abuse of disabled people and of Third World people. The U.S. Senate Committee on Nutrition and Human Needs reported in 1974 that between 75% and 85% of the "mentally defective and retarded children" who are born each year are born into families with incomes below the poverty line. This means that a large number of those who are labeled as "retards" are people of color. The vast majority of people who get diagnosed as being mentally retarded have no definite, identifiable cause for their retardation: they are called the "mildly retarded," the "educable," and those with "cultural-familial" retardation. The same IQ tests which "prove" that Black people as a whole are less intelligent than whites label a far greater percentage of individual Black children as "retarded." (Chase, 1980).

The Eugenics Movement in Nazi Germany. The Model Sterilization Law of Harry Laughlin, which I cited earlier, was never passed in its totality by any state in this country; however a version of it was adopted in Nazi Germany. American eugenicists were often enthusiastic supporters of Hitler's attempt to rid Germany of "defectives."

Nazi ideology stressed purity, fear of disease, and the importance of heredity, intertwining these concepts with racism. In *Mein Kampf,* Hitler calls syphilis "the Jewish disease;" Jewish people (and other "sub-humans") are portrayed as being weak, sickly, and degenerate, in contrast with healthy blonde Aryans. Before the start of World War II, Nazi eugenics courts had forced hundreds of thousands of disabled people to be sterilized. This forced sterilization helped to pave the way for the wartime genocide of Germany's disabled population. (Chase, 1980).

The Reproductive Rights Movement

Many disabled women find involvement in the reproductive rights movement problematic. Not only have many activists in this movement talked about the issues raised by disabled fetuses in ways that are highly exploitative and prey upon fears about disability, the movement also has, by and large, failed to address the denial of reproductive rights to disabled women and men. It has also failed to make itself physically accessible to disabled women.

I often hear an argument in favor of abortion rights that says, "The right-wing would even force us to give birth to a child who was deformed." ("Deformed" is mild in this context. I've heard "defective," "grossly malformed," and "hideously deformed.") This attitude has become so widespread that at a recent conference on reproductive rights I heard disabled infants referred to as "bad babies." *Off Our Backs* parodied a conversation between Nathanson and Hatch on "the joys of having a [sic] mongoloid child."* (Thorne, 1981).

*The term "mongoloid" to describe children with the chromosonal disorder now termed "Down syndrome" originated in the mid-19th century. It was thought that the birth of these children to white parents was a "hereditary throwback" to the "lower race" of Mongols (Asians) from which the white race had ascended. (See Steven Jay Gould, 1981 *The Mismeasure of Man.* Norton & Co., New York.)

No woman should be forced to bear a child, abled or disabled; and no progressive social movemnt should exploit an oppressed group to further its end. We do not need, as Michelle Fine and Adrienne Asch (1982) point out in their article, "The Question of Disability: No Easy Answers for the Women's Movement" to list conditions — such as the presence of a fetus with a disability — under which abortion is acceptable. The right to abortion is not dependent on certain circumstances: it is our absolute and essential right to have control over our bodies. We do not need to use ableist arguments to bolster our demands. There are racist and classist arguments that can be made for abortion: to argue against them does not compromise our insistence on abortion rights.

Issues Raised by Fetal Diagnosis. When we first fought for and won abortion rights, we focused on the situation of the *woman* herself. Most women who choose abortion do so early on in pregnancy, having made the decision that they do not want a child, any child, at the time. Now, however, the availability of techniques for diagnosis of fetal disabilities (such as amniocentesis, ultrasonography, and fetoscopy) means that women can now choose not to give birth to a *particular* fetus. This is a radical shift, one which raises profound and difficult questions. Perhaps some of the kneejerk reaction to the issues of disabled fetuses reflect our unwillingness to fully explore these hard issues.

It is a little too pat to say that decisions about whether to have amniocentesis or to abort a disabled fetus are personal ones. Ultimately, of course, they are and must remain so. But we need to have a feminist, political language and ways of thinking about this issue to aid us in making those personal decisions and discussing these issues.

As Adrienne Asch has pointed out, discussions about whether or not to carry to term a pregnancy where the fetus will be born with a disability are clouded when we think in terms of the "severity" of the "defect." Rather, potential parents need to consider who *they* are and what they see as *their* strengths and weaknesses as parents making these decisions.

In choosing to be a parent, none of us knows what we are getting into: prenatal diagnosis may shed a little light, but everyone who becomes a parent takes a giant leap into the unknown. We need to remember that there is no such thing as a "perfect" child; that all children, abled and disabled, are going to experience suffering and joys in this world.

One thing that feminists should push for is good amniocentesis counseling. Unfortunately, despite my attempts, I haven't been able to witness any such counseling first hand. I was able to interview one disabled woman who had amniocentesis. She was having amnio not because she intended to abort if her fetus had a potential disability, but because she felt that, given her special needs, she needed to be able to make plans if her child was going to have a disability. She was shocked at the assumptions made by the counselors that any woman who was carrying a fetus with Down's syndrome or spina bifida would of course abort. After the group counseling session, she called the clinic to voice her objections about their presentation of disability. She was told by counselors at the clinic that they felt they should provide as *negative* a picture as possible.

Much of this stems from medical attitudes towards physical impairment. One woman did an informal survey in which she asked doctors, "What things would be worse than death?" They answered, being paraplegic, or being deaf, or partially sighted or not having both arms. (Carleton, 1981). I think having attitudes like that is a fate worse than death. Too often, people who see physical and mental limitations as tragedies are counseling women following amniocentesis. Are women who are told they are carrying a Down's fetus told that, due to deinstitutionalization and better educational methods, some people with Down's now go to school in regular classrooms, live in their own apartments and hold jobs? Are they told that 95% of Down's people have moderate to mild retardation? Are they told that if they choose to bear their child, but not raise her or him, the child can be adopted immediately — usually within twenty-four hours? (Ganz, 1983). Do they have anything more to go on than fear, shame, and their own prejudices combined with those of the medical profession? Women who are considering aborting a disabled fetus must have the opportunity to talk to disabled people and the parents of disabled children. Anything less is not real reproductive freedom.

Women considering whether or not to give birth to a disabled child have few, if any, positive role models. Mothers who remain the primary caregivers of disabled children are seen as being either self-sacrificing saints or bitter, ruined women. These popular images get carried into the "objective" scientific literature. Wendy Carlton reviewed the studies done of mothers of disabled children: they were seen as either being "rejecting" or "overprotecting;" they denied the child's condition or had unrealistic expectations; they are "unconcerned or overinvolved." (Carlton, 1981). No matter what they did, they couldn't seem to get it right. One in every twenty children is born with some sort of disability — a quarter of a million children a year. In addition, many become disabled during childhood. There are millions of mothers of disabled children in the U.S., most of whom, I am sure, manage to do a halfway decent job of childrearing, despite stereotypes, social service cutbacks, and the limitations of the nuclear family.

Dealing with Fears. This article grew out of a talk that I gave to a reproductive rights group on this issue. In the discussion that followed, I was very disappointed that women in the audience never once addressed the reproductive rights of disabled women and men, despite extensive presentation of such issues. Instead, the discussion focused on disabled infants and, more specifically, on their personal fears of having a disabled child. The women I talked to are hardly alone.

For instance, Sheila Kitzinger, well-regarded in the alternative birth movement has a chapter on "The Psychology of Pregnancy" in her book, *The Experience of Childbirth.* In the subsection entitled "Fear that the baby will be malformed," she states:

> Any time after about the fifth month of pregnancy, when the child begins to move and becomes a reality to the mother, she may start to think about her baby as possibly deformed... What if this thing I am nourishing and cherishing within my own body, around which my whole life is built now, whose pulse beats fast deep within me — what if this child should prove to be *a hideous deformed creature, subhuman, a thing I should be able to love, but which I should shudder to see?* (emphasis added)

Kitzinger deals with this issue solely on the level of a neurotic fear, never once discussing what happens when a child is actually born with a disability.

The deeply-rooted fears that many women have of giving birth to a disabled child extend to our politics. They need to be worked through. But please don't expect disabled women to sit there and listen to you while you do so.

Killing Babies, Left and Right. Infanticide of the disabled has gone on at least as long as history has been recorded. (Although the Reagan administration would like us to believe that it has gotten worse in the past ten years — *i.e.,* since the legalization of abortion.) Killing of disabled infants continues today —sometimes through denial of nutrition, more often through withholding of medical treatment.

"Baby Doe" is probably the best known case. A Down's syndrome infant, born with a blocked esophagus, his parents and the doctors involved decided to deny him standard live-saving surgery, resulting in his death by starvation. This happened despite the fact that child welfare workers went to court to try to get an injunction to force the surgery to be performed, and despite the fact that there were twelve families ready to adopt the child, and a surgeon willing to perform the surgery for free. (Ganz, 1983). Nearly all Down syndrome children, up to about the age of five, are now adoptable — thanks in large part to the baby shortage caused by legal abortion and the increased number of single women who keep their children.

I believe that it is inconsistent with feminism for us to say that human beings should be killed (or allowed to die, if you prefer) because they do not fit into oppressive social structures. "Anatomy is destiny" is a right wing idea. It is right-wing whether it is applied to women or whether it is applied to disabled children by the people I usually think of as my sisters and brothers.

So-called "right-to-lifers" are among the loudest voices heard in defense of these children's lives, and I have heard the argument made that it is dangerous for us to sound like we are on "their" side. But if we fail to call for full rights for *all* disabled people, we will have allowed right-wing, anti-feminist forces to totally define the terrain on which we struggle. And we can distinguish ourselves from the Right on this issue, by standing for full rights for disabled people — not just the right to live so that we can, in the words of anti-abortionist Nathanson, "evoke pity and compassion" from the abled.

Sexuality, Birth Control,
And Parental Rights

Occasionally, reproductive rights groups make a token mention of disabled women. When we are included, it is usually at the end of a long list. But our particular needs and concerns are rarely addressed, much less fought for. One reproductive rights activist said to me, "We always used to talk about the rights of disabled women, but I was never sure exactly what that meant." Lack of access to our offices, newsletters, demonstrations and meetings remains a barrier, preventing many disabled women from being physically present within the movement to voice their concerns.

Part of this problem lies in the pervasive stereotype of disabled women as being asexual. Disabled women have been asked, "What do you need birth control for?" or "How did *you* get pregnant?" In 1976, SIECUS, the Sex Information and Education Council on the United States, which is a quite respectable organization, prepared a booklet on "Sexuality and the Handicapped" which was sent to the 1976 White House Conference on the Handicapped — and promptly rejected as "inappropriate." (Calderone, 1981).

At least some of this prevalent stereotype of asexuality stems from seeing disabled people as eternal children. Telethons and other charitable activities have played a large role in creating this image. They portray us as being wan, pathetic, pitiful. The Jerry Lewis telethon even showed a series of film clips of adult disabled people saying, "I'm forty-seven years old and I'm one of Jerry's kids," "I'm fifty-five years old and I'm one of Jerry's kids." I won't go into the way that children's sexuality is treated in this society.

This asexual image is often prevalent among doctors and counselors as well. Women who have had spinal cord injury report that when they asked questions about their sexual functioning they were given the information that they could still have children — and nothing more Or else, they received sexist and heterosexist information, typified by the following:

> ... a female paraplegic can have intercourse more easily than a male paraplegic, since she does not have to participate actively. Although

some such women have no subjective feeling of orgasm [as opposed
to an objective feeling of orgasm?] they are perfectly capable of satisfying their husbands. (Becker, 1978)

All human bodies are sexual. People without genital sensation
(which is a fairly common occurence following spinal cord injury)
can have orgasms through the stimulation of other parts of their
bodies, such as their breasts, earlobes, or necks. One measure of the
rigid structure which the medical profession imposes on our bodies
is that these non-genital orgasms are sometimes referred to by
clinicians as "phantom orgasms" These are not genuine, medically-
approved orgasms — they only *feel* like the real thing.

There is an opposite stereotype, in some ways similar to the
madonna-whore dichotomy which women face. Disabled people
(particularly men, although also women) are sometimes seen as
being filled with diseased lusts. Lewis Terman, one of the early
authorities on what was then called "feeble-mindedness" said that
all developmentally disabled women were "potential prostitutes"
since moral values could not "flower" without full intelligence.
Media images portray disabled men — whether they are physically
disabled or "escaped mental patients" — as rapists and potential
rapists. The chilling realities about rape of disabled people, particularly within institutions, has been largely ignored both by the public
at large and within the women's movement.

Disabled lesbians are rarely seen as having made a choice about
their sexuality. Many people see them as having had to take "second best" because of their disability, or as having relationships
which must be asexual. For mentally retarded lesbians the "normal-
ization" which is a part of moving developmentally disabled
people into the community holds pitfalls. "Normal" women are supposed to curl their hair, wear makeup and dresses, giggle, and sleep
with men. Many who argue for the sexual rights of developmentally disabled people point out that if they aren't allowed to
form heterosexual relationships that they will form — horror
of horrors — homosexual ones.

Birth Control. The stereotype of asexuality persists in information that comes from the women's health movement. I have never
seen a discussion of birth control methods — no matter how extensive — that talks about how a particular method works for a woman

who is blind, or has cerebral palsy, or is developmentally disabled. *Our Bodies, Our Selves* (1976), for instance, warns that the pill should not be taken by women who have a "disease or condition associated with poor blood circulation," without mentioning what those diseases or conditions are. Unfortunately, many of us with disabilities are far from fully informed about our medical conditions. I had no idea (and neither, apparently, did any of the gynecologists I saw) that, due to my disability, taking birth control pills put me at great risk of thromboembolism.

When we work for improved birth control, we need to remember that there are many disabled women for whom there is *no* method that comes close to being safe and effective. The pill is contraindicated for most women in wheelchairs because of circulation problems. Many women who have paralysis cannot insert a diaphragm, and these same women may have problems with an IUD, especially if they do not have uterine sensation and cannot be warned by pain and cramping of infection or uterine perforation.

The 1983 hearings in Washington about the possible licensing of Depo-Provera highlight another area of contraceptive abuse of which feminists must be aware. Depo-Provera is an injectable contraceptive. Because it is not user-controlled, it is often recommended for women who have developmental disabilities. (It also has the "beneficial" effect of doing away with menstruation; for developmentally disabled women, this is supposed to be a special plus, since it is more "hygenic". (Is it disability or menstruation that is unclean?)

Part of the problem with this use of Depo is that many of those who are considered severely or profoundly retarded also have physical disabilities. One study found that users of Depo "are several times as likely to undergo thromboembolic (blood clotting) disease without evident cause as non users." (Duffy, 1981). It seems likely that their physical disabilities would put them at increased risk.

Depo-Provera, because of the many side effects that have occurred with its use, is only licensed for use as a treatment for cancer. However, individual doctors can prescribe Depo for any reason they choose; and developmentally disabled women are probably receiving it now, with no method of reporting the side effects and problems they experience. (*Toward Intimacy,* an otherwise excellent booklet about contraception for disabled women, lists only a few of the known side-effects associated with Depo, and candidly notes: "Available only through private physicians until FDA approval is obtained for Depo-Provera's use as a contraceptive. Family planning clinics can often refer you to private physicians if you are interested in this method.")

Parenting, Custody Issues, and Adoption. In preparing this article, I looked for, but was unable to find, any statistics about the number or percentage of disabled people who have children. I did find lots of anecdotal information about disabled people being told they *shouldn't* have children, and heard some chilling stories from disabled women about being pressured into having abortions. There is almost no public image of disabled people as parents, and I do not know of a single book about being a disabled parent — although there are probably hundreds about having a disabled child.

There have been two fairly well-known cases in which a disabled parent fought to win or keep custody of a child. One of these concerned a single mother who had been born without arms or legs: welfare workers attempted to take her child away from her. After demonstrating to the judge that she was able to care for her child's needs herself, she won the right to custody. In the second case, a divorced quadraplegic father won custody of his sons.

It is particularly important that we in the women's movement take up these issues, since too often they are ignored when demands for disability rights are raised. The American Civil Liberties Union puts out a handbook called *The Rights of Physically Handicapped People* which contains no mention of parental rights, sexual rights, rights to adoption, or rights to safe and effective birth control.

The many political issues around adoption are too complex for me to delve into here. We do need to be sure that people are not denied the right to adopt on the basis of their disability. This has a special importance for two reasons: a small percentage of people with disabilities are unable to become biological parents. In addition, there is a growing tendency for disabled people to adopt children with disabilities, so that they can be raised within our community.

Because both the reproductive rights movement and the disability rights movement are rooted in our rights to control our bodies and our lives, there are strong links between the two. Just as there needs to be a realization within the disabled rights movement that the rights of disabled women must be fought for, so there needs to be an awareness within the reproductive rights movement that those of us who are disabled can no longer be exploited and ignored.

References

Bajema, Carl. 1976. *Eugenics Then and Now.* Benchmark Papers in Genetics, 15. Dowden, Hutchinson & Ross, Inc. Stroudsburg, Pennsylvania.

Becker, Elle F. 1978. *Female Sexuality Following Spinal Cord Injury.* Accent Special Publications, Bloomington, Indiana.

Boston Women's Health Book Collective. 1976. *Our Bodies, Our Selves.* Simon and Schuster, New York.

Calderone, Mary S. 1981. Sexuality and disability in the United States. In David G. Bullard and Susan E. Knight, eds., *Sexuality and Physical Disability: Personal Perspectives.* C.V. Mosby Co., St. Louis, Missouri.

Chase, Allan. 1980. *The Legacy of Malthus.* University of Illinois Press, Urbana, Illinois.

Clarke, Adele. Unpublished papers. Compulsory sterilization: past, present, and future.

——————————. Unpublished paper. The double-life of eugenics 1900-1930: pseudo-science and social movement.

Duffy, Yvonne. 1981. *All Things Are Possible.* A.J. Garvin & Associates, Ann Arbor, Michigan.

Fine, Michelle and Adrienne Asch. Fall 1982. The question of disability: no easy answers for the women's movement. *Reproductive Rights Newsletter.*

Friedman, Paul. 1976. *The Rights of the Mentally Retarded: An American Civil Liberties Civil Liberties Union Handbook.* Avon Books, New York.

Ganz, Mary. January 30, 1983. Retarded boy's right to live: who decides. *Sunday San Francisco Examiner and Chronicle.*

Hull, Kent. 1979. *The Rights of Physically Handicapped People: An American Civil Liberties Union Handbook.* Avon Books, New York.

Illich, Ivan. 1976. *Medical Nemesis: The Expropriation of Health.* Pantheon Books, New York.

Kitzinger, Sheila. *The Experience of Childbirth.* Penguin books.

Thorne, Becky, November 1981. "Abortion Battle Intensifies Over Hatch's Amendment." *Off Our Backs.* Washington, D.C.

Suggested Reading

Becker, Elle F. 1978. *Female Sexuality Following Spinal Cord Injury.* Accent Special Publications, ɔmington, Indiana.

Bullard, David G. and Susan E. Knight. 1981. *Sexuality and Physical Disability: Personal Perspectives.* C.V. Mosby, St. Louis, Missouri. Excellent collection of articles, most of which are written by people with physical disabilities. Deals with a broad range of disabilities from differing perspectives.

Califia, Pat. 1980. *Sapphistry: The Book of Lesbian Sexuality.* The Naiad Press, Tallahassee, Florida. Very good chapter on disabled lesbians.

Campling, Jo. 1981. *Images of Ourselves: Women with Disabilities Talking.* Routledge & Kegan Paul, London. While not specifically focused on sexuality or reproductive rights, offers insights in lives of disabled women.

Duffy, Yvonne. 1981. *All Things Are Possible.* A.J. Garvin & Associates, Ann Arbor, Michigan. Compilation of questionnaire responses and interviews with women who are orthopedically disabled.

Fine, Michelle and Adrienne Asch. Fall 1982. The question of disability: no easy answers for the women's movment. *Reproductive Rights Newsletter.* Excellent article which discusses the exploitation of the disabled fetus issue by the abortion rights movement.

Friedman, Paul. 1976. *The Rights of the Mentally Retarded.* Avon Books, New York. Discusses sterilization abuse, parental rights, and rights to sexual expression.

Sex Information and Education Council of the U.S. 1978. *Sexuality and Disability: A Bibliography of Resources Available for Purchase.* SIECUS, New York. Annotated list covering general works and information on specific disabilities. (Available from SIECUS, 80 Fifth Avenue, New York, NY 10011 for $1.00 and a stamped, self-addressed business envelope.)

Task Force on Concerns of Physically Disabled Women. 1978. *Toward Intimacy: Family Planning and Sexuality Concerns of Physically Disabled Women.* Human Sciences Press, New York.

7.

Finding Our Friends

Disabled women want satisfying and reciprocal relationships. To those of us who are disabled, this is neither a profound nor surprising statement. Non-disabled society's image of who we are often ignores the fact that we have relationships at all. But, we are human beings, encircled, surrounded and enmeshed by relationships. These relationships are richly textured and complex.

Added to the intensity of beginning any relationship is the presupposition on the part of the non-disabled person that she will forever be in the role of the ''giver'' and that the disabled woman will be in constant need. This fallacy must be challenged and a balance and exchange must be created. Each must acknowledge her strengths and limitations and ask directly for what she needs. This may be difficult for all of us. We have been taught as women to see only our limitations and to be indirect in our interactions. In our feminist attempts to overcome traditional female sex role stereotypes many of us, disabled and nondisabled, have aspired to the American folklore of the rugged individual. This passing as invulnerable, tempting though it may be, is not constructive for any of us. The concept of independence is a distortion of reality. Disabled women confront the distortion because we cannot afford not to. Of course we are all interdependent.

Disabled women may feel forced to prioritize our needs, asking for only life or death necessities. The causal familiarity of asking for favors from friends becomes a self-conscious act instead of a natural exchange. We fear we will ask for too much and our friends will not be there when we really need them. When community support like reader services for the blind or attendant care are available, there is less pressure to meet all our needs through our friends and lovers.

Our disabilities may force a level of intimacy and honesty that is difficult and challenging to us and our friends. A blind woman may ask a friend to check if she is having her menstrual period. A catherized woman may ask for assistance in changing her collecting bag. A hard of hearing woman may ask how her friend feels about having to speak more loudly and repeat her words often. There is little room for superficiality or hidden agendas. Being open to intimate communication establishes a special bond.

These relationships set off a chain reaction that effects all of society. Instead of perceiving ourselves as "givers" and "takers", we can learn to appreciate each other as full human beings.

October

by nanci stern

*i*t's really cold today. That's what I like about October — that and pumpkins. It took half an hour yesterday at the grocery to slide my hands over every pumpkin in the lot, to find the one with the absolutely weirdest shape. It was a squashed, flat pumpkin with Braille dot bumps all over it which made it look like it had a case of teenage acne. I knew it was just waiting for me to take it home. Wow! As I get further down the hall I can smell that apple-pied kitchen, fresh with yesterday's annual tribute to domesticity. After eating all that pie, I'd better clean my teeth.

Where's that toothpaste? I know I put it on the shelf above the sink last night, but the only paste I can feel up here is old, dried and in blobs.

"Pat! Oh, Pat!" The only sound in this entire apartment is my dog daintily slobbering in her bowl, so I guess my roommate isn't here. Maybe the toothpaste fell on the floor. No, and it's not in the garbage can. But here's that new package of bobby pins I bought yesterday. Where were you last night when I needed you to put those little pin curls in my head? Whoever said a permanent was permanent obviously never had one. I hope no one ever finds out these precious curly little locks are all fake. Ah! This must be the toothpaste, in the medicine chest. Unless I'm about to brush my teeth with the tube of zinc oxide, like I did once in Canada. Oh, you pretty little teeth, I love you, all thirty-two of you. Even if I do own the Stern silver mine, I plan to die with all my own teeth.

Enough, enough with the dental floss. I'm going to be late if I don't hurry. Besides, if I leave early enough I can take a bit of a walk first. It's the perfect night to feel the wind in my face and that little alive sting in my eyes that the cold always gives me. And maybe

I can walk off a little of my nervousness before this date.

I think I'll wear my new mohair sweater. I've been told it will look impressive with grey pants. Dammit, the dots on these Braille labels are so worn down I can barely tell if these are the grey pants or the green ones. Eureka! That is a "Y" at the end. Now if only I remembered to ask Pat to leave out my grey socks. Well, I forgot, so it's potluck again. When I was on a disability panel on TV, the only thing anyone remembered about it was that I was wearing mismatched socks. Maybe I should take my mother's advice and buy all my socks in the same color, then I wouldn't have this problem. I hadn't realized how many of my friends had color televisions.

I'd better go check on the filled insulin syringes Pat left for me in the kitchen. Here they are, taped to a plate. I'm glad we started this new system of leaving two. I got a surprise last night when I sat down at Maria's house to eat dinner. Just before my veggie lasagne was being dished up, I made the awful discovery that the plastic tampon holder had squished in and smashed the needle on my syringe. It was sure a pain in the ass to go home and get another filled syringe while dinner was waiting. I miss the days when I could throw a couple of bottles of insulin and a few syringes in a backpack and take off for my gypsy travels around the country. This plastic box my aunt sent should work better. I hope it will fit in my purse. I won't look too sophisticated tonight schlepping my backpack on our first dinner date.

Before I return to the bedroom for finishing touches I might as well let Tang into the backyard. I understand the guys upstairs have made a really nice garden back there out of that once blackberried jungle. Maybe I'll go out there one of these afternoons and get my hands in the dirt. I grew up wanting to be a gardener until I was eleven or twelve. I was still sighted then and I tried to plant a garden in the shape of Texas in the backyard of my parents' newly rented home in Houston. I was so proud of myself. I brought out a map of the U.S. to get the shape right and staked out the area with string and sticks. Then, I spent the rest of the afternoon digging. When my father came home, he furiously demanded to know who was responsible for digging that huge ugly hole in a backyard that didn't even belong to us. I suppose I could start again in the backyard here, but California is the wrong shape and I don't want to run into Tang's leftovers. "Tang, Tang, come on. I want you to go out. You're going to take me to dinner soon."

How in the world did this bedroom dresser get to be such a mess? All those pictures I covered my mirror with have fallen on top of my hairbrush again. I love to stand right here directly in front of the mirror brushing my hair. I still picture myself with long straight hippie hair like I had when I lost my sight thirteen years ago. It's hard to see my face as it is now, surrounded by these short curls. I used to love brushing that long hair. It's just that when it got caught in car windows and pants zippers that I thought it was time for it to go. I used to be fat. I can still see my round face. Nowadays I just imagine that my face resembles my fantasies and it works. I'm sure I look great unless I can actually feel a pimple or two. I still see myself with big blue eyes the way I last saw them. It was startling last week when Ellen said my left eye had changed again and that it was almost entirely milky white. There were only slight traces of that long ago blue. For a few days I wondered if I looked strange. I asked several friends if my eye looked weird. But most of them had never seen me any other way and didn't really know what I was talking about. I understand I look older, too. I am told there are a few grey hairs here and there, not to mention a couple of new laugh wrinkles. I don't feel any older and I am wearing some of the same sweatshirts and jeans I did when I was twenty. It's an odd feeling not to watch myself change with age.

Where is that jewelry cup? Yuk! There's a used kleenex and that half empty can of Tab from last night. Ah, here are the necklaces. Damn! Now they're all over the floor. I don't have time for all of this. I guess Tang's all right in the backyard. It's dusty under this dresser. They're old bobby pins and that earplug to my tape recorder that I've been missing. Let's see; I don't feel like wearing this little jade heart but here's the amethyst Sara gave me last year for my birthday. I remember the day she gave it to me. I dropped it that day too, and spent time feeling around on the floor for it. She had commented on all the jewelry I was wearing as soon as we met. That is, as soon as she finished playing with my guide dog. That was when it first occurred to me that more people approached me now that Tang is with me than when I carried a cane. Sara is a dog lover. I liked the deep smooth tone of her voice right away. I thought to myself, at least she isn't terribly afraid of blind people or she never would have introduced herself to begin with. After we had talked for a while, she told me that her grandmother had been blind for many years. They had spent a lot of time together reading, going to movies and shopping. It proved to be true that between Sara and me my blindness never seemed to be the problem — everything else did. Maybe if we hadn't been so competitive, jealous and stubborn, things would have worked out better. It's funny, I never expected us to have regular troubles. All that fear I had about my illness never resulted in the kind of relationship problems we couldn't work through.

I remember when Sara and I had that first dinner together. I wanted to seem so entirely independent; never needing anything from anyone else in order to live my life. So here I am, doing it all myself, breathing in the dust under the dresser. Sitting in the restaurant that night I twisted my jade ring round and round. My hands were cold and sweaty. Through the sounds of my pulse beating nervously in my right ear I could hear Sara's voice reading every promise of an excellent dinner from the menu. Then the first question came:

"Have you been blind all your life?"

"No."

"What happened?"

"I have diabetes. In fact, I have an injection I need to give myself before dinner. Will you help me to the bathroom?"

That was the last time I scurried off, inconveniently disrupting a dinner to hide an injection, but back then I was embarrassed about my injections instead of accepting them as part of my daily existence. Sara didn't seem to be squeamish or nauseated, or even fazed by it at all. She stayed with me in the tiny cubicle, describing it to me as I rummaged in my purse.

"Is there a fairly clean sink" I asked, "or something I can put this case on while I take my injection?" I was tentative, concerned that the bathroom was dirty or that someone would walk in while I was injecting and get upset.

"Take my arm and I'll show you." Sara placed my hand on the sink and asked, "How often do you have to take these injections?"

"Three times a day. That's the new philosophy. I take more

injections with less insulin in each to try and meet my insulin needs closer to the way a normal body would." I grabbed onto every ounce of self control when the word "normal" resounded in my mind. I wanted to blurt out all my anxiety and tell her that I am needle-phobic and that I'm always afraid I don't get all my insulin if no one watches me give my injection, but I just wasn't ready to reveal that much wanting or needing of help. After all we had only met a week before at the dance. I didn't need help there; my diabetes wasn't showing yet.

Returning to the table, we dug into our salads with great gusto. I am almost always a happy camper when I'm eating. Along with my shock and displeasure at inadvertantly swallowing a piece of beet, came the next question:

"I don't know much about diabetes except that people take insulin and shouldn't eat sugar. Would you mind talking about it? I mean, what does it have to do with your being blind?"

I started off almost blankly, rattling off the academics: "About ninety percent of adults who become blind in adulthood lose their sight from diabetes. It comes along with the territory."

Sara stopped me, "It must be very hard for you." There was real concern and interest in her voice. I took a deep breath. Where do I begin and just how much do I want to say? Wouldn't she rather talk about herself, our jobs or who we've both slept with? My voice became unfamiliarly quiet, "I never thought having diabetes was a problem for the entire twenty years before I lost my sight. No one used to think it was a problem if you took your insulin." Then my chatter took over. I rambled as though I were reciting effervescent lines from a play:

"I don't mind being blind so much. I wouldn't have chosen it, but I really have a good full life. It's the diabetes that wears me out. Actually, I've been having a great time lately. I've been taking this water aerobics class and I also saw a great new play last week."

Sara broke in, "Hey, slow down! You're talking so fast you'll choke on that hamburger. What do you mean, the diabetes wears you out?"

"Well, each of those three injections I take requires a home blood test to know how much insulin has to be put into the syringe.

In the old days, when there was no blood sugar testing and I could fill my own syringes, I had a lot more freedom. It's harder to travel this way, even though it's safer. I need company to help out with the details. I do find that it's fun travelling with someone else. I always used to travel alone, so that part has been a nice change."

Sara said, "You look great. Do you feel alright most of the time?" I looked down at my throbbing finger. I had twisted my teabag string around my index finger, in tiny little knots. I briefly withdrew into a memory of being in the hospital in 1976. It was the first time I had been hospitalized in my adult life. I had wanted so much to be disconnected from my disease that I didn't even have a doctor when I ended up with strep throat in the city's general hospital. When I got there I found I had water in my lungs, and was also in acidosis, a condition that sometimes occurs in diabetics with serious infections.

I dodged the question, "Would you get more hot water for my tea?" I had lost a friend during and after that illness because she was afraid. Her only communication with me after my hospitalization was a phone call in which she said that she was afraid of hospitals and afraid I would need things from her that she couldn't give. I had never asked her for more than reading occasional mail to me. She was afraid, she said, that I would be sick again. I couldn't answer that. I had just learned that the water in my lungs was from my kidneys. I was beginning to understand that some diabetics had kidney problems. Someday I was going to be sick again. I didn't want to face that any more than she did.

Sara came back. "I brought you a lemon. I don't know if you like them, but they were there with the tea."

"Oh yes, I used to eat them at diabetic camp. We were all on special diets there. The only foods around that didn't seem to affect insulin too much were things like pickles and lemons. I'd put saccharin all over them and eat them. They made my teeth feel clean... anyway, to answer your question, daily, I feel fine. I get a fair amount of exercise. I ride a bicycle that gets me nowhere fast for about forty five minutes a day while watching my favorite soap opera. Other than bouts with low blood sugar, I feel fine. By the way, when you said I looked great, what did you mean? Tell me more."

I soaked up Sara's articulate and charming praises. I felt the beginnings of a connection between us beyond flattery and wanted to be closer. I decided to risk giving further information, opening myself to difficult feelings. "I do have some kidney problems and I take medication to keep my blood pressure down. There's nothing much more I can do but try to keep track of it with various medical tests." I began to feel those damned sneaky tears behind my face, filling my throat and swimming up to my eyes. "The doctors say eventually I'll be on dialysis. It frightens me to think about it."

Crash! Bang! Clatter! The teacup and spoon I'd been playing with hit the floor. Sara and I both bent down to reach for it, clonked heads and ended up sitting on the restaurant floor laughing hysterically. Tang moved in instantly.

"Stop that, you four-footed mobile garbage disposal! There's nothing edible here and you don't need to clean the floor."

At least this jewelry cup didn't break. It was saved by landing on the rug instead of the hardwood floor. Yes, I think the amethyst necklace Sara gave me will be perfect for this evening. It may bring me good luck. After all, she and I certainly weathered a good many growing pains together. The biggest surprise to me was that she never minded helping with my blood tests and insulin. She even stuck around through many of my bad tempered low blood sugar reactions. She did get a bit put out with me when I got back from my four day diabetes course. I had learned new and overwhelming things that I was supposed to be doing for my diabetes. I came home the third night of the course late and tired. I was disgusted because my blood sugars in class had always been so high. I was pained to hear that the people in the most trouble now are those who took a full syringe of insulin a day as teenagers. All I could think over and over was, damn it, that's me. Why didn't I know? Why didn't anyone know?

It was time for my injection and Sara was helping me. I didn't get enough blood from the autolet's pin prick the first time, or the second time. Finally I yelled at Sara, who was trying to get a drop of blood from my ear, "Can't you do any better than that? I'm sick and tired of sticking needles into myself!" With one swoop of my hand I flung the plastic autolet and the syringe across the room. The plastic cracked and broke. The syringe hung limply by its needle, stuck in the kitchen curtain.

Sara yelled back, "I'm angry too. I hate this disease, but I'm not taking it out on you. Do me a favor and don't take it out on me." I was woefully piecing the plastic together to try for another blood test. Tears began rolling down my face. Sara started sniffling too. We sat for a while, first hugging, then crying and finally fighting over who would get the last kleenex in the box. While applying tissues to dripping noses, Sara asked me where I wanted my injection. "In someone else," I said, then we both started laughing and naming all the people we wouldn't mind giving a good poke with an insulin needle. I'm glad we've remained friends.

It's time to get up off this floor and get my dog. "Tang, Tang, come on in. Did you have a nice time outside? You're about to take me to my favorite restaurant, but don't worry, we'll stop at Mr. Bergman's deli first so you can get your bologna treat on the way. Now all I need is my mysterious sophisticated London fog spy coat and your leather harness and leash."

Let's see. I've got my syringes, wallet, keys and dextrosols in case I need a quick sugar fix for emergency low blood sugar. Well, I think I'm ready. I'll just take one more quick swipe with my dental floss before we go. After all, I'm about to meet a new friend.

A special thanks to my readers, Leslie Bergson, Patricia L. Smith, and Sally Gearhardt

Counterpoint

by pennyota ahladas

In my head buzzes the sound of disease
a tiny hiss, a rubble, a roar that haunts me.
A part of me leaves me.
I notice it more each day.

I am left alone
with only the noises in my head.
Perhaps it's time
for me to be alone.

I put my ear to your lips
the whispers on the pillow.
Safe in your arms I cry
because the man in the store repeats himself
three times before I hear him.
I cry because I cannot hear
the bass tones of the Bach Cantatas
or the howling wind outside our bedroom.
I cry for when
I will not hear
whispers on the pillow.

You say it's okay, I love you
think of all the other ways we are.
But will you still love me
when all words are beyond my reach?

At the theater you sit close
and the words of the stage come to me.
What if I did not have you
to speak the world into my ear?

With the sounds that fade away
I am fading too.
Perhaps, I shall disappear into a shell from the sea
a nautilus spiraling inward
to a quiet center point.

A Leg To Stand On

by amber coverdale sumrall

i have been in the hospital for three months. I lie flat on my back, unable to turn over or move my legs. My left leg is in a full cast with twenty-five fractures, major and minor, of toes, foot, ankle, tibia, knee and femur. What remains of my right leg is anchored to a traction device by a metal pin running through my knee, emerging on either side. Where metal pierces flesh, thin scabs have formed. Infection festers underneath. I swab the openings daily with antiseptic, allowing no one to do this for me. It is the one small thing I can do.

A large sign hangs at the bottom of my bed. It reads "Do Not Bump Weight." The weight is a sandbag attached by heavy cord and metal rods to the pin in my knee. Each time it is jolted by people cleaning my room or changing my sheets, the metal pin moves also, tearing open the newly formed scabs.

The skin is stretched taut over the restructured tibia at the end of my stump. My doctors watch it carefully, concerned that the sharp, bony spur will break through. If this happens I will face further surgery, a revision of the amputation. This is my worst fear.

This morning Terry comes in, excited. She is a nurses' aide, full of gentle humor and compassion. We have become friends, comrades in counter-culture. She is a black woman. I am a hippie woman. We both have Indian blood. We each have several cats and are the same age. She brings black-light posters to hang on the walls by my bed.

Terry pulls the curtain around my bed, opens a window and lights a stick of incense. Her dark eyes sparkle with mischief. She takes a small pipe out of her uniform pocket, drops a tiny chunk into it and hands it to me.

"Girl," she says, "take a deep toke. Your cast is coming off today and so is that nasty pin. It's time to celebrate."

I inhale deeply, just once, holding the sweet smoke in my lungs. Trying to imagine how freedom tastes. How it will feel to get out of bed, to bathe, to use the toilet instead of a bedpan. To sleep on my side, to stand on one leg, to leave this room. To go home.

Terry hugs me, then chases the pungent blend of frangipani and hashish smoke out the window with my pillow. She winks, "see you" and is off down the hall to complete her rounds.

I lie back, close my eyes and think about home, the tiny house in Shadow Hills Canyon where Les and I lived together. His clothes still hang in the closet. Home: a place to mourn my lover, to begin the process of letting go. My eyes fill with tears. How much longer must I hold my sorrow?

Ten weeks ago I awakened crying in the night. I felt Les' spirit touch me and knew he had died. He was one floor above me in Intensive Care. He had been in a coma for thirteen days, never regaining consciousness after the accident. A nurse brought sleeping pills to banish my "nightmare." The next morning Dr. Hertl took my hands in his and asked me to be strong. I already knew what he had to tell me. As I wept quietly a nurse arrived with tranquilizers and more sleeping pills. I refused them.

Each time I tried to cry more pills were given to me. I learned to push down the pain until it became a heavy numbness inside. I buried my sorrow, trusting that it would surface when I could release it fully. I could wait for arms to hold me, for hearts to listen. I would not grieve in this place.

The surgery attendants come to take me downstairs. They carefully remove the traction weight and pulleys. They slide me onto the gurney and prepare to leave. "Wait," I say. "I was told I'd get a shot of demerol for this procedure." They have no instructions, tell me I will probably get one in surgery.

Behind the doors marked "Surgery — No Admittance" people are lined up on gurneys like planes waiting to take off. I see Dr. Hertl and ask about the shot. "Oh no, you don't need a shot. After all you've been through! Where's my brave girl?"

He uses the same tone of voice my father uses when he sees me smoking a cigarette in bed. "You mean you still haven't given up smoking? After all you've been through, quitting should be easy."

Dr. Hertl is a short, round, deeply tanned man with a white

moustache. He is from Vienna and speaks with a German accent. He looks like Santa Claus. The nurses are in awe of him. He does not crack jokes or use extraneous words. He is serious, direct and very much respected. I have trusted him implicitly, from the moment I saw tears in his eyes as he told me he'd have to remove my leg.

But now I am afraid, angry at his insensitivity. How dare he patronize me, put me through this ordeal without something to deaden the pain. I swallow my protests.

In the operating room I lie on a table beneath the search-light glare. I smell the harsh disinfectants, see the jars of alcohol holding instruments. The walls are pale green, remind me of grammar school. I feel powerless.

The nurses wear masks. Dr. Hertl puts on green plastic gloves. Fear rises in my throat, there is a metal taste in my mouth. Ice water runs through my veins as I watch him open a large pair of pliers and clamp them to the pin in my leg. He tells me to take a deep breath, asks the nurses to hold me down. I clutch at their hands. In one swift motion he yanks on the pin, pulls it through my knee. I feel an intense burning and am sick to my stomach. The fear and pain take over my breathing and I black out.

When I come to, the cast on my other leg is being cut off and I see this leg for the first time in three months. Lepers have legs like this... yellow, emaciated, protruding bones and peeling skin.

"You will soak in the whirlpool now," Dr. Hertl says. "It will remove the dead skin and increase your circulation. Tomorrow perhaps you can try to stand with a walker."

"But when can I go home?"

"When you have regained maximum flexibility of your foot and are proficient with crutches. You must work very hard these next few weeks."

The nurses lift me into a wheelchair. Both my legs stick straight out in front of me on padded cushions. I wiggle my toes, slowly rotate my foot. There is a crunching sound in my ankle and knee. I think of the Tin Woodsman and his precious oil can. What will I use for lubrication?

Glenda, from Physical Therapy, wheels me down the hall. Familiar faces smile and greet me. She stops at the snackbar to buy us both ice cream. We pass people who have done special things for me: Marguerita, the switchboard operator, who brings homemade wine to my room; Pam, in Admitting, who bakes bread for me and sees to it that I have a private room whenever possible; Brian, from X-Ray, who saves his best jokes for me. And Carrie, from the Lab, who made me a wooden plaque with the inscription, *Ah Life! How like a child you are, you hardly seem worthwhile. You trust in tears but I propose to win you with a smile.*

The trip around the hospital is exhilarating. Glenda shows me how to use the handbrake, how to turn corners and back up. At last I am mobile!

In the Physical Therapy Department Glenda runs hot water into the stainless steel jacuzzi. I tingle with anticipation. This will be my first bath in three months. With the help of another therapist she lowers me into the tub. I sink down, inch by inch, until I'm totally submerged. Bubbles fizz like ginger ale on my skin. There is nothing but this water, swirling around my grateful body.

Traces of phantom pain surface, perhaps activated by the hot water. I feel an intense cramping in the place where my toes and foot used to be. Two months ago, Dr. Ku gave me a series of acupuncture treatments to release the memory of pain my nerves had stored. He put needles in my hands and ears. After three sessions the pain vanished, leaving an annoying itching sensation in my "toes" and a pins and needles feeling in my "foot." My friends sometimes pretend to scratch my "toes" and this often stops the tingling.

Glenda offers to wash my hair. Her fingers are delicious. She wraps a towel around me and lifts me out of the tub. I sit in the wheelchair as she dries my hair. My stump will not bend, it sticks straight out in front of me, frozen in position. I must be cautious not to bump it. The phantom pain recedes. I am suddenly exhausted, want to be back in my room.

She wheels me to the elevator, the one for freight so I won't encounter more people. In minutes I am asleep in my bed. Lying comfortable at last, on my side.

That night, at 11:00, Linda and Diane come into my room. They have just ended their shifts as respiratory therapists. "Jess' truck is parked by the snackbar door," Linda says. "We want to sneak you out for a drink at Los Arcos."

"You're kidding! How will we get away with it?"

"Betty knows and will cover for you. She's the aide on duty tonight."

"How do I get down the hall without being seen?" My room is right next to the nurses' station.

"That's the hard part," Linda giggles. "If anyone sees you, say you're going to the snackbar. But be careful, we can all lose our jobs."

"This is wild but I love it. My first time out of this place! You are amazing."

"Well, it's your first day out of bed and you're way past due for a little fun. So we'll be waiting in the elevator. Good luck!"

Betty brings in a wheelchair, pulls the curtain around my bed. She hands me a pair of jeans, a purple knit shirt. I've kept them here in anticipation of going home. I lie on the bed and slip the jeans on, they are like old friends, very lose and comfortable. No more hospital gowns for me.

"I'll be here when you get back," Betty says as she helps me into the wheelchair. "Off you go now, the nurses are doing rounds. Have a drink for me."

I wheel down the long corridor unnoticed, press for the elevator. The doors open and Linda and Diane push my chair inside. We are laughing in excitement as we descend.

Jess meets us at the pre-arranged door, covers me with a blanket and carries me to his truck. Diane folds the wheelchair and puts it in the back. She and Linda will go in another car. Jess is also a respiratory therapist, a Mexican man with inner wisdom and quiet strength. Many nights he comes to my room to talk. When I first came here, barely conscious, barely alive, he held my hand tightly. Stayed with me. For hours.

Six women, still in their white uniforms, meet us at the restaurant. It is dark and cool inside, candles flicker on our table. I blend into shadow, relax. Here I am free from scrutiny and the glare of harsh light. We order pitchers of margaritas, bowls of chips and salsa. Drink toasts to our bravado, to my imminent discharge from the hospital. Exchange "inside" gossip.

"I hope Hank doesn't hear about this," Diane says. Hank is the head of the department.

"If you're not at work tonight I'll notify the newspapers. We'll create a stink. I'll take all the blame."

"I can just see the headlines," Linda smirks. " 'Staff Members Dismissed Attempting to Aid Disabled Woman.' "

"We'll say you forced us, held that hemostat you use as a roach clip to our throats," Diane banters.

"Maybe they'll expel me and I can go home a few weeks early."

The bar is closing. We drink a final toast and pledge to return one month from tonight. It's 3:00 a.m. when Jess pushes me back through the snackbar doors. I wheel down the bright deserted halls. Safe in my room I push the buzzer. Betty comes immediately. She helps me into bed and I tell her about our adventure. She asks if I want a sleeping pill. "No thanks, I won't need one tonight," I tell her.

"Sweet Dreams," she whispers and closes the door.

In the morning Dan, from Physical Therapy, comes to get me out of bed. He will be the one to teach me how to walk again. I asked for him because I admire his confident manner, his persistence. He has been giving me backrubs three times a week. I'm able to bend down until my head is between my knees and maintain this position comfortably as a result of daily yoga practice.

I am rather hung-over this morning and am feeling capable of great feats of strength. I am also irritable. Mrs. Wright, the Head Nurse, has given me a scolding because I refused breakfast. She believes that hospital food is similiar, in it's properties, to the water at Lourdes.

Dan brings the wheelchair in. "Take it away," I tell him. "I plan on walking down to Physical Therapy. Will you bring me a pair of crutches?"

He humors me. "Oh, I see. Have you tried standing yet?"

"No, but I'm ready."

"O.K.," Dan says. "Let me help you up. Put your elbows in my hands and grab my arms."

I put weight on my foot and attempt to rise. My leg collapses beneath me. I sit on the bed in tears. Dan sits beside me, his hand resting lightly on my shoulder.

"Your fractures may have healed but your leg has forgotten how to bear weight. Your tendons and joints need to be loosened, the muscles developed. Your arms will do most of the work for now, we'll use weights to strengthen them."

"My stump? It won't bend at all."

"It will. With excercise and gentle pressure it'll gradually loosen. You'll be able to wear a prosthesis when it reaches a ninety degree angle."

"My God, is that possible? It will take forever." I see time stretch in front of me, an endless procession of days.

"We'll take one day at a time," Dan says. "And today why don't you just relax. We can begin tomorrow."

"No, I want to start now. The sooner I begin, the sooner I can go home."

Dan lifts me into the wheelchair. Together we begin.

Orthodox Handicapable Chicken Soup

by tzipporah benavraham

i n the paradox I live as a blind Orthodox Jewish woman in my community, I have dealt with some strange attitudinal barriers. One of these has been the typical one that I can't do what everyone else can do. I have to either sit back and bite my tongue and go on, or I have to look upon myself as a survivor.

From a personal viewpoint I have survived many other things: domestic violence, neglect as a child and abuse as a wife, but also DES problems, a slipped disc, a blood clot in my brain, asthma, and epilepsy. The key to my survival is that I come from a people who survive. We survived the Crusades, the Inquisition, Nazi Germany and in every generation some problem which reminds us that "in every generation there are those who would oppress us, but by the faithfulness of the Lord we're still here." That has become an abiding source of my strength.

In dealing with disabled children and their parents, I tell them about a book by a famous rabbi, Moses Maimonides, called *The Guide for the Perplexed,* published in 1539. He wrote that all handicapped conditions are hereditary, and one should avoid a family with a handicapped person because one could inherit that disability. We now know that this is not true, but this is the source for the concept of hiding disabled people. However, in this same book he states that as modern technology reveals itself, an answer will always appear. Where one thing is taken away, another thing will come to be in its place by divine revelation. I can then say it is by divine revelation that modern technology has proven that 98% of handicapping conditions are not hereditary, and that exact remedies are not absolute.

There is much more that a child with a handicapping condition can do. Adaptive techniques and equipment now exist, can be used while accepting the religious premises. One can use a tape recorder to learn Talmudic studies, to enhance the religion.

In doing my job, I am often in the public view and I become a role model for the disabled children. They will often hug me after I have provided a service for them, like helping them mainstream into Yeshivas. They say they want to be like me. This gives me tremendous strength. Although I am only doing my job, they are inspired.

One area I have had difficulty dealing with is this: the Jewish Braille Institute does not have my prayer book in Braille. Although there are 28 Orthdox Jewish prayer books in print, they do not provide my particular one in Braille because we hide our disabled. Because I am blind, I have found other Orthodox Jewish blind people who are also dissatisfied with this situation.

Because the prayer book is not in Braille, and the use of audio cassettes is forbidden on the Sabbath, I have gone to synagogue with my cane, but without my audio cassette. Listening intently to each word of the prayers, I have been kicked out a few times. I want to participate in the synagogue I dearly enjoyed when I was sighted. I am now told I don't belong there, that I should leave because I am embarrassing others. As a disabled person I am not obligated to do anything, so why don't I just go home.

I have never accepted that. I have left with my head hanging and gone home and cried. This is another area of my strength. I know when to cry. It hurts. It is easy to find hurt when I try to be in the mainstream. One place I never expected to find obstacles is in the synagogue, but I have found many there. I do my prayers and learning in my apartment. I follow all the religious precepts taught to me. One will never find me in a non-Kosher store buying non-Kosher food. One will never see me breaking the Sabbath or doing one of the thirty nine forbidden labors. One would never see me in immodest attire. One will never see me doing anything that is outside the mainstream of the community with the exception of being visible and in public.

The emotional problems of dealing with this have left some indelible scars, and a determinism to fight and survive even this. I also teach others to be resilient as I am. I have no right to survive, but I am here. Not only am I here, but I am excelling. Not only am I excelling, I am in the public eye. Not only am I in the public eye, but I am a role model. Here we go, super crip, a common syndrome I am told. But I have become a role model because of my determination. I teach parents to love their children whom they feel so ambivalent about. To love them for their capabilities, not hate them for their handicaps. Often my own ambivalence comes through. If I am in the news people come and tell me you should be married. In Jewish law, people are obligated to marry and have children to replace themselves. They say I should not be in the public eye, and should stop embarassing myself by writing and being written about. I tell them I am pleased being written about, I have nothing to be ashamed of. Just today a friend told me he knew of a man in a wheelchair who would marry me tomorrow and take care of me, so I wouldn't have to worry anymore. I told him I was not worried and not interested in getting married. I will get married at the time I feel I should get married. I am not going to be pressured into that despite the fact that our community holds marriage and the family in the highest regard.

Another precept is that a Jewish person who does not teach a Jewish person a trade is teaching that person to be a thief. I have a vocation in mind for myself. I think I will teach others to teach others to cope with their disabilities. I will not allow people to teach their disabled children to be "thieves". I will not be a "thief" by having no vocation.

I cry a great deal, out of loneliness and frustration that I can't get much farther unless I fight. Fighting is not something I enjoy. Victories I enjoy. I wish I never had to fight any more battles, but am sure I will just to keep on an even keel. The tidal waves of attitudes are overwhelming. However the super woman is going to be there in me as a role model, and who ever heard of Super Woman crying? It would water down the chicken soup I'm supposed to serve as protection against those attitudes.

8.

United We Stand, Sit, and Roll
— Finding Each Other —

Disabled women have worked hard to find each other. There is a great deal of pressure from society to keep us from recognizing that we are disabled and to keep us hidden from the world and each other. Despite the established barriers, we seek each other out. Initially, the drive to do this comes from our loneliness and isolation. We are living with silenced, unacknowledged feelings, each thinking she is the only one involved with the struggles and issues of disability. Sometimes meeting another disabled person provides the first recognition of disability and the first outlet for expression of feelings.

Although our life styles are unique and our disabilities individual, we are drawn to each other by a common thread. When we meet, there is an instinctive connection, a familiarity and an excitement. As we reach out to one another, we develop an atmosphere of sensitivity. We create environments that are physically accessible and emotionally safe places in which to take on the job of breaking down internalized stereotypes of ourselves and each other. We provide a place where we all have permission and freedom to express our feelings, without maximizing or minimizing these feelings, without the fear of being perceived as pathetic, and without creating the assumption that we are asking someone else to "fix" us and make us better. Here we finally have a place to share our common history, to put into context and understand some of the events that have molded our lives. We teach each other how to survive by exchanging the resources which we have acquired from outside or developed within ourselves.

It is a challenge and a struggle for us to face ourselves and each other in depth. Entering this process gives us strength. We become more powerful. *Finding each other is a way to say, "We are here. This is what we need. This is what we want." Disabled women all over the country are finding each other. As a result, here we are,* With the Power of Each Breath, *a beginning.*

The Great Outdoors

by victoria ann-lewis

i stepped gingerly to avoid the poison oak that covered the slope leading to the half-finished cabin where my sleeping bag was laid out. It was hard to keep my footing: I had polio as a kid and I'm missing a significant number of muscles in my legs.

I was camping for a week on the California coast with 15 other disabled women who had come together to train as regional coordinators for a national survey of the educational experiences of women like ourselves. But the project leaders had more than job training in mind. They hoped to forge a tiny community — the beginning of a national disabled women's network — out of these people from very different backgrounds.

When I was invited to "document" the retreat, I hesitated. I'm a loner at work and I live alone — which contents me most of the time. But I was also curious.

Until I moved to California, I had been the only disabled person I had ever known. I was the student carried in the fire drills (when I still wore braces). I was the girl who couldn't wear high heels. While I was growing up, I tried not to think about being disabled (though I secretly poured "Lourdes water" on my leg to restore it to normal fullness). Pimples were more embarrassing.

When I left school, I had no severe mobility problems. I can ride public transport and can enter all buildings and use their bathrooms. So I successfully integrated into nondisabled adult life. I got jobs, had friends, lovers.

Then I moved to California, mainly because I am an actress.

I needed to pay the rent but I passed up the normal actors' jobs — waitressing, cab driving — and took work as a part-time writer for the Center for Independent Living, a disabled rights service and advocacy organization in Berkeley.

Soon after moving, I found a quotation by Dorothea Lange, the world-famous photographer who was disabled by polio:

No one who hasn't lived the life of a semi-cripple knows how much that means. I think it was perhaps the most important thing that happened to me. [It] formed me, guided me, instructed me, helped me, and humiliated me. All those things at once. I've never gotten over it and I am aware of the force and power of it all.

This was the first thing I had ever read that accurately described how I felt. It was a relief. With the relief came the realization of how much energy I was spending *not* looking at my disability. I became curious, if at times uncomfortable, about the role disability had played in my life. It was as if I had overturned a big rock and was going to inspect the subterranean life. It was an investigation I didn't particularly want to make alone. So I agreed to go on the retreat — and I wasn't sorry. We learned a lot about each other, and about ourselves.

Nancy is verbal, ex-Catholic, college-educated, pretty much just like me. Nancy is vision-impaired. Her glasses have a tiny telescopic lens embedded in the regular lens; so when she is looking at you, she appears to be looking past you. In order to read, she holds a book about two inches from her eyes.

Nancy excelled academically in a normal school despite the lack of such learning aids as large-print books. In difficult situations she would push herself to the top. When the typing teacher wanted her out of the class because her posture was incorrect (she had to stoop over the text to read it), she fought to stay and ended up with the top-speed award.

She has mixed feelings about her academic achievement, judging some of it to be a compulsive need to prove herself. And socially it was isolating. "Kids hate the smart kid," she remembers. "I wasn't *that* brilliant. I just went home and studied all the time. I couldn't go out and play basketball: I couldn't see the ball! I never had any fun until I graduated from college. I always had the fear that I was going to be rejected, not because I can't see, but because I can't look people in the eye."

Nancy's idols as a kid were Dag Hammarskjold and Tom

Dooley. She had a fine-tuned sense of justice even as a child due to her own experiences and those of her mentally retarded brother. "He had fifteen broken bones in ten years from kids beating him up and making fun of him. One time he'd been out of a cast for a day and a half and a kid took his arm, twisted it, and broke it again. The principal rationalized, 'That's how kids say hi.' "

Nancy has developed considerable social grace since school. She is very funny and outgoing and everyone wants to spend time with her. Ms. Congeniality of the retreat.

Martha is black, from Kansas City, and she carries herself with a lot of style. Her disability is muscular dystrophy. You can tell from her clothes that she has had trouble finding any grubby camping gear for the trip. Her voice is musical, her fingernails polished.

Although muscular dystrophy is hereditary and had been carried for years in Martha's family, she was the first person to be diagnosed. Her grandmother, who, according to Martha, "went down fast... she went from a cane to crutches to crawling around the house within a few years," was thought to have arthritis.

"Until Medicaid, my family never went to the doctor. We'd buy remedies. One night my fiance and I were watching a muscular dystrophy telethon. As part of the program they described the disease and its symptoms. My fiance said, 'That sounds very familiar.' So I went to a local hospital and was diagnosed."

This was Martha's first trip to California and she was doing her best to appreciate the great outdoors. But too much nature can have a mesmerizing effect on a dyed-in-the-wool city dweller, and it took some effort to rouse Martha out of the lodge and to the beach with a bunch of us to watch the sunset. It was energetic Nancy who eventually persuaded her.

We piled into a modified Checker cab that could easily accomodate a few folded wheelchairs and arrived at the beach at an appropriately gorgeous moment. Martha was wrapped in a turban (and also in what appeared to be every piece of clothing she had brought for the trip) to protect herself from the cold gusty wind. Maria, who is a paraplegic, got in her chair and began to wheel along a trail on the edge of the sea cliff. Carol, who hadn't brought her chair, sank back in the front seat and prepared to watch the sunset.

As I lowered myself over the edge of the cliff, Martha looked surprised. She warned me to be careful. I felt her eyes on me as I went down the cliff in a slow scramble.

Since I've moved to the West some years ago, I've discovered my own climbing techniques. Whenever my balance fails me, I resort to my rump going down and to all fours going up. I get a sort of acrobatic pleasure from moving this way. *Real* climbing situations would be closed to me, but a great deal of the outdoors is accessible.

But I don't use any mobility aids. I had gotten down the beach and was playing in the waves and looked around, and there was Beth propped up on her crutches and braces bending over, picking shells from the wet sand. *How did she get down?* Just like me, I realized: slowly, carefully, enjoying the small shifts in weight precisely placed that led to cool hard-packed sand in the blue shadow from the setting sun.

When we climbed back up, Carol announced that next time she would bring her chair. She hadn't realized how easy it would be.

Meals were raucous affairs. Twenty of us, six in wheelchairs, crammed around one long table. Everyone at the retreat had to serve on a meal crew, with the exception of the two sign-language interpreters who were working 18-hour days. Food preparation and cleanup had the feeling of big family dinners. "I never knew it was possible for so many women to *share* a kitchen," Martha said.

The meal crews were also a way to mix groups smaller than the big training sessions. That's how I first met Carol. Right away I liked working with her. We both know our way around a kitchen and we both enjoy order.

Carol was in a manual chair. She explained that she had been born with dislocated hips and clubfeet. We discovered we were both from the South. Before we knew it, the dishes had been done.

As the week progressed, Carol interested me more and more. She is a big, stately woman. As physical types, we are very different. I'm small and nervous.

But emotionally and experientially, I probably had more in common with Carol than anyone else in the retreat. We had both experienced the alienation that comes from fitting the stereotype of the Southern girl. "I was well liked, lots of friends," she drawled, but it seemed," and her voice quickened, "as if I was always trying to make people like me. And then I always took issues in the community and in the world seriously. I wrote poetry. I was always dying to find someone to share it with.''

I remembered my father counseling me, ''Vicki, you try too hard with people. Relax!'' and my girlfriends sniggering at me as I turned into our school's only beatnik. And the excitement at finding my first friend who wrote poetry.

There's a theory that being disabled confers a negative marginality on one's existence. But there are a few, if only a few, advantages to this. Being disabled, for many of the women I met, removed some of the cultural expectations connected to becoming a woman. We were, for example, the only women in our families to receive a college education. ''Before I got sick,'' one woman explained, ''college was never a serious option for me. Afterward, my parents left no doubt that I was going to college. I had to be able to earn a living, because, unlike my sister, I wasn't expected to marry.'' On the other hand, feminine stereotypes are seen as particularly useful for disabled girls. ''I was taught to be sweet, not sexy. I was going to have to attract not a lover, but a *protector*,'' the same woman continued. She's married now, has a child and a good job.

Adolescence is the time for mastering our sexual identification and thus entering adulthood. Carol flinched when I asked her about those years. Her reluctance was echoed by many of the women I talked to that week. Her first reponse could be taken as an aphorism of life as a disabled teenager: ''Adolescence was real painful for me, but I don't think I realized my disability was the cause of the pain until afterward. Mother had been very supportive of me up until that time, telling me, 'You can do this, you can do that.' I heard now, 'You'll have to accept the fact that you're different.' It was a real blow.''

Carol and I share a love of theater, which in her case had been cruelly crushed in childhood. ''In the second grade I was given one line in the class play: 'Hush, John Adams is about to speak!' I had really wanted a major role so, being a gusty kid, I went to the teacher and told her, '*You* know I can do it, *I* know I can do it, so why don't you *let* me do it?' The teacher called my mother and said, 'Could you please subdue this child?' I went all the way through school thinking I couldn't act.

"Finally in college — I don't know what made me do it, everyone had told me that the drama teacher couldn't tolerate people in wheelchairs — I signed up for drama class. The first day I was the only person in the class who was disabled. The teacher came in, noticed me, and said, 'Well, at least you brought your own chair.' From then on, he encouraged me, had me building sets, working with my hands, crawling around on stage. They made a hoist so I could get up into the lighting booth. Eventually I wrote my first play. It was produced and pronounced a success. Now there are other disabled people in the theater program. I'm proud I was the pioneer."

I loved this story. It mirrored my own early history of breaking into acting and made me feel less lonely.

Carol could look at the dark side of the disabled experience with equal clarity. "I always knew I was disabled," she recalled as she lounged on the sofa one afternoon, "but I don't think it really hit me until I was in college. A woman came out of her room and saw the wheelchair in front of my room and screamed, 'You make me sick!'"

I had never heard the word "cripple" in conversation until one day on the street a few years ago, a kid screamed it at me, "Cripple!" The moment I heard it, it was as if people had been screaming at me all my life, for centuries. The scene was so old. I who have a 'mild' disability and who have heard time and time again, "I didn't even *notice* you were disabled."

Then there was the older man who lived downstairs from me in an apartment I had recently rented, whom I overheard screaming on the phone to the landlady, "She's a cripple, she's always thumping around up there," the edge in his voice sharpened by his lonely, unrecognized life. I was the scapegoat, a ritual object upon which to release his hatred.

Many memories came to me as I talked to Carol, carrying me further and further back. Hospitals. Being a kid and being in a hospital, and not for tonsilitis. Carol had often spent six to nine months a year in the hospital as a child and had found the experience fairly grim. "I was afraid of flies," she recalled. "I was in a cubicle on the children's ward. A fly got in my cubicle and I got hysterical.

When I couldn't stop crying, the hospital staff became impatient with me. They took me and my bed into the bathroom and locked me in for the night. It was a long time before I could cry freely."

After my first major surgery, I awoke in a room with three other children. It was late and only the yellow glow of the night light lit my bed. My mother was there and it was then or the next day that she read me the letter from my adored first grade teacher, Mother Jean Marie. The letter told me she was thinking about me, praying for me. In fact all the nuns were praying for me. And I was supposed to be brave and pray for everyone, and try very hard to be a good girl, *always*. And it was that night or the next day when I saw them offering candy to the little boy in the crib next to mine. Offering candy he was only allowed to grasp with his *right* hand. His parents had beaten him, someone explained to me, and his whole right side was paralyzed. I don't know if I prayed for everyone in the world, but I never forgot that boy.

After the second major surgery (polio kids were always getting their remaining muscles transferred around, steel bars inserted and bones fused to stabilize the body, ball bearings, in my case, sewn in to provide for lost movement), I awoke in the main children's ward, my medal of the Blessed Mother taped to my pillow. Before the operation the nurse made me remove any metal from my body. Through the haze of drugs I asserted my religious convictions and they promised to keep the necklace close to me. Most Catholic girls aged twelve in the 50's aspired to sainthood, particularly in the face of major surgery, when you're knocked out for hours and deep slits are made into your body.

I liked being in the children's ward. All sorts of dramas were enacted around me. I was getting to know the other children and there were group activities. But my parents for some reason, because I was twelve, because it was classier, insisted that I be transferred to a semi-private room. I cried desperately about leaving the ward.

I don't think I ever spoke to the person in the full body cast in the bed next to mine. We were both visited during scheduled hours and the rest of the time passed in silence, for me reading voraciously. Every night I was given a shot to put me to sleep: there was pain I don't remember. And then home the first night, waiting it out in the bathroom till morning, no narcotic to put me to sleep.

As the week wore on, I found myself more and more at ease. This wasn't unusual, given the circumstances. Often on a camping trip my mind and body form a seamless garment and I experience a mild euphoria. But at the retreat, what was usually a solitary experience had become a communal one. How?

Actually, it was more like a summer camp or a high school than a camping trip. But high school with a *big* difference: neither looks nor physical competence separated me from the others. There was *no norm*. For one week, I was nearly a jock.

I had thought that I would have more physical control than the others, because I take dance classes, swim, do aerobics, and am more agile than many of my nondisabled friends. But other women there had also reclaimed their bodies from the sleep imposed by the disabled experience. Beth and her handstands, Maria and her wheelchair dances. They surprised me and gave me courage. I found myself working out more and more each day.

One night a group of us were hanging out in front of the fire. I was doing yoga. The others wanted to try it, and pretty soon we were all doing stretches together and laughing a lot. We drifted back into motionless talk. It came out that every one of us had wanted to be or had greatly admired dancers.

There were women at Pescadero with whom I had very little in common, women who had experienced extreme social isolation or who had received substandard medical care, women whose cultural and ethnic background were based on assumptions totally different from mine.

Gloria Chen was a Chinese woman who had been raised in Peru where her father ran a small business. She contracted polio at the age of 10. From that point until college she studied at home and her social life outside her family was virtually non-existent. "In Latin culture they stare at you if you're different. You feel like a Martian. It was bad enough being Asian, much less disabled. I wouldn't go out during the day. So my father would get off work at night and we'd go to the movies, the 10 o'clock show. My father would wheel me out as soon as the lights came up.

"I had a hard time growing up. I had no one to talk to about being disabled. In Asian culture, there's a stricture against talking about your feelings. Since I've lived in the U.S. I've learned to talk more and open up.''

After an incredible odyssey covering two continents and battle after battle with inaccessiblity, Gloria is now in a doctoral program in advanced linguistics at the University of Texas in Austin. She teaches freshman and sophomore Spanish at the university and says she doesn't know ''if the students are more shocked that I'm in a wheelchair or that I'm Oriental when they arrive for Spanish class.''

Then there was Vivian, a black woman from the deep South. When she was five, much of her body, including her hands, was severely burned and permanently scarred. The streptomycin prescribed against infection left her almost totally deaf. From the age of five until she entered deaf school at 10, she had no language, no way of communication even with her own family. ''When I went to deaf school I knew how to spell my name and count. That was it,'' Vivian recalled. ''I didn't know how to sign and the kids said, 'Boy, you're dumb. What's wrong with your hands?' ''

Vivian lived at the deaf school for ten years. Her family never learned to sign. ''Even by the time I went to college I wasn't told important things like when a relative had died. I'd find out months later. It made me feel totally disassociated.'' But her parents and teachers did encourage her to go to college. She attended Gaulladet College, the only university for the deaf in the world and was one of the first black women to graduate from the school. Vivian married an African man while there and today is a mother who also has a career outside her home.

In the middle of a presentation on outreach techniques, Sandra Wong told us, ''Disabled Asian women will be hard to find because in Asian society a disability is shameful, something you hide. My mother told me, 'Sandra, you should be thankful I'm your mother because if you had been born in old China we'd have thrown you in the river by now.' ''

There was the story from a Native American woman who had been trampled by horses when she was fifteen and her pelvis crushed. There was no hospital on the reservation at the time. The hospital in town refused to take her without the signatures of six white families. Arranging the required signatures took days and, in the meantime, her hips began to mend. By the time the papers were completed the bones had set incorrectly. She spent thirteen years of her life virtually in bed until she received artificial hips in her late twenties and was able to walk again.

When Maria had an accident that left her paraplegic, there was some talk in her Latin community that this disaster had visited her because she was living on her own, away from the family, and had not married.

The stories were endless, even from this comparatively small group of women. In each account, I found clues to myself. I was proud of every victory. I was privileged to record these women's struggles. At the same time, because there were so many of us, because the situation was so normalized, I also experienced a relief and relaxation — being disabled was no big deal.

Pleasures

by diane hugs

e both sat there, two disabled lesbians in our wheelchairs, each on opposite sides of the bed. Sudden feelings of fear and timidness came over us. But once we finished the transferring, lifting of legs, undressing and arranging of blankets, we finally touched. Softly and slowly we began to explore each other, our minds and bodies. Neither could make assumptions about the sensations or pleasures of the other. It was wonderful to sense that this woman felt that my body was worth the time it took to explore, that she was as interested in discovering my pleasure as I was in discovering hers.

From the first touch it was a stream of sensations; to listen to every breath, each sigh, and to feel every movement of our love intermingling. It was so intense, so mutual that I must say this beginning was one of the deepest and most fulfilling that I have ever experienced.

When I was an able-bodied lesbian, my approach to relating sexually had been to find out what moves turned someone on and go from there. Never before have I taken the time or had the opportunity to begin a relationship with such a beautiful feeling of pleasure, not only from the pot of gold at the end of the rainbow, but also from the exploration itself.

Taking Leave

by robyn miller

"Lisa Ann! If you don't get a move on doing this therapy, we'll never get to the movies this afternoon. I don't know why you're so irresponsible; I do twice your therapy and I'm always on time!"

"I don't care about *you!* It's my life and it's my therapy, and I'll do what I want, so just lay off... "

Oh, Lisạ. Please don't let me make you angry. Only a few more months together and we're at it again, spending our time arguing and creating bad memories. It's not that I don't try to understand what you're going through. It's just that I'm sick, but you're sicker, and I haven't learned to let you go.

You know. You comprehend. But lately you are exasperated at my every demand, as if every touch of mine would draw you further into a world you must leave. It's almost as bad as all the weeks you spent taking allergy tests, when you were told it would be best if you gave up chocolate, cold turkey. You never touched a candy bar after those doctor visits, but at times you still walk with me, a little too slowly, past sweet shops. Now you have given up riding your bike. You avoid, even alienate, the people you were close to. If it was hard for the little girl you were to give up chocolate, how much harder is it now, at eleven, to give up life?

Not that you give up completely — not you! I walk with you in the park when I take the dogs out, giving you the slower dog's leash so you will not tire. Still you manage to run wildly through the grass, my spaniel barking as you chase him through the fields. You enjoy the abandon of running so much — what it means to have legs, to have the energy to be free! I never have the heart to stop your play before you cough, and then I curse helplessly in my mind, that you cannot run without pain.

It is something you don't deal with, this feeling of helplessness. Dying is a force you can fight against with your best shot, but watching someone die is a passive thing to do. I can tell you to take your medication and your therapy, but what to do when the medication and the therapy do not heal? If I go into a forest and scream my rage among the trees, will my hysteria help you or will my throat just become sore?

Still, it is your feelings I fight more than my own. You do not open yourself to me as you once did, curling up at a sleepover and telling me your deepest secrets. Once I could make you cry with a glance. Now you are somewhere in a cocoon by youself. You would try, I believe, to draw as far away as possible, because you want no ties to anyone of this world. It is hard because my way of dealing with loss is the opposite: I would have you for my friend every second, while we have time.

So these days, as opposites, we are arguing more and forgiving less. We spend time fighting a disease in different ways, but together, and we grow, but apart, as you start to take leave.

It is not just, this gradual leave-taking of a child. If it were fair it would not be fought by so many doctors, working with science to accomplish what you and I need so much. If I wait for the day I see a medical miracle with eagerness, you must understand I have wished it would have come in time to save *you*.

You will not be here then, when they cure your disease. You will long have been gone, having taken your leave. But you will be a part of the victory, nonetheless, on that day, and then our fight will be over, and something of the world will be at peace.

Robyn Miller died on August 7, 1985.

Remembering Our Past

*by members of the women's reminiscence group
transcribed by marsha ablowitz and tilly schalkwyk*

The Group: "We are nine residents of the Hospital Extended Care Unit. This is a 300 bed facility for people who can't move or care for themselves. About three-quarters are women, with an average age of 87 years. Our group was first organized by a nurse — Tilly, and a social worker — Beryl. Now Marsha has replaced Beryl. None of the women here can walk. Everyone needs a lot of help. Our women's reminiscence group has been meeting for about three years. We share memories of our lives in the past. We also talk about what happens here, problems, parties, pub nights, visits. Sometimes we share our fears and frustrations about having to always wait for help and ask for help. During the last year, we've met before breakfast in Opal's room because Opal can't get up out of bed and because it's so busy here in the day — doctor's visits, exercises, out-trips. Opal is in bed all the time. The rest of us can sit up in our wheelchairs. We can all talk and all tell stories.

The Group Members: We each tell stories about our lives every Thursday morning at 8:30 a.m.

Ella Sibson: "I was born in California in 1897. I remember once we were playing ring-around-the-rosy around a bush and the dog ran into the bush and he picked up a poisonous snake. Another time, my brother wanted to play a trick on us girls. He grabbed a baby pig and climbed a tree and the mother pig was chasing him. He said, "Run girls, run." And then he jumped down and ran for the barn. We ran after him and just made it. The mother pig was mad and she almost bit my leg. I married and had a lovely family. I had three sons and a daughter. The eldest son died. I miss him. I've been in a wheelchair about two years from a stroke. I can't use my hand either."

Gwen says Ella is very kind. Rosina says, "Ella will do anything she can to help you. Nothing seems to be a bother."

Rosina Davies: "I am 93, but I don't feel old. I got married at age 29 and *that* felt old. I was born in Scotland and had lots of boyfriends who used to love to walk me home. They loved my red hair (now I wear a blond wig). After I came to Canada I said I would only return home if I could sail by ship. So, after my marriage, I sailed to Scotland — 21 days on ship — through the Panama Canal, it was lovely."

Rosina looks very fine in her blonde wig. She can still walk a little, and she prefers to take the risk of trying to move by herself even though she's fallen more than once. "I needed to get on the toilet and couldn't wait — so I tried myself and I fell. I was lying on the floor. I couldn't get up. Then Ella called the nurses and they helped me. Sometimes I like to play piano, I hope the others enjoy listening."

Marie Edwards: "I was born in 1898 in Minnesota. I used to live on a farm. I remember when my mother made soap. It sure smelled terrible when it was being made, but we put perfume in it. I like the smell of perfumed soaps. I used to love when my Mom made raisin bread — mmm — that was good. I wish I could stand up and walk. I get tired of this wheelchair. Once I was window shopping with my daughter and I turned around and said, "Look at that handsome man across the street." She said "Oh Mom — that's Dad." I can wheel my own chair so I get around quite well. I used to sing in a choir where my father was the conductor and wrote special music for us to perform. Now I enjoy piano playing."

Mary Green: "I was born in Edmonton in 1906. It was a pretty small town in those days. I was married in Calgary. Frank was a conductor on the trains. I had two girls, and now have seven grandchildren and two great grandchildren. I used to be a pianist. I played in church. I loved all kinds of music, but I can't play now with only one hand. I had the first stroke about 8 years ago and haven't been able to walk for about one year. I learned to drive the electric chair. It was easy to learn since I drove a car. I can't do much now. I read. They use a special lift to get me up out of my bed and into my electric wheelchair."

Merna Jackson: "I love to travel. I've been to California so many times. Three times through the Panama Canal and I'm going again soon. To Alaska and Hawaii ten times and again last year. I get my friend Olive to take me from here. Also Raj took me to Hawaii. Now I'd like someone to take me to Fiji. I was born in Wales in 1903 and came to Canada by boat when I was three years old. I worked as a salesgirl before I got married. Once the other girl and I got down behind the counter and stripped naked. When the next man came in, up we jumped. Was he ever surprised. He ran out!"

Group members say Merna is very lively with a good sense of humor. Now she's busy selling raffle tickets and planning her next trip. She can walk a little bit sometimes and loves to dance as well as she can at our "pub nights". The main problem is she has trouble talking and remembering things.

Gwen O'Kane: Gwen is our Cockney, we love her accent and her laugh. We call her Miss Slip-Slop because of the sound of her shoes dragging along in the wheelchair. Gwen says: "I'm the baby here. I'm only 63. I lived through the war in London which was nothing to sneeze at. I didn't shoot anyone, but I would have loved to take a shot at Hitler or two shots to be sure to get him in the head. After the war I came to Canada. I married and I have one son and one grandson. The little boy, Alexander, is 10 months. He loves to push my wheelchair and run around here. I've made a big list of all the things I can't do with only one good hand, and it's a long list!"

Margaret Stevens: "I was born in Hampshire, England in 1902 and have two children, nine grandchildren and four great grandchildren. I've had arthritis now for 8 or 9 years and can't move very much. Also I'm in a great deal of pain. I've been in hospital for three years now. At age 20, I came to Canada, then returned to England. I got married to Tom Stevens, a Chartered Accountant. We lived in Cyprus for a year after our marriage. I used to shake the poisonous spiders and snakes out of the blankets when we had a picnic. And once, I found a poisonous spider in the bathtub. The second time I came to Canada, I came by boat through the Panama Canal with my six month old son. I used to get very tired and bored here. Now, I've hired a paid companion, Isobel, who is very good. She helps me a lot. I have some very nice friends here. I enjoy our group very much."

Shirley Betts: "I am an artist, a painter. I have sold well over two hundred paintings. I loved painting in the woods in Northern Ontario. The light in the forest was beautiful. When I was young, I used to like to swim across a Northern Ontario lake, we used to go all the way across. Some of my paintings hang on our walls here. Now I have brain atrophy. First, my husband died. I woke up one day and he was dead. Then I got ill, I can't walk or get up. I can't remember things. But the worst thing about my illness is that I can't paint. It sure makes me mad when I wake up at night and think I can't do anything. But that's not true. I can do a little painting and I can swim in the pool."

Lately, Shirley has also been very sick. We miss her and worry about her.

Opal was also a member of the group. She died on September 14, 1983 and the group members miss her. The day after she died was group day and Rosina said a prayer for Opal. "Dear Lord, thank you for our dear friend Opal… Thank you Lord for the time with her. We thank you for her kind words, kind deeds, and her good humor." Gwen said, "I was sad. I hadn't said goodbye to Opal. Then I saw her in a dream. She had on a new dress and I didn't recognize her at first. Then she started laughing — and I knew it was Opal."

Conclusion: We've shared our past accomplishments and problems — we've baked bread together. We've had dinner together and we've enjoyed eating fresh fruit when it's in season. We look out for each other and worry when someone is sick. If one of our friends is sick or dies, we pray for her. At the end of each group meeting, we move the wheelchairs together and all hold hands (which is hard to do). Then, Rosina says our group prayer: "May the Lord watch between me and Thee while we are absent from one another. Amen." Then we all wheel off to breakfast. Another day in Extended Care.

Opal's contribution was unavailable for publication here.

Contributor's Notes

Deborah Abbott was born in 1953, had polio in 1955, started writing in 1959. "Having polio so early compelled me to thrive on struggle, to cultivate my differentness, to write about both." Abbott has been published in various anthologies. She lives in Santa Cruz, California with her two young sons.

Pennyota Ahladas invites those who want to know her better to come visit her in Vermont.

Barbara M. Altman is presently the Undergraduate Coordinator in the Sociology Department at the University of Maryland. As a Medical Sociologist, her area of specialization has been disability and rehabilitation. Her publications in this area include articles on attitudes toward handicapped people and also the mechanisms and management of stigma. Currently her research focuses on the problems of disabled women, particularly their access to rehabilitation and financial assistance in a social structure that favors men.

Lois Anderson is now living in an accessible apartment in Chicago. She attends classes, facilitates groups and volunteers at Access Living, an independent living project. She is the secretary of an accessible housing project, Handicapped Independent People, founded by herself and other participants of Access Living. She will soon be visiting and speaking to handicapped children and student occupational therapists about the barriers she managed to get over as a handicapped woman. She is a happy grandmother who loves photography, hooking rugs and collecting old records.

Victoria Ann-Lewis is an Artist in Residence at Los Angeles' Mark Taper Forum where she developed the award winning television special, *Tell Them I'm a Mermaid,* based on the lives of seven disabled women. Ms. Lewis has toured the U.S. and Europe with Lilith, a Women's Theatre, and the Improvisational Theater Project. She co-authored *No More Stares,* a role model book for disabled teenage girls published by the Disability Rights Education and Defense Fund, Inc., 1982.

Suzanne Beaucher was born and grew up in a suburb just north of Boston. She attended Holy Cross College where she received a B.A. in English. For the last seven years, she worked for a major electronics corporation, most recently as a technical writer. She now lives in the Boston area where she is writing short fiction.

Tzipporah BenAvraham is an Orthodox Jewish disabled woman in Brooklyn, a sightless person with visions of a future. She has her B.S. in Community and Human Service from Empire State College SUNY, and is a M.A. candidate in Urban Administration at Brooklyn College CUNY. She is active in disability issues in her community and is a legislative aide to a state assemblyman.

Maureen Brady, author of *Folly,* The Crossing Press, 1982, and *Give Me Your Good Ear,* Spinsters, Ink, 1979, and The Women's Press, London, 1981, and numerous short stories, wrote "The Field is Full of Daisies..." an autobiographical piece in defiance of those cartoons of her childhood in which women were ridiculed for sharing stories of their accidents, operations or illnesses. She was a co-founder of Spinsters, Ink.

Susan E. Browne grew up raising sheep and riding horses in the country of New Jersey. She has been diabetic since the age of 15. Today she lives in San Francisco and works as a nurse, teacher, counselor and consultant. Susan earned her doctorate in nursing at the University of California-San Francisco. Her dissertation examined social networks, social support and well-being of women with two potentially stigmatizing identities — lesbians with chronic illnesses or hidden disabilities. She dreams of living in the country again some day.

Debra Connors is a political activist, a beach comber, an urban gardener and the surrogate mother of Amanda and Sophie, her elegant old cat and mischievous puppy. She is currently teaching women's studies at San Francisco State University, where she is also a graduate student of Interdisciplinary Social Science. Her research interests include the history of science and technology and the social history of disability. She is a white working class woman who has been diabetic most of her life and now is partially sighted and has arthritis, both as a result of diabetes.

Max Dashu is an artist, a linguist, a folk scholar, and whenever possible, a wilderness backpacker. She has researched international women's history since 1970, and founded the Supressed Histories Archives, independently producing 35 slideshows on women in world cultures. She is writing a book on witches and the witch burnings.

ELB is an English woman currently living in London.

Anne Finger is a socialist-feminist, a writer, and a teacher. She is currently living in exile in Southern California. Her fiction has been published in *13th Moon, Antioch Review, Socialist Review,* and *Feminist Studies.* She received the Joseph Henry Jackson award in 1984 for a collection of her short fiction.

Edwina Trish Franchild is a lesbian, a perpetual student and a part-time telephone worker. She lives in Minneapolis with her two cats, Misty and Nutmeg. She is a member of the Womyn's Braille Press Collective.

Toni Gardiner: "I am a 40-year-old, congenitally blind rehabilitation counselor with an abiding love for animals. As an extrovert, I seek people-oriented activities. My hobbies include reading, handiwork, theater, travel, cooking, cassette correspondence and the telephone. I am deeply sensitive and devoted to my large circle of friends. I live with my guide dog, Ivy, and cats, Disney and Teyve."

Bobbie-Jo Goff is currently the Assistant Executive Director of a Massachusetts agency providing vocational and residential services to developmentally disabled adults. She is also working on her doctoral dissertation entitled "Community Integration and Community Residences" at Boston University.

Rebecca S. Grothaus, born 12-2-40 in Irvine, Kentucky. Bachelor's degree 1978, graduating with highest honors. Developed systemic lupus erythematosus in 1979. Worked for 4½ years as a disability civil rights advocate. Eleven years activism in San Diego County NOW. Founding President, Resource and Education Network for the Equality of Women with Disabilities (RENEWD).

Susan Hansell was born in Stockton, California in 1956. Although she had extensive joint surgery at age 16, she was a serious teen-aged athlete and continues to struggle to be physically active. In 1980 she was diagnosed with systemic lupus erythematosus, an auto-immune disease which has affected her joints and internal organs. She now lives in San Francisco, where she writes poetry, goes to demonstrations and swimming pools, practices yoga, and loves the women and men in her life.

Pam Herbert is a 28 year old quadraplegic with muscular dystrophy. She lives with her husband and 2 dogs in Hays, Kansas. She is a member of 2 disabled groups, and is also an Assistant Girl Scout Leader. She plans to write a book of her own someday.

Diane Hugs is a 30 year old woman with severe multiple sclerorsis. As a writer and activist she does advocacy in many areas including disability, mothering, women's sexuality, health care and human resources.

Donna I. Hyler: "I am 31 years old. I'm still trying to figure out how much of me is my disability and how it affects my view of life and my circumstances. I get angry a lot, and sometimes I'm afraid, but generally I like my life and I'm glad to be here."

Mary Anna Ilves is thirty-six, writes children's stories, and loves to laugh. She has had MS for fourteen years.

Norma James: "I'm Black, Deaf and surviving the slings and arrows of an outrageous fortune. I'm married with 2 sons and live in New York City. After losing my hearing, I worked for many years in Coler Hospital, and then returned to college for an Associate Degree in Science. I am now employed as a Radiology Technologist at Montefiore Hospital. I wish you all the best life can offer.''

JoAnn LeMaistre is a clinical psychologist in Palo Alto, CA. Helping discover the potential for quality living and parenting is both her personal and professional goal. She has completed a book entitled *Beyond Rage* which deals in depth with this process.

Jill Lessing is 42, a Jewish woman from California, born into a liberal, middle-class family. Jill is a human rights activist, artist, writer and counselor. She is post polio from age 8 months and uses a cane when walking.

Emily Levy: ''I am a social change activist, born and still living in San Francisco. I have been a writer since the third grade, when I chose the color orange for my color poem assignment because the others were too easy to rhyme. *Orange* was never published.''

''Frances Lynn'' was born in Kentucky. She became severely physically disabled when she was a child. Presently she lives in a small rural town where her resources are limited but her options growing because of her increasing involvement in her own future. Her story can be followed in *The Disability Rag.*

Robyn Miller is a 20 year old Barnard College junior, planning a writing career. She suffers (and grows!) from cystic fibrosis, a chronic, fatal lung disease. She dedicates ''Taking Leave'' to Lisa Ann who died of cystic fibrosis in 1982. Among her heroes, she counts her friend Danny, and sick children everywhere.

Anita L. Pace: ''I am 33 and have suffered from agoraphobia since age 13. I became housebound and extremely low-functional in my twenties. With years of various therapies, I am getting healthier and increasing my activities, although still hampered by anxiety and panics. During these years, I've discovered an interest in writing.''

Ernestine Amani Patterson: ''I was born to Earnest and Maggie Patterson in 1951 in the small factory town of Flint, Michigan. I am currently a member of the Black Studies Department faculty of San Francisco State University. I proofread braille, write articles for the *New Bayview,* a black community newspaper. For eight years I did reggae Jamaican music programming for alternative radio. I am blind, black and don't have much money and yet, I'm pressing on and enjoying it!''

Elaine Robidoux did, in fact, move into her own apartment in November, 1984 and she feels good about living on her own. She likes doing what she wants and having friends over when she wants. She has traveled to England and Ireland and would go back anytime.

Jill Sager was born in 1957 and raised in a Jewish home in the Bronx. After graduating from Music and Art High School she moved West. She is now a Recreation Therapist, advocate and activist at a non-profit agency run by and for disabled people. She dedicates this to her grandpa.

Carol Schmidt was named "Outstanding Lesbian Journalist" for 1984 by the Gay Press Association. Her first novel, "Child's Play," is about a child sexual abuse survivor who murders her assailant. Her second, "Honeymoon," is on the death of '60s-style politics. She lives on Mt. Washington in Los Angeles.

Nanci Stern arrived in San Francisco in 1967, looking for peace, love and good vibes. She found: a job at the Recreation Center for the Handicapped, a bachelor's and master's degree, the Full Moon Women's Coffeehouse and bookstore, Sha'ar Zahav synagogue, two cats and a guide dog named Tang, a typically freezing S.F. Victorian flat, and her present careers as a writer and counselor. Retrospectively, in 1985, she is beginning again to think about peace, love, and good vibes.

Amber Coverdale Sumrall: "I am a writer, gardener, and singer of bird songs. I live in the Santa Cruz Mountains with John, and seven cats. My poems will appear in *Toward Solomon's Mountain,* an anthology of poetry about disability. My greatest challenge lies in accepting my physical limitations, and in realizing that when certain doors slam shut, others open just ahead."

Julie Taylor: "I go to Lowell High School in San Francisco. I like to write and plan on writing more in the future, maybe even books. I live with four adults which sometimes can be hard. I have no idea what I want to be 'when I grow up.' "

Dai R. Thompson is an attorney serving on the board of RESPOND, a New Haven advocacy agency for people with disabilities. Past affiliations include State Coordinator for the International Year of Disabled Persons; Steering Committee member, National Conference on Women and the Law; and co-founder of a support group for women with disabilities.

Joan Tollifson is a Bay Area photographer/writer. She studies martial arts, has been a political activist for many years. She was born in Chicago in 1948.

Rene Ungerecht: "I am 28, an introspective introvert living in the Lesbian ghetto of Portland, Oregon. Having a touch of agoraphobia, I like cats, movies in dark theatres, science fiction, Holly Near and wheelchair rallies where I look like one of the crowd.

Cheryl Wade: "I am one of the real California girls, not the Pepsi version, but one who has grown cellulite and gray hairs here. I have a master's degree in Psychology, and a decent part-time job that affords writing time and money for Bruce Springsteen concerts. I am working on a book of interviews with disabled persons about maintaining independence called *Comes a Time*, and a book of short fiction for low-level readers called *No Wings*. I am happily in love with a crazy Irishman.

Marjorie Wagner lives in Walnut Creek. After retiring on disability she earned a master's degree at John F. Kennedy University in Orinda. She is now a Marriage, Family, Child Counselor intern with a special interest in counseling disabled people.''

Kathleen M. White: ''At the time of the automobile accident that left me a paraplegic (1965), I had been a special class teacher for 2½ years. I finished a doctoral degree in special education (1970), changed careers to psychology, became a tenured psychology professor (1979). I teach, do research on the family, and write.''

Women's Reminiscence Group — Shirley Betts, Rosina Davies, Marie Edwards, Merna Jackson, Gwen O'Kane, Ella Sibson, and Margaret Stevens are older Canadian women living in a convalescent home. They support each other and meet to share their past and present lives. (Mary Green and Opal were also members of the group before they died.)

Naomi Woronov is a writer and teacher. Her next book entitled *China Through My Window* (Schocken Books, 1985), describes the two years she spent teaching English at Zhejiang University in the People's Republic of China. She is Assistant Professor of English, Manhattan Community College, City University of New York.

Carrie Oyama, the cover artist, was born and grew up in New York City. She moved to California in 1979. She attends San Francisco State University. She plans to do a children's book, teach, and continue doing her art. She has had shows at the Hudson Guild Gallery, and Asian Center in New York City and at the Bacchanal Gallery in Albany.

Books From Cleis Press

LONG WAY HOME
Jeanne Jullion
ISBN: 0-939416-05-0

WITH THE POWER OF EACH BREATH:
A DISABLED WOMEN'S ANTHOLOGY
ed. Debra Connors, Susan Browne, Nanci Stern
ISBN: 0-939416-06-9

THE ABSENCE OF THE DEAD
IS THEIR WAY OF APPEARING
Mary Winfrey Trautmann
ISBN: 0-939416-04-2
8.95

WOMAN-CENTERED PREGNANCY
AND BIRTH
Ginny Cassidy-Brinn, R.N., Francie Hornstein,
Carol Downer & the Federation of Feminist
Women's Health Centers
ISBN: 0-939416-03-4
11.95

VOICES IN THE NIGHT:
WOMEN SPEAKING ABOUT INCEST
ed. Toni A.H. McNaron & Yarrow Morgan
ISBN: 0-939416-02-6
7.95

FIGHT BACK! FEMINIST RESISTANCE
TO MALE VIOLENCE
ed. Frederique Delacoste & Felice Newman
ISBN: 9-939416-01-8
13.95

ON WOMEN ARTISTS: POEMS 1975-1980
Alexandra Grilikhes
ISBN: 0-939416-00-X
4.95